METHODS IN MOLECULAR BIOLOGY™

Series Editor
John M. Walker
School of Life Sciences
University of Hertfordshire
Hatfield, Hertfordshire, AL10 9AB, UK

For other titles published in this series, go to
www.springer.com/series/7651

Drug Safety Evaluation

Methods and Protocols

Edited by

Jean-Charles Gautier

Disposition, Safety and Animal Research, sanofi-aventis, Vitry-sur-Seine, France

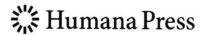 Humana Press

Editor
Jean-Charles Gautier
Disposition, Safety and Animal Research
sanofi-aventis
Vitry-sur-Seine
France
jean-charles.gautier@sanofi-aventis.com

ISSN 1064-3745   e-ISSN 1940-6029
ISBN 978-1-60327-186-8   e-ISBN 978-1-60761-849-2
DOI 10.1007/978-1-60761-849-2
Springer New York Dordrecht Heidelberg London

Library of Congress Control Number: 2010937423

Printed on acid-free paper

Humana Press is part of Springer Science+Business Media (www.springer.com)

Preface

Non-clinical drug safety evaluation is the assessment of the safety profile of therapeutic agents through the conduct of laboratory studies in *in vitro* systems and in animals. The main objectives of drug safety evaluation studies are to differentiate between new drug entities that are unacceptably toxic and those that are not, characterize the potential adverse effects of new drugs, determine animal dosage levels that do not cause toxicity, and to estimate safe dosages to be used in clinical studies. Several types of studies are conducted in drug safety evaluation: acute to chronic general toxicity studies, reproductive toxicity studies, genotoxicity studies, carcinogenicity studies, safety pharmacology studies, and investigative toxicity studies.

General toxicity studies are usually performed in a rodent and in a nonrodent species to determine target organs of toxicity and evaluate doses of a new drug candidate that can be safely administered to man. In this book, specific aspects related to the experimental design of toxicity studies conducted to support drug combinations in humans and pediatric indications are described in the reviews of Chaps. 1 and 2, respectively. In general toxicity studies, the key traditional endpoints evaluated include clinical signs, clinical pathology parameters, along with macroscopic examination of organs at necropsy and light microscopic examination of a comprehensive list of tissues. Chapter 3 details the necropsy and sampling procedures used in rodents, and Chap. 4 highlights the histopathology procedures from tissue sampling to histopathological evaluation. Chapters 5 and 6 describe additional methods, such as immunohistochemistry, tissue microarrays, and digital image analysis, which can be used to complete and refine the traditional histopathological examination of organs.

Genotoxicity studies are carried out to evaluate the potential of new drug candidates to induce mutations and/or chromosomal damages. Chapter 7 presents the method of the micronucleus assay and its combination with centromeric labeling in the fluorescence *in situ* hybridization (FISH) technique to detect aneugenic events. Chapter 8 describes the comet assay, a sensitive electrophoretic method for measuring DNA strand breaks at the level of single cells, together with the use of bacterial repair endonucleases to detect specific DNA lesions.

Safety pharmacology studies are conducted to evaluate the effect of compounds on the cardiovascular, respiratory, and central nervous system functions before the first administration to humans. Chapter 9 describes a manual patch-clamp technique used to study the effect of compounds on the HERG cardiac K^+ channel in order to evaluate the potential to induce "torsades de pointe", an arrhythmic disorder that can be fatal in humans.

When unexpected toxicity arises during these studies, it is important to investigate the mechanisms of toxicity and assess the potential translation to humans. Traditional histopathological examination of target organs and clinical pathology parameters are sometimes in default, and novel 'omics technologies, such as transcriptomics, proteomics, and metabonomics could allow to generate new hypotheses on the mechanisms of toxicity. Detailed protocols related to these 'omics technologies are presented in Chaps. 10–12.

Of note, the gene expression results obtained via transcriptomics experiments need to be confirmed by quantitative RT-PCR. However, accurate interpretation cannot be performed without proper statistical analysis of RT-PCR data. Chapter 13 examines some of the issues concerning RT-PCR experiments that would benefit from rigorous statistical treatment.

In vitro functional assays can be used to elucidate mechanisms of toxicity in the context of drug safety evaluation. Chapter 14 describes an *in vitro* assay used to evaluate the effect of compounds on the mitochondrial respiration chain in cultured rat hepatocytes. Mitochondrial dysfunction is indeed a major mechanism, whereby drugs can induce liver injury and other serious side effects, such as lactic acidosis and rhabdomyolysis, in some patients. *In vitro* assays can also be used during the early phase of drug development to screen compounds for their potential to induce developmental toxicity. This is illustrated with the Fetax and the zebrafish models in Chaps. 15 and 16, respectively. Drug-induced toxicity is often associated with the formation of reactive metabolites that bind covalently to proteins. Chapter 17 describes *in vitro* assays used at the lead optimization stage of drug discovery to evaluate the potential of drug candidates to bind covalently to proteins by incubating a radiolabeled analog of the compound with liver microsomal preparations or whole cells. Sophisticated mass spectrometry-based methods can also be used to identify chemical-adducted proteins both *in vitro* and *in vivo*. This is illustrated with specific examples in Chaps. 18–21.

Another developing field in drug safety evaluation is the identification and qualification of novel safety biomarkers that can be used to better monitor potential toxicity in both preclinical and clinical studies. Ideally, these new safety biomarkers should be more sensitive and/or specific than the traditional clinical pathology parameters and should be measurable in accessible fluids, such as plasma and urine. Chapters 22–24 provide sophisticated methods to discover new safety biomarkers using proteomics and metabonomics approaches. A protocol to quantify potential protein safety biomarkers by mass spectrometry is also described in Chap. 25.

I would like to thank all the contributing authors for providing state-of-the-art procedures, detailed protocols, and tips and tricks to avoid pitfalls. I am grateful to the series editor, John Walker, for inviting me to edit this volume. The result is a compendium of analytical technologies, including some review chapters, with a focus on clarity and applicability in real life laboratory practice. The intended audience mainly consists of pharmaceutical scientists, toxicologists, biochemists, and molecular biologists, and anyone else with a specific interest in methods used in drug safety evaluation that could be translated to other disciplines.

Vitry-sur-Seine, France   *Jean-Charles Gautier*

Contents

viii   Contents

Part I

General Toxicology

Chapter 1

Developing Combination Drugs in Preclinical Studies

Alberto Lodola

Abstract

Although combination drugs have been available for many years, it is only recently that preclinical guidelines have been released by the Food and Drugs Administration (FDA) and EMEA and as yet they are not part of the ICH process. In addition, the World Health Organisation and FDA have issued guidelines for combination drugs developed specifically to treat HIV infections. Depending on the type of combination (marketed drug/marketed drug; marketed drug/NME and NME/NME), the scope and complexity of studies can vary greatly. In all cases, however, a key issue is the potential for pharmacokinetic and/or toxicologic interaction between the components. For a marketed drug/marketed drug combination, a detailed review of the preclinical data available may suffice; particularly when the components have a history of co-administration at about the same dose and ratio as that of the proposed combination. For a marketed drug/NME combination, in addition to a review of the data for the marketed drug, a full ICH programme of studies will be required for the NME, and a study of up to 90 days duration (in one species) for the combination. With an NME/NME combination, each component will require a full ICH battery of studies and a combination study in one species. In all cases, additional studies may be needed to address data gaps. Given the many novel and complex issues that arise when developing combination drugs, we recommend that, whenever possible, the preclinical study strategy is discussed with the regulatory authorities.

Key words: Combination drugs, Regulatory guidelines, Preclinical issues, Study design, Dose selection, Development strategies

1. Introduction

The US Food and Drugs Administration (FDA) defines "Combination Drugs" (1) as follows:

- Co-packaged products (two or more separate drugs packaged together);

- Adjunctive therapy (when a second drug is used together with the drug for primary treatment);

Jean-Charles Gautier (ed.), *Drug Safety Evaluation: Methods and Protocols*, Methods in Molecular Biology, vol. 691,
DOI 10.1007/978-1-60761-849-2_1, © Springer Science+Business Media, LLC 2011

- Fixed dose combinations (two or more drugs combined in a single pill).

These drugs should not be confused with "Combination Products" which are defined in 21 CFR3.2(e) (2). A brief description of the development of "combination products" has been provided by Segal (3) and Portnoy and Koepke (4).

In this chapter, we discuss the preclinical development of "combination drugs." These drugs have been available in our pharmacies for many years; for example in 1975 in West Germany greater than two-thirds of the drugs on the official list were fixed combinations (5). In 1982 it was reported that about half of all marketed drugs in the USA were fixed combinations (6). Combination drugs are used in the treatment of a range of illnesses (7–10). Their major disadvantage is that neither the dose nor the ratio of the individual components can be varied by the physician. However, for patients on multiple medication, a combination drug simplifies treatment and hence compliance, given that fewer pills are taken there may also be a cost advantage (11). Combination therapy may also be more effective than monotherapy or have an improved safety profile. In Stage-I or -II hypertension, monotherapy may only produce a modest effect on blood pressure while a combination drug can produce a more significant reduction, given that each component blocks different effector pathways. Similarly, the incidence of peripheral oedema, linked to the use of calcium channel antagonist therapy, is reduced when co-administered with an ACE inhibitor (7).

2. Regulatory Guidance

The "International Conference on Harmonisation of Technical Requirements for Registration of Pharmaceuticals for Human Use" (ICH) (12) has defined the preclinical data requirements for monotherapy development. These requirements are an essential backcloth when assessing the preclinical needs for combination drug development.

2.1. Guidance for Monotherapy Development

Current guidance for monotherapy development is described in a range of guidelines (12) which are detailed in Table 1. In addition to data from these studies, "special studies," developed in the light of the emerging preclinical and clinical data, may also be needed to address specific issues. The relevance of these documents to combination drug development is twofold. First, for marketed drugs they are the reference against which the preclinical data for the marketed drug, often produced pre-ICH, are judged. Second, they define the studies and data needed for the

Table 1
List of current preclinical guidance documents available for the development of monotherapies (12)

ICH guideline	Topic
S1A	Need for carcinogenicity studies of pharmaceuticals
S1B	Testing for carcinogenicity of pharmaceuticals
S1C(R1)	Dose selection for carcinogenicity studies of pharmaceuticals and limit dose
S2A	Guidance on specific aspects of regulatory genotoxicity tests for pharmaceuticals
S2B	Genotoxicity: a standard battery for genotoxicity testing of pharmaceuticals
S3A	Note for guidance on toxicokinetics: the assessment of systemic exposure in toxicity studies
S3B	Pharmacokinetics: guidance for repeated dose tissue distribution studies
ICH	Single dose toxicity tests
S4	Duration of chronic toxicity testing in animals (rodent and non-rodent toxicity testing)
S5(R2)	Detection of toxicity to reproduction for medicinal products and toxicity to male fertility
S6	Preclinical safety evaluation of biotechnology-derived pharmaceuticals
S7A	Safety Pharmacology studies for human pharmaceuticals
S7B	The non-clinical evaluation of the potential for delayed ventricular repolarisation (QT Interval prolongation) by human pharmaceuticals
S8	Immunotoxicity studies for human pharmaceuticals
M3(R2)	Guidance on Non-Clinical Safety Studies for the Conduct of Human Clinical Trials and Marketing Authorization for Pharmaceuticals

novel component of a combination drug and guide the choice of studies with the combination.

2.2. Guidance for Combination Drug Development

Currently guidelines for combination drugs are nationally based and not part of the ICH process. The FDA provides specific guidance based on the preclinical requirements for three combination drug scenarios; combinations of marketed drugs, combinations of marketed drugs and new molecular entities (NME) and combinations of NMEs. Data requirements are summarised in Table 2.

In general, for marketed drugs, and if the components have a history of concomitant use at about the projected ratio little, or no, preclinical work is needed. For combinations involving NMEs, a full ICH package of studies is needed for the NME (see Subheading 2.1) and additional studies with the combination.

Table 2
Summary of the key points from the FDA Guidance for Industry (2006) Nonclinical Safety Evaluation of Drug or Biologic Combinations (1) for combinations involving NMEs

Study	Combination type		Comment
	MD/MB + NME	NME + NME	
Genetic toxicology	On the NME	On the NME	Not required for MD/MB if data consistent with modern requirements
	Combination	Combination	Generally not required
PK/ADME and toxicokinetics	On the NME	On the NME	Per ICH-M3 and/or ICH-S6
		Combination	If same target organ/system
Safety pharmacology	On the NME	On the NME	Per ICH-M3 and/or ICH-S6
	Combination	Combination	If same target organ/system
General toxicology	On the NME	On the NME	Per ICH-M3 and/or ICH-S6
	Combination	Combination	Study of up to 90-days duration
Reproductive and development toxicology			
Fertility (Study 1)	On the NME	On the NME	Per ICH-M3
Implantation/early development (Study 2)	On the NME	On the NME	Per ICH-M3
Embryo-foetal development (Study 3)	On the NME	On the NME	Per ICH-M3
	Combination	Combination	Unless the MD or NME is pregnancy category "D" or "X"
Carcinogenicity	On the NME	On the NME	Generally not needed for the combination if NMEs tested
Animal models of efficacy	Generally not needed	Generally not needed	
Further studies	As required to address data gaps/specific issues	As required to address data gaps/specific issues	

Abbreviations: *MD* marketed drugs, *MB* marketed biologics, *NME* new molecular entity

Liminga and Silva Lima (13) have discussed the background to the EMEA's guidance documents (14, 15). These guidelines provide general guidance to preclinical requirements; the key elements are summarised in Table 3. Overall, the position adopted by the EMEA is consistent with that of the FDA, although the general nature of the guidance suggests a more flexible approach than that of the FDA.

While no formal guidance is available from the Japanese authorities, their position has been summarised by the "English RA Information Task Force, International Affairs Committee" of the Japanese Pharmaceutical Manufacturers Association (16). An extract of the preclinical requirements in Japan for combination

Table 3
Summary of the key points in the EMEA's Guideline on the non-clinical development of fixed combinations of medicinal products (CHMP/EMEA/CHMP/ SWP/258498/2005) and Note for guidance on fixed combination medicinal products (CPMP/EWP/240/95)

Study type	Comment
Pharmacodynamic	Required to assess any unexpected or undesirable interactions between components
Pharmacokinetic	Required to assess effects on respective pharmacokinetic patterns or to demonstrate lack of interaction
Genotoxicity	Studies with the combination are not needed for combinations of non-genotoxic components Studies with individual components may be needed to address data gaps or specific issues, e.g. possibility of potentiation
General toxicity	Usually not needed for a combination which corresponds closely to monotherapies that are already in widespread concomitant use A study of up to 3-month duration, in one species, is recommended for approved compounds indicated for long-term use but with no experience of concomitant use. Studies of longer duration or with additional species may be needed in the light of the data
Reproductive toxicity	Generally not needed if single components have been adequately tested Studies may be needed depending on the componets used and potential interactions
Carcinogenicity	Not needed for combinations of approved compounds previously shown not to be carcinogenic For combinations containing one NME recommend adding an additional group to the NME carcinogenicity study for the combination. Deviations from this approach considered on a case-by-case basis

Table 4
Data to be submitted with an Application for
Approval to Manufacture/Distribute in Japan
for a new prescription-based combination drug.
The data are a summary from a report by the
Japanese Pharmaceutical Manufacturers
Association (16)

Data type	Required/not-required
Single dose toxicity	Required[a]
Repeated dose toxicity	Required[a]
Genotoxicity	Not required
Carcinogenicity	Not required
Reproductive toxicity	Not required
Local irritation	Required[a] in some cases
Other	Not required
Absorption	Required
Distribution	Required
Metabolism	Required

[a]Toxicity data for the combination and each component are required

drugs is presented in Table 4. The Australian Therapeutic Goods Administration (TGA) has adopted the EMEA's guidance (17) as the basis for regulating combination drugs, and recently Hunt (18) has discussed the Australian perspective. The Canadian Therapeutic Directorate (TPD) in a guideline relating to hormone replacement therapy in menopause (19) makes reference to "fixed combinations." The principal data requirements are for bioavailability, pharmacokinetics, pharmacodynamics and metabolic studies in all species studied. It is accepted, however, that when there is substantial information already available for the monotherapies, then there may only be a need for "abridged toxicology," that is a reduced programme of studies. Moreover, with the agreement of the Therapeutic Products Programme staff the need for toxicology testing will in certain cases be waived.

Once more, while not providing a high level of detail the position taken in Japan by the TGA and the TPD is aligned with those of the FDA and EMEA.

2.3. Guidance
for Special Cases

In 2005, the World Health Organisation's (WHO) "Expert Committee On Specifications For Pharmaceutical Preparations" published guidelines for the registration of "combination medicinal products" (20). This document is focused on the regulatory needs for the development and marketing of combination drugs to treat HIV infections, tuberculosis and malaria. The information provided by the WHO is highly detailed describing preclinical, clinical and marketing requirements for the specific indications listed above. They consider the following four scenarios:

1. A generic copy of an existing combination;
2. The combination is composed of established monotherapies which have been used in combination;
3. A combination composed of established monotherapies which have not previously been used in combination;
4. The combination contains one or more NMEs.

The data requirements for each scenario are summarised in Table 5. For scenarios 1 and 2, no additional experimental work is required relative to the individual monotherapies. While there is no specific description of the preclinical data which is required for Scenarios 3 and 4, it is made clear that the WHO guideline is not "stand-alone" and has to be used in conjunction with current national and ICH guidelines (see Subheadings 2.1 and 2.2).

The FDA has also released specific guidelines for the development of fixed dose combinations for the treatment of HIV infections (21). This wide ranging document is focussed on combinations developed using only marketed drugs. Two scenarios which are discussed are of interest to us, and we have summarised the data requirements in Table 6.

Table 5
Summary of non-clinical data requirements developed in the WHO Guidelines for registration of fixed-dose combination medicinal products (20)

	Scenario			
Requirement	**1**	**2**	**3**	**4**
Type of FDC	Generic copy	Approved components previously used in combination	Approved components not previously used in combination	Contains one or more NCEs
Analysis of literature	Not required		Required	
Bioavailability data	Not usually required		Sometimes required	Required
Pharmacology and safety data	Not usually required		Sometimes required	Required

Table 6
Summary of preclinical data requirements from the FDA's Guidance for Industry: Fixed Dose Combinations, Co-Packaged Drug Products, and Single-Entity Versions of Previously Approved Antiretrovirals for the treatment of HIV (21)

Requirement	Scenario 1	Scenario 2
FDC components	Two- or three-drugs which have are separately approved	
Data from human usage	Data available to show components are safe and effective when used together	No support data for concomitant use
Type of FDA application	Stand-alone NDA Applicant/s own or have a right to reference underlying preclinical and safety and efficacy data	NDA
Preclinical data	No new preclinical data for the components or FDC	No new preclinical data for the components Safety data for the FDC either from studies or from the literature are required
Bioavailability	For the FDC need to show efficacious blood levels of each component are achieved	

Abbreviations: *NDA* new drug application

3. Preclinical Safety Issues for Combination Drugs

The issues that underpin the need for the wide range of preclinical ICH studies associated with monotherapy development also apply for combination drug development. These issues have been discussed in detail elsewhere (22). In addition, however, particular attention is focused on the potential for Pharmacokinetic and/or Toxicologic Interaction when developing combination drugs.

If we consider a two drug combination containing components "A" and "B," component-A may affect the pharmacokinetic (PK) profile of component-B (or vice versa). This can result in circulating levels of "B" being increased or decreased, altered tissue binding and/or distribution or altered rates of metabolism and elimination. These changes in PK profile can result in reduction of the No Observed Effect Level (NOEL) and No Observed Adverse Effect Levels (NOAEL), hence the safety margin (for specific toxicities) and the overall risk assessment of the combination relative to that of the individual components when used in monotherapy.

Similarly, a PK-interaction can produce a pharmacodynamic effect; that is, component "A" increases or reduces the response of the organism to the pharmacological effects of component "B." It should be noted that in some instances, this effect is the pharmacological basis for the combination: for example, Kaletra, a combination of Lopinavir and Ritonavir used in the treatment of HIV infections. Ritonavir inhibits the metabolism of Lopinavir, thus improving the PK profile of Lopinavir increasing its pharmacological effectiveness (23). In other cases, both drug components could have a common target organ of toxicity; this could result in an aggravation of this toxicity with a potentially reduced safety margin and an altered risk assessment for the combination relative to that of its components.

4. Preclinical Study Issues for Combination Drug

There are a number of tactical issues that need to be considered when developing combination drugs. Primarily, these issues relate to the increased complication of defining the dose response and the effects of component ratio changes on safety for a "chemical mixture."

4.1. Dose Selection for Preclinical Studies

Genotoxicity studies with the drug combination are usually not required. However, this is not the case for safety pharmacology, general toxicology and developmental toxicology studies. In studies with a combination, dose selection is complicated by the need to consider two factors. The first is the dose itself; this is made up of the dose of the individual components (A mg/kg and B mg/kg) and the combined dose [total (A+B) mg/kg]. The second is the ratio of the components which will be used (i.e. 1:10 vs. 1:1 vs. 10:1 of A and B, respectively) at a given dose.

In safety pharmacology studies dose selection is not, in our view, problematic. In general, the doses used are small multiples of the expected therapeutic dose, so it is unlikely that severe toxicity will occur with a combination (24). Nevertheless, if there are fears about the severity of adverse effects the approach described below can be adopted.

In toxicity studies (general and reproductive), the high dose should produce toxicity or be a limit dose (12). For studies with a combination of marketed compounds, to answer a specific question or resolve a specific issue, the dose and component ratio used in studies will most probably be defined by the data available. In this instance, the dose/ratio used may not need to produce adverse effects. For novel combinations or combinations involving one or more NMEs, this is not the case. If for each component its toxic dose is used in the combination, there is a strong possibility that the combined toxicity of the components will be excessive (compromising the relevance of the study) or lethal for the test animals (compromising the integrity of the study). In our view, a more rational approach is to identify the high dose on the basis of the "total dose," then as for monotherapy development, the mid- and low-doses can be set accordingly.

In the early stages of the development programme, the ratio of components for optimal pharmacological/therapeutic effect is usually uncertain. However, preclinical studies must fully characterise the safety profile of the combination while providing flexibility in clinical studies to vary the total dose and component ratio. The "Factorial Study" described in the Draft ICH-E12A guideline (25) is a good basis with which to address this issue. Since the optimal (pharmacological) ratio of the components is unclear in the early stages of development, a reference ratio can be set using the best estimate of a clinically relevant ratio (e.g. 1:1). This ratio can then be bracketed with ratios that favour one component than the other. (e.g. 10:1 and 1:10). In preclinical studies as the ratio is altered the *same* total dose is maintained. Thus, a study with total doses of 100, 40 and 10 mg/kg and a reference component ratio of 1:1 could use a dosing regimen as shown in Table 7. The choice of total dose must clearly be based on data from studies with the individual components (A and B) and possibly (small scale) preliminary studies with the combination.

4.2. Species Selection for Combination Studies

For studies with a single NME or the marketed drug component, species selection should not be a major issue. It is likely that the rodent used will be the rat or mouse and the non-rodent will be the beagle dog, rabbit and less often the non-human primate. For studies with a marketed drug, the species used will almost

Table 7
Possible dosing regimen for early studies in the development of a combination drug. Based on the "Factorial Study" described in the Draft ICH-E12A "Consensus Principal" (25)

		Component ratio (A:B)		
Total dose (mg/kg)	Component	10:1 Dose (mg/kg)	1:1	1:10
10	A	9.1	5	0.9
	B	0.9	5	9.1
40	A	36.4	20	3.6
	B	3.6	20	36.4
100	A	90.9	50	9.1
	B	9.1	50	90.9

certainly be that used in the original study which generated the issue that needs to be investigated.

Species selection can become more problematic for studies with the combination, however. The species used must be "the most appropriate species" and problems may be heightened if studies must also be conducted in a second species (1). Problems are due principally to two factors:

- poor toleration of one species to one component
- different species being optimal from PK/ADME considerations for each component.

If toleration is a problem and the use of an alternate species does not resolve the issue, then the dose of the combination drug used should be lowered to ensure that the adverse events produced are acceptable (1). If PK/ADME is an issue and changing dose levels of the combination and or the test species does not produce PK/ADME profiles for each component which are broadly similar to that in humans, the best compromise in terms of dose and species should be adopted.

In general, in cases where species selection is a major problem, a pragmatic approach should be adopted. Where such cases arise, it is imperative that a clear set of arguments is developed, ideally supported by experimental data, for the choice that is made. Given the uncertainty in such cases whenever possible, it is advisable to discuss species selection with the regulatory authorities.

4.3. Study Structure

For monotherapies, preclinical studies usually follow a standard design. In general, male and female animals are used with four dose levels; control, low-, mid- and high-dose. As shown in Table 7, with combination drugs the number of groups needed in a study is greatly increased. Even if individual components have been characterised in separate studies, studies with the combination should include groups treated with the highest dose of the single components. This insures that there is a bridge to studies with the individual components, and they are internal references for the source of any adverse events in the study.

A single study composed of all these groups would be of significant size and complexity. This is not to say that it is not feasible. However, at an early stage in the project, it must be decided whether to conduct a single study or a set of overlapping studies. There is no right answer; the response is conditioned by the specific characteristics of the combination drug being developed and the emerging data. This problem of complexity primarily affects the early stages of the preclinical programme at a time when the final clinical dose and component ratio is ill-defined. As the programme unfolds, preclinical studies can be simplified. Once the effective clinical dose and ratio of the combination have been defined, preclinical studies can be conducted at a single ratio.

5. Scenarios for the Preclinical Development of Combination Drugs

To facilitate discussion we will consider three main development scenarios, and while we will focus on a two component combination the rationale we develop applies equally to combinations with greater numbers of components; only the complexity increases.

Overall, given the level of detail provided by the FDA's guidance (1), we recommend this as the base case for establishing a preclinical strategy for a combination drug; given the breadth and scope of this document, it will, in our view, also be consistent with needs of the European and Japanese regulatory authorities. However, we recommend that, if possible, as soon in the development process as feasible the preclinical strategy is discussed with the regulatory authorities.

5.1. Combination of Established (Marketed) Drugs

The simplest case is for a combination of marketed drugs *with* a significant history of concomitant use of the components in humans at about the same ratio as that of the intended combination. In this instance, the first key step is a rigorous review of all the preclinical data available; this should include regulatory submission documents and publications in the open literature and, ideally, original study reports. The objectives of this review are:

- To identify any issues with the quality of the data relative to current (ICH) standards;

- To determine the potential for interaction between the components and any actual or potential overlapping toxicities;

- To identify any unresolved preclinical issues;

- To review the safety assessment of the individual components and the combination to ensure that the safety margins for the components are acceptable (for both dose and duration of treatment!).

If there are no significant issues or data gaps, this review should fulfil the preclinical needs for the combination. If data gaps are identified, then studies with the individual components and/or the combination may be needed; these studies would fall within the scope of the ICH studies for monotherapies or be specifically designed in the light of the data/issues.

For combinations of marketed drugs *with no* significant history of concomitant use in humans, the initial approach is identical to that described above. In addition, data from a toxicity study of up to 3 months duration in one species may be required (depending on the duration of treatment in humans). Usually, unless one or both of the components have been assigned pregnancy category "D" or "X," then an embryo-foetal development study (in one species) should also be conducted. However, depending on the target population and/or therapeutic indication, it may not be necessary to conduct such a study; this underlines the importance of discussing key development issues with the regulatory authorities.

5.2. Combination of an Established Drug with an NME

The preclinical requirements for the marketed drug component have been described in Subheading 5.1. For the NME, a complete ICH programme of studies is required to evaluate the safety profile of the new molecule (see Subheading 2.1). Additional preclinical studies will be required with the combination. As a minimum a study of up to 3-months duration will be required and depending on the developmental toxicity of each component possibly a developmental toxicity study. The value of an additional combination group(s) in the carcinogenicity study for the NME (using the most appropriate species) should be considered. If it is decided that carcinogenicity data on the combination are not required, then a literature argument should be developed to justify this decision.

Finally, in the light of the emerging data additional studies may be needed to address data gaps or emerging safety issues. Designs for these studies could be based on standard ICH studies or may need to be developed specifically to address the question under investigation.

5.3. Combination of NMEs

In general, a choice has to be made between conducting preclinical studies only with the combination or with the single components and the combination. The latter is probably the best option since this allows the components to be changed while retaining the ability to exploit the data generated for the other component/s. In addition, this also supports the option to develop one (or both) of the NMEs as a monotherapy or indeed its use in other combinations.

For each NME, a complete ICH programme of studies is required to evaluate the safety profile of the new molecule (see Subheading 2.1). Additional preclinical studies will be required with the combination. As described above, as a minimum a study of up to 3 months duration will be required and depending on the developmental toxicity of each component possibly a developmental toxicity study. A choice must also be made between conducting a carcinogenicity study with the combination or additional combination group(s) in the carcinogenicity study for one NME component (using the most appropriate species). As in all the scenarios described, additional studies may be needed in the light of the emerging data.

References

1. FDA (2006) Nonclinical Safety Evaluation of Drug or Biologic Combinations. At URL http://www.fda.gov/downloads/Drugs/GuidanceComplianceRegulatoryInformation/Guidances/ucm079243.pdf

2. Office of Combination products (2007) At URL http://www.fda.gov/oc/combination/definition.html

3. Segal, S.A. (1999) Device and Biologic Combination Products. Understanding the Evolving Regulation. *Medical Device and Diagnostic Industry* January, 180–184.

4. Portnoy, S., and Koepke, K. (2005) Regulatory Strategy. Preclinical Testing of Combination Products. *Medical Device and Diagnostic Industry* May, 152–157.

5. Herxheimer, H. (1975) The danger of fixed drug combinations. *Int. J. Clin. Pharmacol. Biopharm.* **12**(**1–2**), 70–73.

6. Shenfield, G.M. (1982) Fixed combination drug therapy. *Drugs* **23**(**6**), 462–480.

7. Sica, D.A. (2002) Rationale for fixed-dose combinations in the treatment of hypertension: the cycle repeats. *Drugs* **62**(**3**), 443–462.

8. Moulding, T., Dutt, A.K., and Reichman, L.B. (1995) Fixed-dose combinations in antituberculous medications to prevent drug resistance. *Ann. Intern. Med.* **122**(**12**), 955–956.

9. Majori, G. (2004) Combined antimalarial therapy using artemisinin. *Parasitologia* **46**(**1–2**), 85–87.

10. Fechtner, R.D., and Realini, T. (2004) Fixed combinations of topical glaucoma medications. *Curr. Opin. Ophthalmol.* **15**(**2**), 132–135.

11. Wertheimer, A., and Morrison, A. (2002) Combination drugs. Innovation in pharmacotherapy. *P&T.* **27**(**1**), 44–49.

12. ICH guidelines (2007) At URL http://www.ich.org/cache/compo/276-254-1.html

13. Liminga, U., and Silva L. (2004) Non-clinical development of fixed combinations. A European regulatory perspective. *Int. J. Pharm. Med.* **18**(**3**), 135–138.

14. EMEA (2005) Draft Guideline on the non-clinical development of fixed combinations of medicinal products. CHMP/EMEA/CHMP/SWP/258498/2005. At URL http://www.ema.europa.eu/docs/en_GB/document_library/Scientific_guideline/2009/10/WC500003975.pdf

15. EMEA (1996) Note for guidance on fixed combination medicinal products. CPMP/EWP/240/95. At URL http://www.ema.europa.eu/docs/en_GB/document_library/Scientific_guideline/2009/09/WC500003689.pdf

16. Japanese Pharmaceutical Association (2010) At URL http://www.jpma.or.jp/english/parj/pdf/2010.pdf

17. Australian Therapeutic Goods Administration. *TGA News* (1998) Issue 28, December.

18. Hunt, L. (2003) Fixed-combination medicines: an Australian perspective. *WHO Drug Inf.* **2**, 110–112.

19. Therapeutics Product Directorate (2000) Guidelines for preparation of New Drug Submissions for Products Used for Estrogen–Progestin Replacement Therapy in Menopause (HRT). At URL http://hc-sc.gc.ca/dhp-mps/prodpharma/applic-demande/guide-ld/hrt-ths/hrt_ths_e.html

20. WHO Expert Committee on Specifications for Pharmaceutical Preparations (2005) Guidelines for registration of fixed-dose combination medicinal products Technical Report Series. *WHO Tech. Rep. Ser.* **929**, 93–142.

21. FDA (2006) Fixed Dose Combinations, Co-Packaged Drug products, and Single-Entity Versions of Previously Approved Antiretrovirals for the Treatment of HIV. At URL http://www.fda.gov/RegulatoryInformation/Guidances/ucm125278.htm

22. Rogge, M.C., and Taft, D.R. (Editors) (2005) in Preclinical Drug Development. Taylor & Francis Group, Boca Raton, FL, USA.

23. CDER Medical review for Kaletra. International Conference on Harmonization Toxicology Guidelines. At URL http://www.accessdata.fda.gov/drugsatfda_docs/nda/2000/21-226_Kaletra_medr.pdf

24. ICH Guidelines (2007) Safety Pharmacology Studies for Human Pharmaceuticals. At URL http://www.ich.org/LOB/media/MEDIA504.pdf

25. FDA (2000) Draft ICH Consensus Principal. Principles for Clinical Evaluation of New Antihypertensive Drugs E12A. At URL http://www.ich.org/LOB/media/MEDIA488.pdf

Chapter 2

Preclinical Evaluation of Juvenile Toxicity

Paul C. Barrow, Stéphane Barbellion, and Jeanne Stadler

Abstract

A pediatric assessment is now a required component of every New Drug Application in North America or Marketing Authorization Application in Europe, unless a waiver has been granted previously. Nonclinical juvenile toxicity studies are usually required as part of this assessment. The protocols for juvenile toxicity studies are devised in consultation with the FDA or EMEA. It is important to approach the regulatory authority well in advance in order not to delay the marketing authorization of the drug and to confirm the need or not to perform a preclinical evaluation in juvenile animals. The choice of species and the design of juvenile studies are based on a series of complex considerations, including: the therapeutic use of the drug, the age at which children will be treated, the duration of treatment, and potential age- or species-specific differences in pharmacokinetics or toxicity.

Key words: Juvenile animals, Toxicology, Pediatric, Safety testing

1. Introduction

1.1. Pediatrics as a Recent Science

In many civilizations, children were considered as miniature adults for centuries. In Europe, the dual vision of the child, inherited from the Greek and Roman eras, persisted until the nineteenth century. A child was, on one hand, the symbol of innocence and pureness and, on the other hand, an imperfect and disabled person. Familial care and medical practices were largely influenced by this vision of hyper-fragile miniature adults.

It was only at the beginning of the twentieth century that the science of pediatrics emerged and the physiological differences between adults and children were first recognized. Pediatrics recognized that childhood is divided into stages with specific medical needs evolving with age. This led to the emergence during the second half of the twentieth century of sub-specialities including specific focus on prematurity and adolescence.

Jean-Charles Gautier (ed.), *Drug Safety Evaluation: Methods and Protocols*, Methods in Molecular Biology, vol. 691,
DOI 10.1007/978-1-60761-849-2_2, © Springer Science+Business Media, LLC 2011

In modern times, pharmaceutical companies have been reluctant to study medicines in children because of concerns about toxicity, the difficulty in organizing clinical trials, and limited financial returns (1). Due to a lack of effective medicines approved for use in children, unlicensed and off-label use of drugs in children is still widespread today. In the late 1990s, a large proportion (50–90%) of medicines given to children had only been studied in adults, and not necessarily for the same indication or same disease as in children (2, 3). In addition, according to the American Academy of Pediatrics, a majority of marketed drugs were not labeled, or were insufficiently labeled, for use in pediatric patients (4).

This forced unregulated use of adult drugs and of adult dosage forms in children posed an obvious risk of adverse effects or of under- or overdosing. A consensus was finally reached, first in the USA and then in Europe, on the need to reinforce the existing international regulations with incentives for the pharmaceutical companies to perform specific safety studies when developing pediatric medicines.

1.2. Functional Immaturity

Many organs are not fully functional at birth and must continue to mature during postnatal development. This functional immaturity may have complex and far-reaching consequences on the effects of drugs in children. For instance, the absorption of a drug following oral ingestion may differ between the child and adult due to differences in the permeability of the intestinal wall or due to differences in the pH of the gastrointestinal tract. The distribution of the drug following absorption or parenteral administration may then be influenced by differences in membrane permeability. The blood–brain barrier, for instance, is incomplete up to the age of about 5 years, which may result in adverse CNS effects in children with drugs that do not cross the adult blood–brain barrier. The bioavailability and the distribution of drugs may also be influenced by differences in the composition of body tissues and fluids between children and adults (e.g., water content of organs or the binding affinity of plasma proteins). Drugs are often metabolized more slowly or via different pathways in children due to a reduced enzyme activity related to immaturity of the liver. Likewise, a drug may be eliminated more slowly from the circulation in the child due to the relative inefficiency of the immature kidney. Finally, the pharmacological efficacy of the drug may be enhanced or diminished due to differences in the relative numbers of excitory or inhibitory receptors present in the target tissue of the immature organism compared with the adult.

2. Legislative Environment

In 1986, the World Health Organization (WHO) issued a report on the need to adopt a special approach when evaluating risks from chemicals during infancy and early childhood (5). Then, the

International Life Sciences Institute (ILSI) studied in detail the similarities and differences between children and adults and their implications for risk assessment (6).

The Food and Drug Administration Modernization Act (FDAMA) passed in the USA in 1997 offered an additional 6 months protection from generic competition on all juvenile and adult applications of a drug in return for the additional work to develop the product for pediatric use. The carrot was then followed by the stick...

In 1998 (7), the FDA issued the Pediatric Rule, which obliged pharmaceutical companies to assess the safety and effectiveness of all new drugs likely to be of therapeutic value in children. The rule presumed that all new drugs will be studied in pediatric patients, but allowed the manufacturers to obtain a waiver for drugs with no therapeutic use in children. It also allowed the FDA to require pediatric studies for existing drugs known to be used off-label in children. To complete this rule, the FDA issued a list of drugs for which additional pediatric information was at that time considered necessary (8).

The incentive was renewed in the Best Pharmaceuticals for Children Act (BPCA) in 2001, which also authorized the National Institutes of Health (NIH) and the FDA to undertake pediatric studies of approved drugs that do not benefit from other types of pediatric development incentives. After a suspension by court in 2002, the Pediatric rule was re-enacted by the Pediatric Research Equity Act (PREA) in 2003. This requires a pediatric assessment as part of all NDAs and biologics licensing applications (or supplements to applications) for new active ingredients, new indications, new dosage forms, new dosing regimens, or new routes of administration, unless the applicant has obtained a waiver or deferral. It also authorizes FDA to demand a pediatric assessment for previously approved marketed drugs and biological products, even if no change to the existing license has been requested (9).

As a result of this legislation, labeling changes have been made to nearly 200 drugs studied in children under the BPCA or PREA (10). Of the more than 150 drugs studied under the exclusivity incentive program within the BPCA, 133 have new pediatric labeling information including:

- 39 drugs with new or enhanced pediatric safety data
- 25 drugs with new dosing or dosing changes
- 29 drugs with information stating that they were not found to be effective in children.

European initiatives followed on from the American process. A round table of EMEA experts in 1997 recognized a need to strengthen the legislation and to develop incentives. In 1998, the European Commission supported the ICH project of a specific guideline, the ICH Topic E11. This guideline became the European guideline and is in force since 2002 (11).

A memorandum was presented under the French European Presidency to the Council of Health Ministers in December 2000 demonstrating that a regulation on evaluation of drug for pediatrics was a public health priority. A Resolution was then adopted on 14 December 2000.

In February 2002, the European Commission published a consultation paper on "Better Medicines for Children – proposed regulatory actions in pediatric medicinal products." After an in-depth analysis of the economical, social and environmental impacts, a draft regulation was issued on 29 September 2004. The final Regulation was agreed on 1 June 2006 by the European Parliament and entered into force in January 2007. This legislation comprises two texts (12, 13) and encompasses three objectives:

- Facilitate the development and availability of medicines for children

- Ensure the quality and ethical environment of the research

- Improve the availability of information on the use of medicines in children.

The additional requirements must not subject children to unnecessary tests and should not delay the authorization for use of the drug in adult patients.

This legislation brings Europe in line with the PREA in the USA, with 6 months additional exclusivity in return for pediatric testing. A Pediatric Investigational Plan (PIP) is required even for adult medicines and has to be agreed with a Pediatric Committee (PDCO) of the European medicines agency (EMEA) prior to the clinical phase 2 studies. This Committee comprises members of the Committee for Medicinal Products for Human Use (CHMP), health care professionals and representatives of patients' organizations.

In December 2007, the European Medicines Agency (EMEA) adopted a list, established by its Pediatric Committee, of medical conditions that do not occur in children. Companies developing medicines intended to treat any condition on this list will be granted a waiver from the requirement to submit the results of pediatric studies when seeking a marketing authorization for their product (14).

3. Preclinical Guidelines

The emergence of new pediatric regulations raised questions on the need for improvement of the preclinical studies which support these trials in children. The existing ICH guidelines for the reproductive toxicity testing of medicinal agents were issued in 1994 (15). These identified the potential specific risks incurred when treating immature individuals, but did not propose postnatal testing other than the classical pre- and postnatal study, where juvenile animals are exposed in utero and through the milk. There was an obvious gap in the international regulatory requirements regarding risk evaluation of direct exposure during postnatal life until sexual maturity (see also Note 1).

Indeed, most of the pharmaceutical companies involved in the development of drugs for pediatric use had been testing their molecules in juvenile animals for years, long before the implementation of the new pediatric regulation (16–18). However, the results of these studies were rarely included in marketing submissions. The reason for this was that it was commonly accepted, and published in the regulatory guidance documents, that data collected from humans were more relevant than those from studies in juvenile animals.

Both the FDA (19) and the EMEA (20) issued guidance documents on the need for juvenile toxicity studies, with the dual aim of testing whether the juvenile is more susceptible than the adult to the general organ toxicity of the drug and of testing the drug for adverse effects on postnatal development. The two guidance documents are essentially similar in content and manufacturers generally aim to comply with both.

Both guidance documents require attention to effects of the test compound on development of the nervous, renal, reproductive, immune, and pulmonary systems; the FDA text insists as well on the detection of potential effects on the development of the skeleton and gastrointestinal system. On the other hand, the European text is slightly more detailed regarding the need and design of specific studies addressing potential neurotoxic, immunotoxic, or nephrotoxic effects. In addition, the American guidance document provides examples of human-to-animal comparison of developmental periods and considerations for application of juvenile animal data in risk management. Both guidance documents also indicate circumstances, however, where juvenile animal studies would be neither informative nor necessary (see Note 2).

The ICH "M3" guideline (21) on nonclinical safety studies for the conduct of human clinical trials for pharmaceuticals requires that general toxicity studies, reproductive toxicity studies, and genotoxicity tests should be completed before the initiation of clinical trials in children. However, this requirement is not essential if risks resulting from exposure before sexual maturity have been evaluated in relevant juvenile animal studies. For example, the ICH pre- and postnatal study design can be adapted to adequately fulfill the present regulatory requirements (see above). The FDA and EMEA are open to these initiatives and expect manufacturers to develop their strategies in partnership with the respective pediatric committees, even if this is not always clearly stated.

4. Submission Strategy – Instructions

4.1. Consult with the Regulatory Authority

Seek the agreement of the regulatory authority on the proposed pediatric program as early as possible. This is done by submitting a draft Pediatric Investigation Plan (PIP) to the pediatric committee of the EMEA or a Proposed Pediatric Study Request (PPSR) to the FDA. The results of any requested juvenile studies will be a requirement of the NDA or MAA submission (unless a deferral is granted) (see Notes 3 and 4). It is possible to commence preliminary juvenile studies before agreement has been reached on the design of the main studies to save time and anticipate possible difficulties.

4.2. Request a Waiver if a Pediatric Program is Not Warranted

Clearly, juvenile studies are not necessary for drugs that have no therapeutic use in children (e.g., Alzheimer therapies). If a pediatric program is not warranted, seek the agreement of the FDA, or a formal waiver from the EMEA, well before the time of submission.

4.3. Decide Whether Juvenile Animal Studies are Necessary in Support of the Proposed Clinical Program in Children

Juvenile animal studies serve no purpose when sufficient human data are already available from off-label use of the drug in children. Note, however, that reliable data are rarely compiled for off-label drug use.

If the drug is only of therapeutic value in older children, the relevant developmental periods may have already been covered in the existing toxicology studies (see Note 1).

According to the ICH M3 (and US and EMEA guidelines on Nonclinical testing in juvenile animals), animal studies may be omitted or deferred for life-threatening diseases for which there is no current effective therapy (see Note 2).

4.4. Should the Pediatric Assessment be Deferred?

The potential therapeutic benefit of the drug in children may be in doubt pending the initial results on efficacy and/or safety in the adult. In such cases, the FDA or the EMEA should agree to defer the pediatric assessments until more data are available in adults. Again, the agreement of the agency should be sought well in advance.

4.5. One or Two Species?

According to the FDA and EMEA guidance documents, juvenile studies in a single species may be sufficient to complete a NDA or MAA submission. At present, however, some divisions of the FDA tend to request studies in two species, one rodent and one non-rodent, applying the same principle as that used for the general toxicity safety testing in adult animals. This decision will ultimately be based on the relevance of the available models. If a single animal model can adequately address the considerations given below, then a second species is unnecessary. For practical purposes, a non-rodent study (e.g., dog) may be used for a detailed evaluation of the direct short-term consequences of juvenile exposure to the drug, in addition to a rodent study (e.g., rat) to evaluate the long-term developmental consequences of exposure.

5. Testing Strategy

5.1. Considerations Influencing Study Design

Each study is designed case-by-case, based on the following considerations:

- Therapeutic use of drug
- Timing and duration of treatment in children
- Potential age- or species-specific differences in pharmacokinetics or toxicity
- Interspecies differences in the timing of development
- Known organ toxicity of the drug.

5.2. Devising a Testing Strategy – Steps to Follow

1. Review the available human data (including pediatric data, if available) alongside the toxicology data in adult animals.
2. Identify the potential target organ(s) in the juvenile.
3. Select the most appropriate juvenile animal model(s) that show a similar pattern of postnatal development of the identified target organ(s).
4. Perform preliminary studies to evaluate the tolerance of the drug in the juvenile under the anticipated conditions of the main study and also to generate any required data on pharmacokinetics and metabolism in the juvenile animal.
5. Adapt the treatment period in the main juvenile studies to encompass all of the relevant developmental stages of the animal with respect to the therapeutic use of the drug in children.
6. Consider specific endpoints for inclusion in the study design to monitor the function and development of the identified target organs.

A comparison of the ages of the different developmental stages of various species with respect to the human is given in Table 1. This summary is relatively vague, however, and the timing of the treatment period and examinations in a juvenile study should be based on the comparative timing of development of the specific potential target organs in the species in question (see Note 5).

Table 1
Age comparison between humans and various animal models. Adapted from Barrow 2007 (38)

Species	Preterm	Newborn	Infant	Child	Adolescent
Human	–	0–28 days	1–23 months	2–12 years	12–16 years
Monkey	–	0–15 days	0.5–6 months	0.5–3 years	3–4 years
Dog	–	0–21 days	3–6 weeks	6–20 weeks	5–7 months
Pig	–	0–15 days	2–4 weeks	4–14 weeks	4–6 months
Rabbit	0–4 days	0–10 days	1.5–5 weeks	5–12 weeks	3–6 months
Rat	0–4 days	0–10 days	1.5–3 weeks	3–6 weeks	7–11 weeks
Mouse	0–4 days	0–10 days	1.5–3 weeks	3–5 weeks	5–7 weeks

5.3. Objectives of Juvenile Toxicity Studies

Regulatory juvenile toxicity studies are designed to detect two distinct types of hazard:

- Increased vulnerability of the immature organism to general organ toxicity of the drug
- An adverse influence of the drug on the development or maturation of the organism.

The detection of general toxicity in the juvenile can usually be detected at the end of the period of exposure, though a recovery period may be necessary to investigate the persistence of any induced lesions.

The detection of developmental toxicity, on the other hand, requires monitoring of the development of the animal until the target organs reach maturity. Developmental insults may result in latent defects that are only manifest much later in development, thus necessitating an extended follow-up period in juvenile studies. Such lesions may, for instance, result in functional defects in the adult animal.

Juvenile animal studies should also aim to provide information on the following:

- Identification of biomarkers for use in the clinic
- Extrapolation of clinical exposure levels
- Evaluation of the risk–benefit ratio in children.

5.4. Selection of Juvenile Animal Models

The choice of species to be used for the juvenile studies is influenced by the following factors:

- Data from adult toxicology studies
- Pharmacokinetics of the drug in the adult versus the juvenile

- Species differences in pharmacology and pharmacodynamic responses
- Physiological similarities to human
- Developmental similarities to human (i.e., timing of organ development)
- Practical considerations.

5.4.1. Rodents

The rat is the most practical and most commonly used species for juvenile toxicology studies. It is also the most commonly used species for general and reproductive toxicology.

The mouse is more difficult to handle because of its smaller size and greater activity, but is a feasible alternative to the rat.

The short, compressed lifespan of rodents allows the evaluation of many life stages in a relatively short experiment (e.g., 3 months).

The small size and low cost of rodents are also obvious advantages over larger species.

Rodents are very immature at birth: a rat pup of 4–7 days old is roughly equivalent to a preterm infant.

5.4.2. Non-rodents

The dog is the second most common species for juvenile studies. It is also the most used non-rodent species for pharmaceutical safety testing, so a great deal of toxicology data is usually available in the adult dog prior to commencement of the juvenile studies.

The minipig is the most practical non-rodent species for juvenile studies and is the species of choice when the general toxicity studies have been performed in a non-rodent species other than the dog. All routes of administration are feasible in the minipig except intravenous and inhalation.

Rabbits are rarely used for juvenile studies, since general toxicity data are rarely available in this species (despite being routinely used for embryotoxicity studies). Handling of the litters without due caution may result in maternal cannibalism or rejection. Nonetheless, juvenile studies are feasible in the rabbit.

Juvenile toxicity studies in monkeys are problematic in part due to the poor availability of suitable animals and in part due to the technical complexities of handling baby monkeys and their mothers.

Juvenile studies have been successfully, but rarely, performed in other species, such as cats, sheep, and goats.

5.5. Parameters

The regulatory guidance documents define a series of standard endpoints that should be routinely determined in all juvenile toxicology studies. Other non-routine parameters should be devised case-by-case for each study to better characterize the anticipated effects of the drug and to identify possible biomarkers of toxicity that could serve as an alert in the clinic.

6. Study Design

6.1. Number of Animals

There is no clear regulatory guidelines on the number of animals required per dose group. As a general rule, the group sizes for juvenile studies are based on the requirements for other types of toxicology studies (i.e., general toxicology studies, neurotoxicity studies for protocols including behavioral tests or reproductive toxicology studies for protocols with a mating phase).

1. *Rodents and rabbits*: each subgroup should include at least 16 males and 16 females (i.e., the minimum numbers considered necessary to interpret the findings from behavioral tests and mating). Most rodent studies comprise two subgroups (see below), so 32 pups of each sex per group are allocated to the study.

2. *Non-rodents*: the usual group size for dog and minipig studies is eight males and eight females per treatment group.

6.2. Split-Litter or Entire-Litter Design?

Before weaning, the experimental data need to be collected and analyzed in such a way as to take into account the genotypic similarity of the pups within the same litter and their dependence on the health and behavior of the mother. No definitive regulatory guidance has been provided to indicate which approach should be used.

Two basic study designs may be used:

1. Split-litter design: different pups within each litter are allocated to different experimental groups, such that each dam raises a mixture of treated and control pups (see Note 6).

2. Entire litter design: all of the pups in each litter are allocated to the same experimental group.

Advantages and disadvantages of split-litter design:

+   Comparison of treated and control pups within each litter, thus controlling for genotypic and maternal influences.

+   Increased statistical power for low group sizes, since each pup may be taken as an individual experimental unit.

+   Less risk of death due to treatment-related hypothermia, with the few affected high dose pups kept warm by their littermates.

–   High risk of cross contamination between pups of the same litter (possibly via the milk following contamination of the mother).

Advantages and disadvantages of entire-litter design:

+   Little risk of cross contamination.

+   Lower risk of treatment error due to confusion of littermates.

– Increased risk of maternal toxicity at high dose levels, due to the mother grooming greater numbers of treated pups.

– Poor statistical power with smaller group sizes, since the litter has to be taken as the experimental unit. This problem is avoided in larger studies, where different pups from each litter are allocated to different subgroups for several panels of examinations.

In practice, this choice of study design is taken based on the group sizes and the perceived importance of cross contamination.

6.3. Age at Start of Dosing

1. Oral: rodent pups are frequently dosed by the oral or subcutaneous routes from 4 days of age. It is possible to start treatment earlier after birth, but this is usually not necessary, the newborn rodent being very immature by comparison with the human. Dogs and minipigs may be orally dosed from 7 days of age.

2. IV: intravenous administration is possible in the rat from about 10 days of age. Dogs may be injected from birth. IV administration is difficult in the minipig at all ages, though juvenile studies have been successfully performed using implanted vascular access ports. Rabbits may be injected from 2 weeks of age.

3. SC: Subcutaneous administration is feasible in all species from birth.

4. IM: Intramuscular administration to rodent pups is limited to very small volumes before weaning owing to the low muscle mass. Dogs and minipigs can be injected from birth. Rabbits may be injected from 2 weeks of age.

5. Inhalation: Rodent litters may be exposed with the mother using whole body exposure. Dogs may be exposed via mouth breathing or nose-only from 2 weeks of age using an adapted mask. Inhalation studies are not normally conducted in juvenile minipigs or rabbits.

6.4. Duration of Treatment

Dosing will be continued until all of the relevant developmental stages have been covered. This may involve treatment up to the adult age or up to the age at which treatment commenced in the general toxicity studies in the same species.

6.5. Need for a Post-treatment Follow-Up or Reversibility Period

It is necessary to retain at least a proportion of the animals from rodent studies up to maturity to detect any latent defects, such as neurobehavioral defects or influences on reproductive development. These examinations are not usually required for non-rodent species.

6.6. Subgroups in Rodent Studies

Rodent studies usually comprise two subgroups of at least 16 animals of each sex within each treatment group:

1. Subgroup 1: necropsied 1 day after the last dose (e.g. at 7 weeks of age)

2. Subgroup 2: retained after the end of the treatment period for further developmental and behavioral monitoring and mating at 12 weeks of age.

All non-rodents are usually necropsied at the end of the treatment period.

7. Study Performance

7.1. Animal Supply

1. Rodents: many breeders will supply lactating rats or mice with litters from about 1 day post partum. Otherwise, it is also possible to order time-mated females and allow them to give birth in the lab. Large numbers of animals are required to give birth at the same time to provide enough pups for the purposes of a full juvenile study. The females may be mated in house, but logistical challenges need to be overcome to provide the large numbers of animals that are required to give birth at the same time.

2. Non rodents: it is not normally considered ethical to transport neonatal dogs, minipigs, or rabbits. It is therefore necessary to either order pregnant females or to mate the females in-house. As for rodents, it is important to ensure that a sufficient number of pups are born within a short period.

7.2. Cross Fostering

Cross fostering is used to optimize the number of pups available by exchanging pups between mothers to obtain litters of the required size. This is easily accomplished in rodents and minipigs and is also possible in dogs.

All of the pups born over a period of about 24 h are pooled and then randomly redistributed with equal numbers of each sex in each litter.

7.3. Identification of Pups

Rodent pups are best identified by tattoo on the paws (16).

Dogs and minipigs may be tattooed on a pinna or implanted with a transponder. Rabbits are tattooed on a pinna.

7.4. Clinical Condition and Body Weight up to Weaning

All pups are examined frequently during the study to observe any clinical reactions to treatment.

Rodent pups are weighed every 2 or 3 days.

Dogs and minipigs are weighed at least twice per week.

7.5. Monitoring of Preweaning Growth and Development

1. Rodents and rabbits: the growth and development of rodent pups is assessed by individual daily monitoring of developmental milestones and reflex testing using similar techniques as those routinely used in developmental toxicity studies (*22*). In addition, specific growth measures, such as manual external measurement of tibia length, are determined every 2 or 3 days.

2. Dog: growth measures, such as standing shoulder height and external tibia length, are recorded at least twice per week for each dog. The puppies are examined daily to determine the days of tooth eruption and eye opening. The auditory, fossorial, labial, and perineal reflexes may be evaluated at various ages. The days of acquired locomotion are noted, i.e. crawling, standing, walking, and running are noted.

3. Minipig: growth measures, such as standing shoulder height and external tibia length, are recorded at least twice per week for each piglet. The piglets are examined daily to determine the days of tooth eruption and eye opening. The papillary and auditory reflexes may be evaluated at various ages.

4. Rabbits: each rabbit kit is examined daily to determine the days of incisor eruption and eye opening. Tibia length is recorded twice per week. The surface righting, papillary, and auditory reflexes may be evaluated at various ages.

7.6. Blood Sampling for Toxicokinetics or Clinical Pathology

1. Rodents: blood sampling may be performed in rats from 4 days of age from a mandibular vein, but the volume of blood that can be withdrawn is severely limited before the age of 2 weeks. For this reason, satellite animals are usually used for toxicokinetic sampling in rodent studies, allowing the use of terminal sampling methods.

2. Dogs: blood may be withdrawn from a jugular vein of dogs under anesthesia from 1 week of age.

3. Minipigs: blood may be withdrawn from the cranial vena cava of minipigs without anesthesia at any age (*23*).

4. Rabbits: blood sampling may be performed from an ear artery from about 2 weeks of age.

7.7. Pre-weaning Cardiovascular Examinations

Cardiovascular parameters may be determined in dogs and minipigs from 1 week of age.

A standard ECG trace is recorded with the puppy or piglet lightly restrained in a net hammock, allowing the determination of the heart rate. The ECG wave-form is difficult to analyze before regularizing at around the age of weaning.

Blood pressure is measured using a limb cuff.

7.8. Weaning

Rodents are weaned at 3 weeks of age, dogs at 7 weeks, minipigs at 5 weeks, and rabbits at 5 weeks.

7.8.1. Considerations for Postnatal Juvenile Studies

The practical organization of juvenile studies in all species is considerably simpler if dosing can be commenced after weaning. The litter origin of the pups nonetheless needs to be taken into account in the allocation of pups to the treatment groups. Pups from the same litter should preferably be spread across all treatment groups, or failing this, randomized.

7.8.2. Considerations for the Post-natal Component of Perinatal Juvenile Studies

For studies in which dosing was started before weaning, the animals are rehoused following separation from the mother. The same treatment regime will normally be continued during the post-treatment period, though the dosing regime may be adjusted to allow for age-dependent differences in pharmacokinetics or metabolism.

7.8.3. Individual Versus Group Housing After Weaning

Group housing is preferred for the housing of juvenile animals, since social contact is necessary for normal neurobehavioral development. Aggressive behavior is rarely a problem between immature animals that have been housed together from weaning. Cage-mates should be of the same sex, the same approximate postnatal age and, if possible, derived from different litters.

7.9. Animal Identification After Weaning

After weaning, the animals of all species are individually identified by tattoo on a pinna and/or tail or using an implanted transponder.

7.10. Routine Post-weaning Examinations

The routine examinations, as described for the preweaning phase, are continued after weaning. The frequency of body weights and growth measurements may be reduced to twice-weekly in view of the slower rate of growth.

7.11. Specific Post-weaning Examinations

The food consumption of each cage of animals is recorded.
Other post-weaning examinations include the following:

1. Vaginal opening in females
2. Balano-preputial separation in males
3. Clinical pathology (hematology, serum clinical chemistry and coagulation): determined at intervals for non-rodents and at termination for rodents (see Note 7).
4. ECG examinations are performed during the last week of the treatment period (and during the recovery period if applicable) in dogs and minipigs.

7.12. Neurobehavioral Tests in Rodents

Various divisions of the FDA frequently request complex neurobehavioral tests in juvenile rodent studies (see Note 8). These tests are typically performed once during the treatment period (in the subgroup terminated at the end of dosing) and once after the end of the treatment period. The types of test requested include the following:

1. Motor activity (total activity and stereotypy).

2. Cognitive function using a complex maze test.

3. Auditory startle reflex, including habituation and pre-pulse inhibition.

7.13. Mating and Fertility Assessment

Rodents:

1. Rodents are paired at approximately 12 weeks of age.

2. One male and one female from the same treatment group (avoiding siblings) are housed in the same cage until copulation occurs, as detected by the presence of sperm in a vaginal smear.

3. The pregnant females are submitted to cesarean section at mid-pregnancy. The numbers of live and dead embryos in the uterus are counted.

Non-rodents:

Mating assessments are rarely performed in non-rodent species. Nonetheless, a detailed histopathology evaluation of the reproductive organs may be expected to reveal any adverse effects of the drug on reproductive capacity (provided that the animals are sufficiently mature at the end of the study).

7.14. Necropsy and Histopathology

All animals (whether terminated at the end of the treatment period or at maturity) are submitted to routine necropsy. Organs are weighed, sampled, and examined microscopically following similar procedures as those used for the general toxicity studies in the same species.

In addition to routine histopathology, some divisions of the FDA frequently request detailed examinations of the CNS (neuro-histopathology) and the reproductive organs.

7.15. Non-routine Endpoints after Weaning

Additional endpoints may be incorporated into the study design to evaluate the development and integrity of potential target organs, for example:

1. Serum samples for hormone determinations.

2. Skeletal examinations: periodic X-ray imaging or bone densitometry at termination.

3. Periodic or terminal sperm analysis.

4. Immune evaluations (see Note 9): immunoglobulin and cytokine serum determinations, lymphocyte subset determinations, primary antibody response to sheep red blood cells, or keyhole limpet hemocyanin. The objectives of immune evaluations within the context of juvenile studies are essentially limited to the detection of effects leading to immune depression. There are no validated tests available at the present

time for the evaluation of adverse effects resulting in immune stimulation, which may make the child more vulnerable to autoimmune disease or hypersensitivity (24).

8. Notes

1. In practice, the animals used for many subchronic and chronic studies are not sexually mature at the start of the study. It is quite usual, for instance, to commence a 3-month general toxicology study with rats of 6 weeks of age, roughly corresponding to the stage of development of a 10-year-old child.

2. According to the US guidance, juvenile animal studies might not be necessary when: (1) data from similar therapeutics in a class have identified a particular hazard and additional data are unlikely to change this perspective; (2) there are adequate clinical data and adverse events of concern have not been observed during clinical use; (3) target organ toxicity would not be expected to differ in sensitivity between adult and pediatric patients because the target organ of toxicity is functionally mature in the intended pediatric population and younger children with the functionally immature tissue are not expected to receive the drug. The EU guidance indicates medicinal products under development for specific pediatric indications or in life-threatening or serious diseases without current effective therapies warrant a case-by-case approach. In some cases, some studies may then be adapted, deferred, or omitted.

3. In the USA, a pediatric assessment, or justified reason for its absence, is a required component of the NDA. The FDA is open to discussion on the design of the proposed juvenile studies and should always be consulted to avoid delays in the NDA approval arising from requests for additional studies.

4. In Europe, the results of studies according to the agreed PIP (or waiver) is a required component of MAA, so the plan needs to be submitted to the Pediatric Committee (PDCO) of the EMEA as early as possible. The agreement procedure currently takes at least 4 months. Aim to submit the PIP during Phase I, or at the latest, during the Proof of Concept Phase.

5. The Development and Reproductive Toxicology Technical Committee of the ILSI Health and Environmental Sciences Institute (HESI) has issued a series of reviews on comparative organ development for use in the design of juvenile studies (25–35).

6. Also called "within-litter design" (all dosage groups equally represented in each litter) or "between-litter design" (all dosage groups in the litter).

7. Clinical pathology endpoints may be monitored as indicators of anticipated organ toxicity (e.g., liver hypertrophy or renal tubular dilatation). Other parameters, such as differential blood cell counts, are also used to monitor the postnatal development of the bone marrow or immune organs. In rodent studies, clinical pathology is often only included as an apical measure at the end of the study, due to the limited volume of blood that can be sampled from the young pups. A larger volume of blood can be withdrawn from puppies or piglets, allowing clinical pathology parameters to be monitored regularly throughout the study. Reference data for rats and dogs at various ages are available (36).

8. Behavioral and cognitive tests are generally only performed in rodents. A battery of tests is used to assess sensorimotor function, locomotor activity, reactivity, learning, and memory. The battery used in juvenile studies is usually based on that already in place for developmental toxicity studies. The most common tests include: motor activity monitoring, open field activity, learning and memory tasks in a water-filled maze, passive avoidance, performance on a rotating rod, grip strength, and startle habituation (37).

9. An initial screen for immune effects in a juvenile study may be limited to histopathological examination of the lymphoid organs/tissues (including organ weights) and routine clinical pathology. If necessary, tests are available for the detection of immune depression in juvenile rodents (26).

References

1. Choonara, I. (2000) Clinical trials of medicines in children: US experience shows how to ensure that treatment of children is evidence based. *Br. Med. J.* **321**, 1093–1094.

2. Conroy, S., McIntyre, J., and Choonara, I. (1999) Unlicensed and off label drug use in neonates. *Arch. Dis. Child.* **80**, F142–F145.

3. Conroy, S., Choonara, I., Impicciatore, P., Mohn, A., Arnell, H., Rane, A., Knoeppel, C., Seyberth, H., Pandolfini, C., Raffaelli, M.P., Rocchi, F., Bonati, M., 't Jong, G., de Hoog, M., and van den Anker, J. (2000) Survey of unlicensed and off label drug use in pediatric wards in European countries. *Br. Med. J.* **320**, 79–82.

4. Committee on Drugs, American Academy of Pediatrics. (1995) Guidelines for the Ethical Conduct of Studies to Evaluate Drugs in Pediatric Populations. *Pediatrics* **95**(2), 286–294.

5. WHO (1986) Principles for evaluating health risks from chemicals during infancy and early childhood: the need for a special approach. International Programme on Chemical Safety. Environmental Health Criteria 59. World Health Organization, Geneva.

6. Guzelian, P.S., Henry, C.J., and Olin, S.S. (1992) *Similarities and differences between children and adults: Implications for risk assessment.* ILSI Press, Washington, D.C.

7. FDA (1998a) Regulations requiring manufacturers to assess the safety and effectiveness of new drugs and biological products in pediatric patients. *Fed. Regist.* **63**, 66632–66672.

8. FDA (1998b) List of drugs for which additional pediatric information may produce health benefits in the pediatric population. *Fed. Regist.* **63**, 27732–27733.

9. FDA (2005) Draft guidance for industry: How to comply with the pediatric research equity act. September 2005 (http://www.fda.gov/cber/gdlns/pedreseq.pdf).

10. FDA (2007) Should your child be in a clinical trial?http://www.fda.gov/consumer/updates/pediatrictrial101507.html. Consulted 19 May 2008.

11. ICH (2000b) E11: Clinical investigation of medicinal products in the pediatric population. *Fed. Regist.* **65**, 19777–19781.

12. EU (2006) Regulation (EC) No 1901/2006 of the European Parliament and of the Council of 12 December 2006 on medicinal products for paediatric use and amending Regulation (EEC) No 1768/92, Directive2001/20/EC, Directive 2001/83/EC and Regulation (EC) No 726/2004 – Official Journal of the European Union. 27 December 2006, pp. L378-1-19.

13. EU (2006) – Regulation (EC) No 1902/2006 of the European Parliament and of the Council of 20 December 2006 amending Regulation 1901/2006 on medicinal products for paediatric use – Official Journal of the European Union 27 December 2006, pp. L378- 20-21.

14. EMEA (2007) European Medicine Agency decision of 3 December 2007 on a class waiver on conditions in accordance with Regulation (EC) 1901/2006 of the European Parliament and of the Council as amended – EMEA/551894/2007 P/1/2007.

15. ICH (1994) Step 4 tripartite harmonised guidelines. Detection of toxicity to reproduction for medicinal products, in *Proceedings of the second international conference on harmonisation Orlando* (D'Arcy, P.F., and Harron, D.W.G., eds.), Queen's University: Belfast. pp. 557–578.

16. Barrow, P. (1990) Technical procedures in reproduction toxicology. Laboratory animals handbooks 11. Royal Society of Medicine, London.

17. Baldrick, P. (2004) Developing drugs for pediatric use: A role for juvenile animal studies? *Regul. Toxicol. Pharmacol.* **39**, 381–389.

18. Hurtt, M.E. (2004) Workshop Summary. Juvenile animal studies: Testing strategies and design. *Birth Defects Res. B Dev. Reprod. Toxicol.* **71**(**4**), 281–288.

19. FDA (2006) Guidance for industry: nonclinical safety evaluation of pediatric drug products, February 2006 (http://www.fda.gov/cder/guidance/5671fnl.htm).

20. EMEA (2008) Guideline on the need for non-clinical testing in juvenile animals on human pharmaceuticals for paediatric indications. Ref. EMEA/CHMP/SWP/169215/2008.

21. ICH (2000a) M3(R1): Maintenance of the ICH guideline on non-clinical safety studies for the conduct of human clinical trials for pharmaceuticals.

22. Barrow, P. (2000) Reproductive and developmental toxicology safety studies, in *The laboratory rat.* (Krinke, G.J., ed.), Academic Press, London, pp. 199–225.

23. NCR3S (2008) Blood sampling microsite. http://www.nc3rs.org.uk/bloodsampling-microsite/page.asp?id=346, consulted 16 May 2008.

24. Barrow, P.C., and Ravel, G. (2005) Immune assessments in developmental and juvenile toxicology: Practical considerations for the regulatory safety testing of pharmaceuticals. *Regul. Toxicol. Pharmacol.* **43**, 35–44.

25. Hurtt, M.E., and Sandler, J.D. (2003) Comparative organ system development: Introduction. *Birth Defects Res. B Dev. Reprod. Toxicol.* **68**, 85.

26. Beckman, D.A., and Feuston, M. (2003) Landmarks in the development of the female reproductive system. *Birth Defects Res. B Dev. Reprod. Toxicol.* **68**, 137–143.

27. Hew, K.W., and Keller, K.A. (2003) Postnatal anatomical and functional development of the heart: A species comparison. *Birth Defects Res. B Dev. Reprod. Toxicol.* **68**, 309–320.

28. Holsapple, M.P., West, L.J., and Landreth, K.S. (2003) Species comparison of anatomical and functional immune system development. *Birth Defects Res. B Dev. Reprod. Toxicol.* **68**, 321–334.

29. Marty, M.S., Chapin, R.E., Parks, L.G., and Thorsrud, B.A. (2003) Development and maturation of the male reproductive system. *Birth Defects Res. B Dev. Reprod. Toxicol.* **68**, 125–136.

30. Walthall, K., Cappon, G.D., Hurtt, M.E., and Zoetis, T. (2005) Postnatal development of the gastrointestinal system: A species comparison. *Birth Defects Res. B Dev. Reprod. Toxicol.* **74**, 132–156.

31. Watson, R.E., DeSesso, J.M., Hurtt, M.E., and Cappon, G.D. (2006) Postnatal growth and morphological development of the brain: A species comparison. *Birth Defects Res. B Dev. Reprod. Toxicol.* **77**, 471–484.

32. Wood, S.L., Beyer, B.K., and Cappon, G.D. (2003) Species comparison of postnatal CNS development: Functional measures. *Birth Defects Res. B Dev. Reprod. Toxicol.* **68**, 391–407.

33. Zoetis, T., Tassinari, M.S., Bagi, C., Walthall, K., and Hurtt, M.E. (2003) Species comparison of postnatal bone growth and development. *Birth Defects Res. B Dev. Reprod. Toxicol.* **68**, 86–110.

34. Zoetis, T., and Hurtt, M.E. (2003) Species comparison of anatomical and functional renal development. *Birth Defects Res. B Dev. Reprod. Toxicol.* **68**, 111–120.

35. Zoetis, T., and Hurtt, M.E. (2003) Species comparison of lung development. *Birth Defects Res. B Dev. Reprod. Toxicol.* **68**, 121–124.

36. Beck, M.J., Padgett, E.L., Bowman, C.J., Wilson, D.T., Kaufman, L.E., Varsho, B.J., Stump, D.G., Nemec, M.D., and Holson, J.F. (2006) Nonclinical juvenile toxicity testing, in *Developmental and reproductive toxicology: A practical approach*, 2nd ed. (Hood, R. D., ed.), CRC Press, Boca Raton, pp. 263–328.

37. Meyer, J.S. (1998) Behavioral assessment in developmental neurotoxicology, in *Handbook of developmental neurotoxicology* (Slikker, W., and Chang, L.W., eds.), Academic Press, San Diego, pp. 403–426.

38. Barrow, P. (2007) Toxicology testing for products intended for pediatric populations, in *Nonclinical drug safety assessment: Practical considerations for successful registration,* (Sietsema, W.K., and Schwen, R., eds.) FDA News, Washington, D.C., pp. 411–440.

Part II

Pathology

Chapter 3

Necropsy and Sampling Procedures in Rodents

Laurence Fiette and Mohamed Slaoui

Abstract

Necropsy is a major step of most studies using laboratory animals. During necropsy, tissue and organ changes noticeable grossly can be recorded, and important tissue samples can be stored for subsequent evaluation. It is therefore important that the personnel in charge of this key experimentation step be adequately trained and aware of the study endpoints.

Key words: Necropsy, Histology, Macroscopy, Sampling, Rodents, Mouse, Rat

1. Introduction

Necropsy is a postmortem procedure that consists of observation of macroscopic changes of tissue and organ *in situ* with naked eyes and of collection of key organs and tissues samples for further analyses.

Necropsy techniques have been developed to diagnose diseases in animals and are classically used in health status monitoring of domestic and laboratory animals. These postmortem procedures are also considered as an important step in biomedical research using laboratory animals and in particular in toxicity studies where histopathology is a major endpoint. In all cases, necropsy is the ultimate examination of the animal body. It allows detecting, describing, and reporting of any gross finding that could be key to understand changes noted during the *in vivo* part of the experiment. It is therefore important that the personnel in charge of the postmortem procedure have access to the animal history including clinical examination and behavioral changes that preceded necropsy as well as to the results of any imaging or laboratory investigations. On the other hand, the necropsy personnel should have access to the experiment study plan to harvest tissue important samples to meet the objectives of the study.

Jean-Charles Gautier (ed.), *Drug Safety Evaluation: Methods and Protocols*, Methods in Molecular Biology, vol. 691,
DOI 10.1007/978-1-60761-849-2_3, © Springer Science+Business Media, LLC 2011

Since necropsy can be performed only once, it is crucial to follow a precise procedure that allows identification of gross abnormalities and adequate sampling of organs.

The necropsy procedure consists of a series of systematic operations that allow examining all body organs and cavities without altering the characteristics of any tissue or organ of the animal. The collection of samples for histology or other complementary analyses also follow precise rules.

Histopathology is a major endpoint of many experiments. It is therefore crucial that tissues be sampled and preserved in a standardized manner especially when the microscopic findings need to be compared group wise. The amount of tissue that needs to be sampled should be representative of the whole organ since the probability of detecting lesions is primarily dependent on the amount of the tissue examined. For large organs of the body, such as the lungs or the liver, it is therefore necessary to define the number of sections and the specific lobe/area to be sampled. The anatomic characteristics of each organ should be considered. For example, the kidney is composed of a cortex, a medulla, and a pelvis. Each of these anatomical regions has distinct histological characteristics that need to be evaluated, as microscopic changes may reside only in one or two of these structures. For organs comprising a lumen or a cavity (such as intestines, urinary bladder, uterus, or heart), the amount and type of structures present on a transversal section may considerably vary and may subsequently compromise and sometimes irreversibly hamper adequate microscopic evaluation. Therefore, the plane of section should be considered and carefully standardized during sampling. For tissues with multiple or complex anatomical structures (such as the brain, nasal cavity, or intestines), it is advised to collect multiple sections to examine all structures of interest.

The probability of detecting lesions in the histological slide is also influenced by the technical procedures such as method of preservation and preparation. It is essential that the postmortem degradation process (otherwise termed as autolysis) be controlled. This is achieved by thorough immersion of tissue samples in a fixative like formalin. Other fixation techniques are available and should be always considered depending on each experiment-specific endpoints.

The purpose of this chapter is to describe the different steps of the necropsy, and to give general guidelines for sampling procedures in Rodents although these can be easily adapted to other laboratory animal species. As the knowledge of anatomy basics and species differences is required to perform the necropsy, a basic anatomical description will also be given. It is extremely useful to be aware of the subsequent histological processing of organs/tissues for histology to understand the rules of sampling and trimming. Hence, this chapter is intimately linked to the next one dedicated to Histopathology procedures: from sampling of tissues to histopathological evaluation.

Well-illustrated descriptions of necropsy protocols are available (1–5), some of them on the Web (6, 7) that would complement this chapter. Handbooks on the anatomy of Rodents are also useful (8, 9). The reader is also strongly encouraged to refer to the three excellent publications from the RITA/NACAD group about organ sampling and trimming in rats and mice that give guidelines in a very attractive manner, with excellent full-color macrophotographs and microphotographs from the corresponding Hematoxylin and Eosin (H&E)-stained slides (10–12).

2. Materials

1. Fume hood.
2. Rubber gloves (vinyl gloves in case of allergy to latex), protective clothing, eyeglasses, and mask.
3. Dissecting board preferentially in plastic, which could be easily cleaned and autoclaved.
4. Blunt ended forceps. Serrated forceps should be avoided as they may damage small animal tissues.
5. Small dissecting scissors, surgical scissors, and microsurgical (ophthalmologic type) scissors (These are very useful especially during extraction of the central nervous system).
6. Syringes (1 mL, 5 mL, 10 mL) and needles (a 21-gauge needle is suitable for infusion of the lung with fixative).
7. Scalpels (new blades and handle).
8. Plastic bags and paper towels.
9. Containers for histological specimens, cassettes, and labels. All containers should be adequately identified before start of necropsy.
10. Specific containers for other specimens (bacteriology, virology, mycology, parasitology, chemistry) should be available.
11. Tubes for liquid samples.
12. Euthanasia solution or suitable source of CO_2 and container.
13. Fixative (usually 10% neutral buffered formalin). Unless otherwise specified, the fixative mentioned in the text will be 10% neutral buffered formalin. Ready-to-use 10% neutral buffered formalin is commercially available from major suppliers. However, this fixative can be easily prepared. A detailed procedure is described in Table 1. Formalin is now included

in the list of human carcinogens and will be abandoned in the near future. Different commercial alternatives are proposed and are currently under testing in many laboratories.

14. Decalcifying solution (in case bones should be examined). There are several decalcifying solutions. A 26% formic acid solution (TBD2® Shandon Lipshaw) is routinely used in histopathology laboratories.

15. Ethanol 95% and 70%.

Table 1
Protocol for preparation of formalin and modified Davidson's fixatives

Protocol for preparation of formalin 10%, buffered	
Formaldehyde (37–40%)	100 mL
Distilled water	900 mL
Monosodium phosphate anhydrous	4 g
Disodium phosphate anhydrous	6.5 g
Final solution 3.7–4% formaldehyde	
To be used preferentially within 6 months after preparation. Keep at room temperature	
Protocol for preparation of paraformaldehyde 4% (PFA 4%)	
Paraformaldehyde (powder)	4 g
Distilled water	80 mL
Put 6 μL of sodium bicarbonate	
Put 10 mL of PBS ×10	
Filtrate on a paper	
Add PBS to obtain 100 mL	
Adjust the pH to 7.2–7.4	
The solution should be heated to facilitate the dissolution of the PFA, but below 65°C and in a fume hood	
Store at 4°C up to 24 h	
Can be also frozen in aliquots	
Protocol for preparation of modified Davidson's fixative	
30% of a 37–40% solution of formaldehyde	
15% Ethanol	
5% Glacial acetic acid	
50% Distilled H_2O	

16. Saline solution or Phosphate Buffer Solution (PBS).

17. Weigh scale.

18. Material to take photographs.

19. Metric scale.

20. Recording necropsy cards.

During necropsy, it is recommended to place the instruments in a stainless steel instrument holder with 70% ethanol. Used needles and scalpel should be placed in a special container for harmful material.

There are several hazards related to handling and dissection of laboratory animals during necropsy that should be considered. The chemical risk is one of them. For example, formalin causes eye, skin, nose, and respiratory tract irritation; it is also classified as a strong skin sensitizer and carcinogen in humans. Therefore, formalin should not be handled without gloves or outside a fume hood (13, 14).

Laboratory Rodents can spontaneously carry and transmit several diseases to man (also called zoonoses) (15). Although laboratory Rodents are usually tested for these agents, there is always a risk to contract one of these diseases. In addition, the allergic risk remains important especially for people with known animal allergies. Working with laboratory animals can lead to exposure to allergens via inhalation, direct skin and eye contact with animal dander, hair, urine, serum, or saliva. It is therefore essential that all necropsy personnel uses protective equipments (16, 17) and that cadavers and all waste be eliminated appropriately.

3. Methods

3.1. General Recommendations

3.1.1. Necropsy Protocol and Specimen Collection

It is strongly recommended to carefully read the experimental study plan or protocol. The list of organs that should be examined and sampled differs from one study to another depending on the aim and duration of the study. The following procedure allows examining and collecting most tissues and organs in Rodents with the main purpose of histopathology evaluation of tissue samples. It is very much inspired from necropsy performed in toxicity studies. The major steps are as follows:

- Examination of the live animal
- Euthanasia
- Exsanguination
- Opening of the abdominal cavity
- Opening of the thoracic cavity

- Opening of the skull
- Examination of muscles and skeleton.

This protocol should be followed step by step. It is the more convenient way to remove, examine, and sample each organ or tissue. Alternative methods are available; they will be mentioned in the notes.

Organs should always be immersed in the fixative immediately after their removal, macroscopic examination, or weighing. It is sometimes required to perform necropsy on animals found dead. Variable degrees of autolysis will inevitably take place, but it is still useful to perform the autopsy. Carcasses of found dead animals can be placed in a refrigerator (but NOT frozen). Necropsies should be performed as soon as practicable (if possible within the same day).

3.1.2. Weighing of Organs

One important part of necropsy is to describe the size of organs. This requires that the dissector has in reference the normal size of the organ. Small variation in size can be challenging even for experienced pathologist especially when organ sizes need to be compared among several individuals and groups. To accurately compare organ sizes, it is most helpful to record individual organ weights. These can be compared either as absolute organ weights or as ratios of organ weight to total body weight or to brain weight. Following the recommendations from the Society of Toxicologic Pathology (STP) (18) liver, kidneys, heart, brain, adrenal glands, testes, spleen, and thymus should be weighed routinely in all general toxicology studies with multi-dose administration in Rodents (Table 2). Thyroid and pituitary gland should be weighed in rats but not in mice, as handling of these minute tissues may induce artifacts that can complicate microscopic assessment. Epididymides and prostate weighing is recommended in rat studies but only on a case-by-case basis in mouse as well as other organs including female reproductive organs in Rodents. Organs weights are not recommended in carcinogenicity studies.

In all cases, organs should be weighed free of surrounding fat and connective tissues. It is important to remove these tissues in a standardized manner and without inducing any damage or artifact to the tissue.

3.1.3. Organ Sampling for Histology

Most of the tissue samples will be immersed in the fixative. Small tissues can be kept in histology cassettes at the time of dissection. The same cassette, adequately identified, can be used for the paraffin embedding and paraffin block preparation. The number of cassettes and hence paraffin blocks can be considerably reduced by combining a few tissues and organs in one cassette. For example, several small and large intestines can be grouped (19, 20) (Table 3).

Table 2
List of organs for weighing

Rat	Mice
Liver	Liver
Kidney	Kidney
Heart	Heart
Adrenal glands	Adrenal glands
Brain	Brain
Testes	Testes
Prostate	Spleen
Epididymes	Thymus
Spleen	Thyroid/parathyroid
Thymus	Pituitary gland
Thyroid/parathyroid	
Pituitary gland	

Sellers, R., et al., in *Toxicologic Pathology* **35**, 751–755 (2007)

3.1.4. Examination and Recording of Macroscopic Observations

The description of macroscopic findings should be sufficiently detailed to give a mental representation of gross changes. Therefore, all criteria should be used to describe the gross changes of an organ: location, appearance (color, shape, consistency), demarcation from surrounding tissues, number, distribution and severity, size, which should always be measured in two or three dimensions (cm or mm), or in volume (mL).

3.1.5. Orientation

It is critical for the necropsy personnel to correctly use the terms that define the orientation of an organ or a section (Fig. 1):

1. Dorsal refers to the back of the animal whereas ventral refers to the abdomen.
2. Cranial refers to the skull, whereas caudal refers to the tail.
3. Rostral refers to the organs or structures situated toward the front of the head.
4. Lateral pertains to a side, medial is related to, situated in, or extending toward the middle, closer to the body's midline.
5. Proximal is located nearer to a point of reference; distal is located far from a point of reference (origin, point of attachment, or midline of the body).

Table 3
Example of blocking scheme

Cassette	Tissues
1	Heart Aorta Vena cava
2	Muscle skeletal (diaphragm, tongue and soleus)
3	Lung: entire (all lobes)
4	Thyroid with trachea (specimen immediately caudal to larynx, cross section)
5	Kidneys (cross-sections of left and right kidneys) Urinary bladder
6	Ureters
7	Adrenal glands
8	Stomach: glandular and nonglandular portions Duodenum Jejunum
9	Ileum (with Peyer's patch) Cecum Colon Rectum
10	Salivary glands (Mandibular, sublingual and parotid) Cervical lymph nodes
11	Pancreas Mesenteric lymph node Thymus Spleen
12	Liver: left lateral (largest) lobe (one section cut from hilus to periphery), median lobe (one section to include gall bladder)
13	Ovaries Oviducts Uterus (two cross sections through horns and one longitudinal section through body and cervix) Vagina (cross section)
14	Testes (cross sections, left and right) Epididymides Seminal vesicles with coagulating glands (cross sections or longitudinal sections depending on size) Prostate (cross section)
15	Skin ventral inguinal specimen (one section parallel to hair growth, to include mammary glands)
16	Clitoral or preputial glands
17	Femur with knee and tibia with bone marrow
18	Sternum with bone marrow
19	Brain (2 transversal sections through cerebrum including olfactory lobes and hippocampus, and one through cerebellum and pons)
20	Spinal cord
21	Pituitary
22	Eyes with optic nerves and lacrimal glands

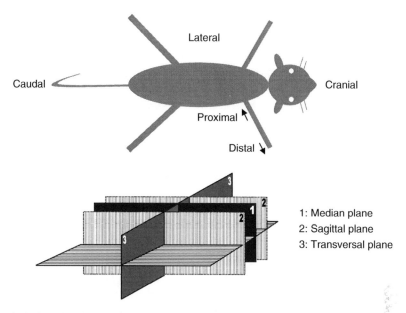

Fig. 1. Anatomical orientation descriptors usually used at necropsy.

The major planes of sections are defined as follows:

1. Median plane, passing longitudinally through the middle of the body from front to back, dividing it into left and halves right.

2. Frontal (coronal) planes, passing transversally through the body from side to side, perpendicular to the median plane, dividing the body into front and back parts.

3. Sagittal planes are vertical planes passing through the body parallel to the median plane dividing the body into left and right portions.

4. Transverse plane (dorsoventral), passing vertically through the body, perpendicular to the sagittal planes, and dividing the body into front and back portions.

5. Horizontal plane, passing through the body, perpendicular to both the frontal and median planes, dividing the body into upper and lower parts.

6. Vertical plane, perpendicular to a horizontal plane, dividing the body into left and right or front and back portions.

3.2. Examination of the Live Animal

1. Observe the behavior of the animal and check its response to external stimuli.

2. Observe the fur and the skin to detect any changes.

3.3. External Examination

1. Weigh the animal. As indicated in Subheading 3.1.2, this will be useful to calculate organ weight to body weight ratios.

2. Examine the animal before proceeding to the necropsy.

3. Assess the general condition of the animal (emaciated, thin, adequate/good condition, obese).

4. Check and record any external lesions (skin lesions, fur loss or discoloration, and subcutaneous masses). Record sizes and surfaces whenever possible and record their gross appearance and precise location.

5. Check and record the color changes of the skin and mucosae (gingival, genital mucosae, conjunctiva).

6. Examine the eyes, mouth, teeth, and nasal openings and record any abnormality.

7. Examine the ano-genital region to look for signs of diarrhea, rectal, or vaginal prolapse and record any abnormality.

8. Gently palpate the abdomen to reveal abdominal masses or presence of fluid.

9. If the abdomen is distended by fluid, take a sample with a sterile needle and syringe for further evaluation.

10. Palpate any mass and record its consistency (soft, fluctuant, firm, or hard).

3.4. Euthanasia

Various methods of euthanasia are available for Rodents. The selected method should induce death quickly with minimal animal pain or distress and should not interfere with the gross observation and microscopic evaluation of the tissues. Euthanasia protocols should be approved by the local ethical committee.

We describe in this chapter the euthanasia method which is commonly used in toxicological studies: exposure to carbon dioxide (CO_2). This method requires only a source of CO_2 and a polycarbonate box of a size that is well-matched with the size of rodents. The euthanasia procedure is as follows:

1. Place a wet sponge in one of the corners of the box.

2. Place the lid with the CO_2 tube attachment on the box.

3. Charge the chamber with CO_2 gas for 1–2 min.

4. Place animals in the box.

5. Turn gas on low so as not to frighten the animals.

6. Administer CO_2 until deep sedation is observed.

7. Death is induced by maximal exsanguination from the abdominal aorta (this can be the occasion to collect blood for hematology, coagulation, and clinical chemistry parameters).

8. Check heart beat and respiration to verify death.

3.5. Incision of the Skin and Examination of the Subcutaneous Tissues/Organs

Skin, subcutaneous tissue, mammary glands, salivary glands, superficial cervical lymph nodes, extraorbital lacrimal gland, clitoral glands, preputial glands, penis, and prepuce.

3.5.1. Incision of the Skin and Examination of the Subcutaneous Tissue

1. Pin the animal on the dissection board, ventral side up and head in front of you. Remember that from this point, the left side of the animal is on your right side and vice versa.

2. Moisten the skin and hairs with 70% alcohol.

3. Incise the skin with a scalpel on the midline, from the mandibles to the pubis. In males, incision should end on both sides of the penis.

4. Reflect the skin on both sides of the incision.

5. Examine the skin and the subcutaneous tissue. Record any lesion; confirm skin changes observed in the previous step.

3.5.2. Examination and Sampling of the Mammary Glands

1. Examine the mammary glands: the mouse has five pairs of mammary glands (three thoracic and two abdominal), while the rats have six pairs (three thoracic and three abdominal). There are six or seven pairs in hamsters (21, 22). In females, the mammary tissue extends from the salivary gland region to the base of the tail. When lactating, the mammary gland occupies almost all the abdominal and thoracic ventral subcutaneous area in the mouse and in the rat.

2. Harvest the mammary gland from the inguinal region where the mammary tissue is abundant in both rats and mice. Take a transverse section (1 cm × 3 cm) including the associated nipple and skin (see Note 1). This applies to males as well as to females.

3.5.3. Examination and Sampling of the Superficial Lymph Nodes

Examine the superficial lymph nodes. Under normal conditions, lymph nodes are grayish organs, bilateral, and have the size and shape of a small pea. Major superficial lymph nodes, located in the subcutaneous area are the cervical superficial, *axillary* in the axillary fossa, *brachial, inguinal,* and *popliteal.* The peripheral lymph nodes that are most often examined are the *mandibular, axillary,* and/or *popliteal lymph nodes* (see Note 2). The location of these lymph nodes is detailed in Table 4 (23).

3.5.4. Examination, Removal, and Sampling of Salivary Glands, lacrimal glands, clitoral or preputial glands

1. Examine the three pairs of salivary glands located on both sides in the cranioventral region of the neck: *mandibulary glands, sublingual glands,* and *parotid glands* (24, 25). The mandibulary gland is the largest one, located in the ventral region of the neck. Sublingual glands are situated on the top of mandibulary glands. Parotid glands are the most lateral ones; they extend to the base of the ear.

2. Collect salivary glands by gently grasping the tip of the closest salivary gland to the thorax with forceps. Then slowly pull toward cutting the surrounding tissues with scissors and immerse in fixative.

Table 4
Nomenclature and location of major lymph nodes

	Name	Location
Superficial	Mandibular	Rostromedial to the sublingual and mandibular salivary glands
	Axillary	Axillary fossa
	Brachial	Proximity to the angle of the capsula, upon the biceps, underneath the pectorals
	Inguinal	Adherent to the skin of the groin
	Popliteal	Between the adductor muscle and the semimembranous muscle behind the knee
Deep	Deep cervical	Behind the salivary glands hidden in the connective tissue encircling the trachea
	Lumbar, caudal	Anterior to the bifurcation of the abdominal aorta
	Mediastinal	Posterior face of the thymus
	Mesenteric	Lengthened shape, with the mesentery, close to the ascending portion of the colon
	Pyloric (pancreatic)	Anterior end of the pancreas, near the pylorus
	Renal	Between the aorta and hilum of the kidneys
	Sacral	Posterior to the bifurcation of the abdominal aorta
	Sciatic	Below the sciatic nerve on the back

3. Examine extraorbital lacrimal glands. These glands are located on the ventro-lateral aspect of the head. They appear as flat, brown-gray glands next to the parotids.

4. Remove extraorbital glands on both sides by gently grasping the tip of the gland with forceps, isolate the gland from its attachment in the eye socket using scissors, and immerse the two glands in fixative (see Note 3).

5. Examine clitoral glands in females or preputial glands in males. Clitoral/preputial glands are modified sebaceous glands that are included in the subcutaneous adipose tissue. They can be found cranial to the vulva in females and lateral to the penis in males. Preputial glands are leaf-shaped and dark-gray color with a soft consistency.

6. Remove whole glands on both sides by gently grasping the tip with forceps to isolate them from the surrounding tissue. Immerse the clitoral/preputial glands in fixative.

3.5.5. Examination of the Penis

Examine the penis and the prepuce in males. These organs will be harvested with the remaining genital organs.

**3.6. Opening
of the Abdomen
and Examination
of Abdominal Organs**

Abdomen is opened and abdominal organs such as peritoneum, spleen, mesenteric lymph nodes, pancreas, digestive tract, liver, adrenal glands, kidneys, and genital organs are examined.

3.6.1. Opening of the Abdominal Cavity

1. Grasp the abdominal wall with forceps near the sternal xyphoid appendix and lift firmly.

2. Make a small incision to let air into the abdomen. This will allow abdominal viscera to be separated from the abdominal wall.

3. Cut the abdominal wall on the midline with scissors from the pelvis to the xyphoid appendix. Make sure not to cut any of the abdominal organs that lie underneath.

4. Reflect the abdominal wall on the sides.

5. Examine the abdominal serous membrane (*peritoneum*) and look for the presence of abnormal contents such as serous fluid, blood, or fibrin as well as to any adhesion between abdominal wall and abdominal organs.

6. Check the position of the different organs *in situ*.

7. Check fat deposits and score the nutritional conditions (1. Obese, 2. Good nutritional condition, 3. Poor nutritional condition, 4. Bad nutritional condition, 5. Emaciation, absence of fat in the body deposits). The amount of fat is dependent on the age and strain of the animal: adults and aged animals tend to have more fat deposits in the abdominal cavity.

3.6.2. Removal, Examination, and Sampling of the Spleen

1. The spleen is situated on the left superior abdominal quadrant. To remove it, grasp the connective tissues and fat surrounding the spleen with the forceps. Cut them along the hilus of the spleen and cut the gastrosplenic ligament as well.

2. Examine the spleen. It is a lengthened, oval, slightly curved shape organ, has a dark-red color, and is soft in consistency with a thin transparent capsule (26). It is attached to the stomach by the gastro-splenic ligament.

3. Should spleen be weighted, it should be carefully freed from all remnants of connective and adipose tissues, in particular along the hilus.

4. The entire spleen can be sampled and immersed in fixative although a 2-mm thick transverse mid-section can be sufficient.

3.6.3. Removal of the Digestive Tract and Mesenteric Lymph Nodes

Abdominal part of the esophagus, stomach, small intestine (duodenum, jejunum, ileum), large intestine (cecum, colon, rectum), and mesenteric lymph nodes.

1. Dissect the anus free from the surrounding skin.

2. Insert the tip of heavy duty scissors between the colon and the pelvis to cut the pelvic arch on both sides. Take off the resulting bone chip to facilitate the subsequent removal of the genital tract and rectum.

3. Hold the rectum with forceps and lift it upwards.

4. Isolate the rectum from the vagina in females.

5. Gradually extract the intestines in a caudal-cranial direction, while cutting the insertion of the mesentery as close to the intestines as possible.

6. Cut the esophagus just below the diaphragm in the abdomen leaving a small portion of esophagus connected to the stomach.

7. Isolate the whole digestive tract together with the pancreas.

8. Examine the deep abdominal lymph nodes (23, 27) for nomenclature and location before unzipping the intestines. The mesenteric lymph nodes are usually the largest lymph nodes of the abdominal cavity. They drain the duodenum, ileum, cecum, and colon.

9. Starting at the rectum, progressively unzip the coiled intestines by pulling gently with scissors.

10. Samples of intestine segments as well as mesenteric lymph nodes should be immersed in the fixative as soon as possible.

3.6.4. Examination and Sampling of the Pancreas

1. In Rodents, the pancreas is very diffuse and completely enclosed in the mesentery. It is tan in color and therefore easily identifiable from the surrounding fat. It has one *left lobe* located close to the spleen in the great omentum, and one *right lobe* adjacent to the duodenum.

2. Lift up the pancreas attached to the spleen and separate them from the intestines by cutting its insertion with scissors.

3. Isolate the spleen from the pancreas with the scissors.

4. Take a sample from the *left pancreatic lobe* to have the largest surface. The *right pancreatic lobe* will be sampled with the duodenum.

3.6.5. Examination and Sampling of the Stomach

5. In small Rodents (mice, rats, hamsters, and gerbils), the stomach has two distinct regions: the proventricular or anterior region that has a white appearance, and the glandular region which has a reddened and thicker wall (28, 29). Both are clearly demarcated by a limiting ridge in these species but not in the guinea pigs.

6. Isolate the stomach from the esophagus and the intestines.

7. In mice, open the stomach along the greater curvature, mount on a plastic card, fix it with pins, and immerse it in the fixative. In rats, open the stomach of the rat along or para-median

to the greater curvature and placed on a corkboard. Remove the gastric content and, if necessary, clean carefully the mucosa with saline solution or fixative. Spread out the stomach and pin it on the cardboard. This procedure avoids folds in the mucosa and therefore is essential for the macroscopic orientation and allows reproducible microscopic evaluation of the thickness of gastric mucosa.

3.6.6. Examination and Sampling of the Intestines

1. The small intestine has three different regions: *duodenum*, which is very short (1 cm) in Rodents, *jejunum* and *ileum* that are not recognizable grossly. The large intestine is composed of the *cecum, colon,* and *rectum* (short segment in Rodents, included in the pelvis) (30). Lymphoid tissue associated with the small intestine (jejunum and ileum) is also called gut-associated lymphoid tissue (GALT) or Peyer's patches. These appear as slightly elevated lighter fields in the intestine's wall and can be discernible as prominent areas when activated.

2. Separate carefully the intestines from the mesentery during necropsy (or after fixation).

3. Examination of Intestines should comprise at least the content, wall thickness, color, aspect of mucosa, or any noticeable lesion in each intestinal segment.

4. If the microscopic evaluation of the whole intestine and GALT on a single section is preferred, the so-called "Swiss roll method" can be performed (31, 32) (see Note 4).

5. Routine intestine samples for histopathology evaluation usually consists of one transverse section (2–3-mm thick) from each part of the bowel without opening it: duodenum (1 cm distal to the pyloric sphincter), jejunum (central section), ileum (1 cm proximal to cecum), cecum, colon (central section), rectum (2 cm proximal to the anus). For small intestines, it is also essential to sample the GALT. Standardized sampling procedure of the bowel segments is necessary to guarantee examination of each required segment.

6. After sample collection for histopathology, the remaining intestine should be opened longitudinally and examined for abnormalities. To better examine the mucosa, a gentle rinse of the ingesta with saline solution may be necessary. This latter procedure is time consuming and should be considered on a case-by-case basis only.

3.6.7. Removal, Examination, and Sampling of the Liver

1. The liver has four lobes: *medial lobe, right medial lobe, right lateral lobe, caudate lobe*, plus a *papillary process* (see Note 5). There is no gallbladder in the rat. The liver is normally dark-reddish and has a hard, but friable consistency. A thin transparent capsule covers the liver.

2. The liver is a fragile organ that should be handled with caution.

3. Remove the liver gently out the way with the forceps.

4. Grasp the xyphoid process firmly with the forceps.

5. Puncture the diaphragm with scissors and trim it completely away from the ribs.

6. Pull upward to create a negative pressure in the thorax.

7. Using the diaphragm as a handle, pull the liver out of the abdominal cavity. Separate the liver from the diaphragm by cutting the falciform and coronary ligaments that attach the liver to the diaphragm.

8. Before weighing the liver, remove all remnants of the diaphragm and ensure that the small lobes are present to weigh the entire organ.

9. Sampling of the liver (see Note 6). In the rat, take a piece from the left lateral lobe (transverse) and the right medial lobe (transverse); in the mouse from the left lateral lobe (transverse), from the left and right medial lobe including gall bladder (longitudinal-vertical preferentially to keep the gallbladder with the liver). In both species, a transverse section from the caudate lobe is optional. Size of samples should be as large as possible, but all pieces should fit into one cassette.

10. Immerse the two or three liver samples in the fixative. It is advised to keep the remaining liver tissue in fixative.

3.6.8. Removal, Examination, and Sampling of the Kidneys and Adrenals Glands

1. Remove the kidney and adrenals, grasp the caudal part of the ureter with forceps near its opening, and keep the adrenals attached to the kidneys. Adrenal glands and kidneys are located deep in the retroperitoneal space; they should be recognized as early as possible during the process.

2. Separate the adrenals from kidneys.

3. Examine each adrenal gland. These glands are small white structures within the perirenal fat. In male, adrenal glands tend to be large, often rose-colored and translucent while in females, they are smaller and, due to high lipid content, have an opaque pale color (24, 33, 34). Adrenals have an external *cortex* and central *medulla*.

4. Check their shape, volume, as well as the presence of nodular formations.

5. Before weighing adrenal glands, remove carefully all remnants of fat and connective tissues. As for all paired organs, unless otherwise specified in the study plan, the weight of the pair is recorded.

6. Immerse the adrenal glands in the fixative. Due to their relative small size in Rodents, they will be embedded *in toto*.

7. Examine the kidneys. Kidneys are located on the dorsal wall of the abdominal cavity. They are bean-shaped pair organs, with a hilus in the concave margin from which main vessels, nerves, and ureters exit. Their color is brownish red and their consistency is firm. The right kidney is the more cranially located, usually larger and heavier than the left one (35, 36). The kidneys are surrounded by a capsule and have three different regions: *cortex*, *medulla*, and *papilla*.

8. Before weighing, kidneys must be freed of all remnants of connective and adipose tissues.

9. Kidneys can be immersion fixed *in toto* or after trimming (e.g., take a longitudinal section from the left kidney and a transverse section from the right kidney).

3.6.9. Removal, Examination, and Sampling of the Urinary Bladder

1. Examine the urinary bladder (12, 37).

2. The urinary bladder can be freed of urine after incision of the wall and then sampled *in toto*. Alternatively, the bladder can be sampled after instillation of the fixative. In the mouse, instill the fixative (0.05 mL) through the bladder wall after ligation of the urethra with a ventral knot. In the rat, it is more convenient to instill the fixative (0.2 mL) with a needle inserted via the urethra. In both rats and mice, fixative instillation should not be performed when the bladder is distended with urine.

3. Then continue the fixation by immersion in a container of fixative.

4. It may be helpful also to mark the ventral side of the bladder with a stick of silver nitrate.

3.6.10. Removal, Examination, and Sampling of the Male Genital Organs

1. Remove the testes. They are oval-shaped paired organs, a few millimeters in diameter that lay inside the scrotum. They are covered by a smooth and transparent membrane *(tunica albuginea)*. They are grayish-white with a soft elastic consistency. When the abdominal cavity is opened, testes are often found outside the scrotum, in an intra-abdominal position. Grasp them delicately by the inguinal fat pad and cut them away from the viscera. If the testes are still in the scrotum, open the scrotum and extract the testes with the epididymides by cutting the fibrous ligaments anchoring the tail of the epididymis to the scrotum. Cut the vas deferens.

2. Examine the testes (38–41). Check the shape, volume, weight, consistency, and presence of masses.

3. Weigh the testes individually or as a pair. Weigh the epididymis (in rats only) separately if needed. Before weighing the testes

and epididymes, all remnants of connective and adipose tissues should be removed.

4. Place the testes with the epididymis on a piece of cardstock. Orient testis and epididymis in the same plane so that they can be trimmed simultaneously later (see Note 7). Fix the testes and epididymis as a whole, without cutting the testes before fixation to prevent them from rupturing (see Note 8).

5. It is suggested to fix testes and epididymis in Davidson solution instead of formalin (Table 1).

6. Remove the male accessory glands: *seminal vesicles, coagulating glands* (dorsocranial lobe of the prostate), *prostate* (two ventral lobes and two dorsolateral lobes). The dorsolateral and ventral lobes lie in a vertical axis above each other with urinary bladder and seminal vesicles in between.

7. Remove the group of adjacent organs consisting of prostate, urinary bladder, seminal vesicles, and coagulating glands.

8. Examine the male accessory glands (38, 39, 42, 43). Check any size or color changes or presence of nodular masses.

9. Before weighing the prostate (rats only), all remnants of connective and adipose tissues should be carefully removed.

10. Immerse these organs into the fixative *in toto* if weights are not required to prevent leakage of the glandular secretions.

11. Remove the penis, prepuce, and urethra.

3.6.11. Removal, Examination, and Sampling of the Genital Organs in Female

1. Dissect the vulva and vagina free from the skin and cut the supporting ligaments of the vagina, uterus, and oviducts.

2. Cut the ligaments and isolate the ovaries with the oviduct and the whole genital tract.

3. Examine the ovaries and oviducts. Ovaries are small oval reddish organs found within the fat tissue caudally to the kidneys and attached to the inferior poles of the kidneys, and to the posterior wall of the abdomen by ligaments. Check the shape, volume, consistency and presence of any gross lesions (24, 38, 44, 45).

4. If ovaries are to be weighed, isolate them from the oviducts before weighing.

5. Examine the uterus and the vagina. Record any enlargement, fluid, or mass (24, 38, 44, 45).

6. If uterus has to be weighed, uterine horns and the cervix should be weighed together but separated from the vagina.

7. The *uterine body* (fused part of the uterus) and the vagina should be placed with their dorsal aspect on cardboard before fixation.

3.7. Opening of the Thorax and Examination of Thoracic Organs

The thorax is opened and the thoracic organs such as tongue, larynx, trachea, thymus, mediastinal lymph nodes, lungs, heart, and thyroid gland (with parathyroids) are examined.

3.7.1. Opening of the Thorax

1. Open the thorax by first lifting the sternal xyphoid process with forceps. Then cut the ribs starting from the xiphoid process and up to the first rib to remove the sternum and rib cage to reveal the thoracic organs.

2. The sternum is a convenient organ for bone marrow examination after decalcification. Take a piece containing two to three sternebrae and immerse this sample into fixative.

3. Examine the thoracic serous membrane (*pleura*) and presence of abnormal contents such as serous fluid, blood, fibrin, or adhesions between organs.

4. Check the position of the different organs *in situ*.

3.7.2. Removal of the Tongue, Trachea, Esophagus, and Thoracic Organs

1. Cut the muscles of the lower jaw with a scalpel.

2. Cut the soft palate and pharynx.

3. Grasp the tip of the tongue with forceps and retract gently to remove the tongue, larynx, trachea, and esophagus from the head and neck.

4. Continue retracting to remove the heart and the lungs from the thorax. Use scissors to perform a blunt dissection to free these tissues.

5. Cut the thoracic aorta and posterior vena cava at the level of the diaphragm

3.7.3. Isolation, Examination, and Sampling of the Heart and Aorta

1. Isolate the heart from the lungs by delicately cutting the main vessels with scissors.

2. Examine the heart without opening the inner cavities (*atria* and *ventricles*) (24, 46, 47). Before weighing the heart, all blood should be removed. In Rodents, this can be easily achieved by placing the base of the heart over a piece of cleaning paper.

3. Immerse the heart *in toto* in the fixative.

4. Take a section from the *thoracic aorta* (in the middle of the last 1 cm caudal segment). This region is closely attached to dorsal vertebrae and can easily be removed.

3.7.4. Isolation, Examination, and Sampling of the Thymus

1. Isolate the thymus by gently grasping one of the two lobes in its inferior part and cut the ligament connecting it to the pericardium.

2. Examine the thymus (48). In rodents, the thymus is an oval-shaped lobulated organ with a whitish-translucent color. With age, the thymus shrinks but remains grossly visible.

3. Before weighing the thymus, all remnants of connective and adipose tissues should be carefully removed.

3.7.5. Examination and Sampling of the Tongue

1. Examine the tongue (28).

2. Make a transversal incision to sample half the tongue and immerse it in the fixative (see Note 9).

3.7.6. Examination and Sampling of the Thyroids (Parathyroids), Trachea, and Esophagus

1. Examine the thyroid gland. Thyroid gland has two symmetric oval lobes, adherent to the lateral and dorsal surfaces of the trachea and has a translucent, tan yellowish color. The parathyroids are located around or within the thyroids but *are not visible grossly* (49, 50), (see Note 10).

2. Take the *larynx* including *epiglottis, ventral pouch,* and *cricoid cartilage* (rats only) and immerse it in the fixative.

3. If the thyroid is weighed (rat only), carefully remove all remnants of connective and adipose tissues. Immerse the thyroids in the fixative. It is advised to weigh the thyroid gland after 1 or 2 min of fixation.

4. Then take a transverse sample section of trachea and esophagus. If the thyroids are not weighed, leave them on the trachea. Take a transverse section of the esophagus, trachea, including the thyroids (and parathyroids) (oral studies). Tracheal content should be noted and reported.

3.7.7. Examination and Sampling of the Lungs

1. Examine the lungs (51, 52). In Rodents, lungs have three right lobes (*right cranial lobe, right middle lobe, right caudal lobe*), an *accessory lobe,* and one *left lobe* (see Note 11).

2. The lung parenchyma has normally a smooth surface, a nice light pink color (but that depends on air and blood present if not inflated), and a spongy consistency. Examine all lung lobes and note any changes.

3. For optimal microscopic evaluation, instillation of the lung by the fixative is strongly recommended. This can be performed easily through the trachea. A 21-gauge needle is placed on a 3-mL syringe filled with the fixative. The needle is introduced in the trachea at its open end. Clamp gently around the needle with forceps and inflate the lung by depressing the plunger of the syringe very slowly until excess fixative refluxes up the trachea. The lung with the trachea should be then immersed in the fixative. If the procedure is correctly executed, there is no need to place a ligature on the trachea (see Note 12).

3.8. Head and Central Nervous System

Brain, cerebellum, spinal cord, pituitary gland, eyes, Harderian glands, nasal cavities, and Zymbal's gland.

The most optimal way the fix to central nervous system is intracardiac perfusion of fixative (see Note 13). However, fixation of the nervous system by immersion allows acceptable preservation of tissues and is routinely used in toxicity studies.

3.8.1. Removal of the Brain and Spinal Cord

1. Cut the skin over the head with a median-longitudinal incision from the nape to the snout.

2. Reflect the two edges of the skin and pull them to better observe the entire skull.

3. Remove any excess tissue or muscle from the cranium and neck.

4. Keeping the head firmly with large forceps, insert the tip of heavy duty scissors in the left eye socket (avoid any damage to the eyeball), and cut the nasal bone transversely at the level of the nasal septum between the two orbital cavities. The used scissors for this operation should be exclusively dedicated to this step.

5. Then, with the ophthalmologic scissors, cut progressively the parietal, interparietal, and occipital bones in a craniocaudal direction on both sides to isolate a bone cap and reveal the brain. Be very careful to avoid damaging the brain beneath the skull bones during this operation.

6. Pull the skullcap caudally with forceps and take it away.

7. Use the small ophthalmologic scissors to cut the vertebrae. Start from the occipital bone level and then, with the tip of the scissors, alternate right and left side cuts of the vertebral bodies to progressively remove the vertebral arches. In this way, the spinal cord will be uncovered in the vertebral canal.

8. Raise the brain by gently introducing forceps under the frontal lobe of the encephalon, then cut intracranial vessels and nerves at the brain base.

9. Gently handle the brain between the thumb and forefinger and cut successively the spinal nerves coming from the ventral aspect of the spinal cord on each side of the brain, and hold the detached segment of the spinal cord. In the area of the cauda equina (where nerves are numerous), cut the spinal cord transversely (see Note 14).

10. Isolate the brain and the spinal cord by a scalpel frank transversal section at the junction between the medulla oblongata and the brain.

3.8.2. Examination of the Brain and Spinal Cord

1. Examine the brain (cerebrum and cerebellum) (53, 54). The brain is covered by the meninges: the *dura mater* is fibrous and in direct contact with the skull, the *pia mater* is highly

vascularized and adheres intimately to the surface of the brain, the *arachnoid* is a transparent membrane located between the *dura* mater and the *pia* mater, but too thin to be visualized grossly.

2. The cerebrum has two *cerebral hemispheres*, separated by a longitudinal fissure. There are no cerebral circumvolutions in Rodents that have a lissencephalic brain. Rodent brains have two large *olfactory bulbs* located in the front. The cerebellum shows thin convolutions and lays in the caudal part of the brain.

3. On the ventral part of the brain, the *optic chiasma*, the *median eminence* (representing a part of the hypothalamus), the *pons*, and the *medulla oblongata* can be observed.

4. The brain is a very fragile tissue, especially if not fixed. It is therefore important not to handle this organ with the forceps but rather lift it carefully using the scalpel blade.

5. Before weighing the brain, carefully remove all remnants of connective tissue (see Note 15). To achieve accurate brain weights, the spinal cord should be cut off at a consistent level.

6. It is preferable that the brain (undetached from the cerebellum) be immersion fixed *in toto*. The brain is an anatomically complex tissue. Therefore, microscopic examination of the brain should be performed at standardized section levels: transverse section of the cerebrum at the optic chiasma, cerebrum at the base of the posterior hypothalamus, midcerebellum, and medulla oblongata (12). Therefore, the brain slices are routinely prepared after fixation.

7. Examine the *vertebral canal* on the cadaver.

8. Examine the spinal cord.

9. Take three transverse sections of the spinal cord for microscopic examination at the upper cervical, mid-thoracic, and lumbar levels. Put all three segments in a cassette and immerse in the fixative (see Note 16). As for the brain, spinal cord is a very fragile tissue and should not be handled with the forceps.

3.8.3. Examination, Removal, and Sampling of the Pituitary Gland

1. Examine the pituitary gland (24, 55). The pituitary gland can be easily seen on the ventral aspect of the cranial cavity after removal of the brain. It appears as a small spherical gland, covered by a thin layer of *dura matter* and located behind the optic chiasma in the *sella tursica*, a small depression of the sphenoid bone.

2. The fixation *in situ* of the gland is recommended before removal or weighing. Weighing after fixation provides accurate weight measurements and improves morphology. Fixation can be performed by a few drops of fixative on the ventral aspect of

the cranial cavity or by immersion of the remaining skull in the fixative; the gland can be removed later (11) (see Note 17).

3. Weighing of the pituitary gland is not required in mice and usually performed after fixation.

3.8.4. Removal, Examination, and Sampling of the Eyes, Optic Nerve, Harderian Gland, and Lacrymal Glands (Internal/External)

1. Remove the eyes by sinking a pair of curved forceps behind the orbit. Gently grasp the optic nerve, isolate the eye by pulling it outward and cutting its attachments to the socket (see Note 18).

2. Examine the eyes (56).

3. Immerse the eyes with the optic nerve in the fixative (see Note 19).

4. Examine the Harderian glands (or retroorbital gland). The Harderian gland lies intraorbitally behind the eyes and embraces the back of the ocular globe. It is a gray-colored gland under normal conditions, cone-shaped in the rat, and horseshoe-shaped in the mouse.

5. Remove the Harderian glands and immerse them in the fixative.

3.8.5. Sampling of the Nasal Cavity and Zymbal's Glands

1. Remove the skin and muscles and immerse the head in the fixative if further histological examination of the nasal cavity and paranasal sinuses, nasal cavity, nasopharynx, and paranasal sinuses is needed (57, 58).

2. Zymbal's glands are modified sebaceous glands located at the base of the external ear in anterio-ventral position (59). A section through the base of the skull after gentle decalcification will allow histological examination of these glands.

3.9. Muscles and Skeleton

Bone (femur, sternum), skeletal muscle (biceps femoris), peripheral nerve (sciatic nerve), bone marrow (femur, sternum).

1. Remove the skin from the hind leg.

2. Transversally cut the biceps femoris with a scalpel (12, 27, 60). Gently grasp one edge with the forceps and immerse it into the fixative.

3. Take a sample of the sciatic nerve (1 cm long) (12) (see Note 20). Gently grasp one edge with forceps and fix it on a card board.

4. Remove the distal portion of one femur, the knee joint with the proximal portion of the adjacent tibia. This will allow microscopic examination of the bone, joint tissues, and bone marrow (12, 61, 62). For routine bone and bone marrow microscopic examination, a sternum section should be sampled (see Note 21).

5. Immerse the samples in the fixative.

4. Notes

1. A longitudinal section, vertical to the direction of the hair flow can be taken to examine the skin and mammary glands; in this case, the nipple is not included if the lymph node is enclosed.

2. In case of parenteral application, one lymph node draining the application site and another distant one could be collected.

3. The extraorbital glands can be removed and embedded together with the salivary glands.

4. "Swiss roll" technique: this technique allows examining the whole intestine and the GALT on a single section. However, these transverse sections when they are made properly will often provide a better morphology. Strip the intestines off the mesentery, open it with a pair of scissors, and gently rinse the intestine to remove the content. Then recoil the intestine except cecum on cotton swabs and put in the fixative. After fixation, detach the spooled intestine and proceed to embedding. This procedure is not required in routine microscopic examination of the intestines. Bear in mind that with this technique, the intestinal mucosa and the lymph follicles will often be cut tangentially.

5. Nomenclature of hepatic lobes can differ. We have elected to use the anatomical terms we recommend: medial lobe, right medial lobe, right lateral lobe, caudate lobe, and papillary process.

6. If major bile duct is required, take a section through the left lateral lobe of the liver.

7. Optionally epididymides can be isolated from the testes, fixed, and trimmed separately

8. In short-term studies, fixation of the testes with modified Davidson's or Bouin's solutions is highly recommended to detect less extensive early and subtle changes (63).

9. The longitudinal vertical section of the tongue covers a large part of the dorsum including the dorsal prominence. The section also includes the lingual lesser salivary glands and should be slightly lateral to the median sulcus. A transverse section of the tongue is recommended if blood sampling from the tongue is performed.

10. There are variations in position and number of parathyroids in Rodents. In the rat, there is one pair of parathyroids, with a variable position but usually on the anterior lateral aspect of the thyroid lobes. In the mouse, there are usually two parathyroids (sometimes more than two), situated bilaterally just under the capsule near the dorsolateral border of each thyroid

lobe. They are rarely at the same level and may be deeply embedded in the thyroid tissue.

11. Nomenclature of lung lobes can differ. We have elected to use the anatomical terms that we recommend: right cranial, right middle, right caudal lobe, accessory lobe, and left lobe.

12. Alternative procedure for the lung in oral studies in the rat: right lobes embedded, ventral surface down and in the mouse: whole lung embedded, ventral surface down.

13. The optimal way to fix the central nervous system is to perfuse it *in situ* while the animal is deeply anesthetized. The procedure is as follows: anesthetize the animal (for example) with intraperitoneal injection of Nembutal working solution (1.6 mL stock solution with 8.4 mL PBS), 0.1 mL/10 g body weight. Then, pin the mouse on a dissection board ventral side up. Trim back the skin from the thorax to the mandible. Open the thorax following the necropsy protocol (herein described). If blood is needed, collect it by cardiac puncture at this time. With small scissors, cut the right auricle (64). Blood will start to flow from the heart. Insert a 23-gauge needle within the left ventricle, with the syringe containing PBS. Perfuse the PBS with steady pressure, strong enough to wash the blood out from the body, but not so much that it causes damages. The liver (and other organs) would normally go pale very quickly. The lungs should not bulge; if they do, your syringe has perfored the interventricular septum. Slowly remove the needle and repeat the perfusion. After injecting 15 mL of PBS, change the syringe and perfuse 4% paraformaldehyde in the same way. If fixation is successful, the body will stiffen from the tip of the tail to the tip of the nose. Proceed as usual for tissue collection.

14. Alternatively remove the vertebral bodies with the spinal cord.

15. Changes in brain weights are rarely associated with neurotoxicity. The utility of brain weight rests in the ability to calculate organ to brain weight ratios which is helpful when terminal body weights are affected or to normalize organ weight data.

16. To avoid artifactual vacuolation in the white matter, do not store specimens from nervous tissue in alcohol.

17. The pituitary gland can be trimmed *in situ* as transverse section of skull. This procedure is not recommended.

18. Each eye can be removed from the socket together with the optic nerve and the Harderian gland after fixation of the head.

19. For long-term studies, formalin fixation of the eyes is generally sufficient. For other study types, fixation in Davidson's fixative is recommended to avoid detachment of the retina.

20. Alternatively, the skeletal muscle and sciatic nerve can be sampled together. In this case, the gracilis, adductor, semimembranous,

and semitendinous muscles are removed from the medial aspect of the thigh to get access to the sciatic nerve running along the medial surface of the biceps femoris muscle. After fixation, transverse and longitudinal sections are prepared.

21. The bone marrow is generally examined concurrently with the bone tissue after decalcification. On this specimen, it is possible to evaluate the cellularity, the number of megakaryocytes, and the stromal compartment. If evaluation of the iron content and more precise cytology are needed, examination of a bone marrow smear of a core sample from the femur may be useful. This method requires training to obtain satisfactory results. Prepare bone marrow smears as fresh as possible to avoid blood clotting. Cut off the proximal and distal epiphyses with scissors. Then blew air from one end into the marrow cavity and collect the marrow cast onto a glass slide. The smear is prepared conventionally with a cover glass. A smear of adequate quality contains grossly visible particles. Alternatively, aspiration with a pipette containing anticoagulated serum or a small paint brush or a cotton bud from the longitudinally opened femur can also be performed (this procedure implies that the contro-lateral femur, knee joint, and proximal tibia should be sampled).

References

1. Olds, R.J., and Olds, J.R. (1979) *A color atlas of the rat-dissection guide*. Wolfe Medical Publications Ltd, London.
2. Feldman, D.B., and Seely, J.C. (1988) *Necropsy guide: rodents & the rabbit*. CRC Press, Boca Raton.
3. Walker, W.F. Jr, and Homberger, D.G. (1998) *Anatomy and dissection of the rat*. W.H. Freeman and Company, New York, USA.
4. Bono, C.D., Elwell, M.R., and Rogers, K. (2000) Necropsy techniques with standard collection and trimming of tissues, in *The laboratory rat* (Krinke, G.J., ed), Academic Press, San Diego San Francisco New York, pp 569–600.
5. Relyea, M.J., Miller, J., Boggess, D., and Sundberg, J.P. (2000) Necropsy methods for laboratory mice: biological characterization of a new mutation, in *Systematic approach of mouse mutations* (Sundberg, J.P., ed), CRC Press, Boca Raton, pp. 57–89.
6. EULEP, European Late Effects Project. Covelli's Necropsy protocol & pictures. http://eulep.pdn.cam.ac.uk/Necropsy_of_the_Mouse/printable.php.
7. Virtual Mouse Necropsy, National Institute of Allergy and Infectious Diseases (NIAID), National Institute of health, USA: http://www3.niaid.nih.gov/labs/aboutlabs/cmb/InfectiousDiseasePathogenesisSection/mouseNecropsy/.
8. Cook, M. (1965) *Anatomy of the Laboratory Mouse*, Academic Press (Web version) http://www.informatics.jax.org/cookbook/.
9. Krinke, G.J. (ed) (2000) *The laboratory rat*. Academic Press, San Diego San Francisco New York.
10. Ruehl-Fehlert, C., Kittel, B., Morawietz, G., Deslex, P., Keenan, C., Mahrt, C.R., Nolte, T., Robinson, M., Stuart, B.P., and Deschl, U. (2003) Revised guides for organ sampling and trimming in rats and mice – Part 1. *Exp. Toxicol. Pathol.* **55**, 91–106.
11. Kittel, B., Ruehl-Fehlert, C., Morawietz, G., Klapwijk, J., Elwell, M.R., Lenz, B., O'Sullivan, G., Roth, D.R., and Wadsworth, P.F. (2004) Revised guides for organ sampling and trimming in rats and mice – Part 2. *Exp. Toxicol. Pathol.* **55**, 413–431.
12. Morawietz, G., Ruehl-Fehlert, C., Kittel, B., Bube, A., Keane, K., Halm, S., Heuser, A., and Hellmann, J. (2004) Revised guides for organ sampling and trimming in rats and mice – Part 3. *Exp. Toxicol. Pathol.* **55**, 433–449.

13. Formaldehyde: Health-based recommended occupational exposure limit Dutch expert committee on occupational standards (DECOS): Health Council of The Netherlands (Gezondheidsraad). Vol. 02 osh (2003) 124.

14. Woods, A.E., and Ellis, R.C. (1994). *Laboratory histopathology, a complete reference.* Vol. I and II. Churchill Livingstone.

15. Fox, J.G., Cohen, B.J., and Loew, F.M. (ed) (1984) *Laboratory animal medicine.* Academic Press, Orlando, USA.

16. Bush, R.K., and Stave, G.M. (2003) Laboratory animal allergy: an update. *ILAR J.* **44(1)**, 28–51.

17. Figler, N. (2004) Laboratory animal allergies: overview of causation and prevention. *Lab. Anim.* **33(10)**, 25–27.

18. Sellers, R.S., Morton, D., Michael, B., Roome, N., Johnson, J.K., Yano, B.L., Perry, R., and Schafer, K. (2007) Society of Toxicologic Pathology Position Paper: Organ Weight Recommendations for Toxicology Studies. *Toxicol. Path.* **35(5)**, 751–755.

19. Leblanc, B. (2000) Pathology and tissue sampling protocols for Rodent carcinogenicity studies, time for revision. *Toxicol. Path.* **28**, 628–633.

20. Bregman, C.L., Adler, R.R., Morton, D.G., Regan, K.S., and Yano, B.L. (2003) Recommended tissue list for histopathologic examination in repeat-dose toxicity and carcinogenicity studies: a proposal of the society of toxicologic pathology (STP). *Toxicol. Pathol.* **31(2)**, 252–253.

21. Russo, I.H., Tewari, M., and Russo, J. (1989) Morphology and development of the rat mammary gland, in *Monographs on pathology of laboratory animals. Integument and mammary glands* (Jones, T.C., Mohr, U., and Hunt, R.D., eds), Springer, New York, pp 233–252.

22. Boorman, G.A., Wilson, J.T., Van Zwieten, M.J., Wilson, J.T., and Eustis, S.L. (1990) Mammary gland, in *Pathology of the Fischer rat. Reference and atlas* (Boorman, G.A., Eustis, S.L., Elwell, M.R., Montgomery, C.A., and MacKenzie, W.F., eds), Academic Press, San Diego New York, pp 295–313.

23. Van den Broeck, W., Derore, A., and Simoens, P. (2006) Anatomy and nomenclature of murine lymph nodes: descriptive study and nomenclatory standardization in BALB/cAnNCrl mice. *J. Immunol. Methods.* **312(1–2)**, 12–19.

24. Hebel, R., and Stromberg, M.W. (1986) *Anatomy and embryology of the laboratory rat.* Worthsee: BioMed Verlag.

25. Botts, S., Jokinen, M., Gaillard, E.T., Elwell, M.R., and Mann, P.C. (1999). Salivary, harderian, and lacrimal glands, in *Pathology of the mouse* (Maronpot, R.R., ed), Cache River Press, Boca Raton, pp. 49–79.

26. Dijkstra, C.D., and Veerman, A.J.P. (1990) Spleen. Structure and function. Normal anatomy, histology, ultrastructure, rat, in *Monographs on pathology of laboratory animals. Hemopoietic system* (Jones, T.C., Mohr, U., Hunt, R.D., Ward, J.M., and Burek, J.D., eds), Springer, New York, pp 185–193.

27. Popesko, P., Rajtova, V., and Horak, J. (1992) *A colour atlas of the anatomy of small laboratory animals. Vol. 2. Rat, mouse, golden hamster.* Wolfe Publishing, Bratislava, p 89.

28. Brown, H.R., and Hardisty, J.F. (1990) Oral cavity, esophagus and stomach, in *Pathology of the Fischer rat. Reference and atlas* (Boorman, G.A., Eustis, S.L., Elwell, M.R., Montgomery, C.A., and MacKenzie, W.F., eds), Academic Press, San Diego New York, pp 9–30.

29. Matsukura, N., and Asano, G. (1997) Anatomy, histology, ultrastructure, stomach, rat, in *Monographs on pathology of laboratory animals. Digestive system*, 2nd edition (Jones, T.C., Popp, J.A., and Mohr, U., eds), Springer, New York, pp 343–350.

30. Elwell, M.R., and MCConnell, E.E. (1990) Small and large intestine, in *Pathology of the Fischer rat. Reference and atlas* (Boorman, G.A., Eustis, S.L., Elwell, M.R., Montgomery, C.A., and MacKenzie, W.F., eds), Academic Press, San Diego New York, pp 43–61.

31. Moolenbeek, C., and Ruitenberg, E.J. (1981) The "Swiss roll": a simple technique for histological studies of the Rodent intestine. *Lab. Anim.* **15**, 57–59.

32. Soul, N.W. (1987) Gut rolls: a better technique for GI tumor assessment. *Toxicol. Pathol.* **15**, 374.

33. Paget, E.G., and Thomson, R. (1979) *Standard operating procedures in pathology.* MTP Press, Lancaster, pp 134–139.

34. Nyska, A., and Maronpot, R.R. (1999) Adrenal Gland, in *Pathology of the mouse. Reference and atlas* (Maronpot, R.R., Boorman, G.A., and Gaul, B.W., eds), Cache River Press, Vienna, pp 509–536.

35. Liebelt, A.G. (1998) Unique features of anatomy, histology and ultrastructure, kidney, mouse, in *Monographs on pathology of laboratory animals. Urinary system*, 2nd edition (Jones, T.C., Hard, G.C., and Mohr, U., eds), Springer, New York, pp 37–57.

36. Khan, K.N.M., and Alden, C.L. (2002) Kidney, in *Handbook of toxicologic pathology*, Vol. 2, 2nd edition, (Haschek, W.M., Rousseaux, C.G., and Wallig, M.A., eds), Academic Press, San Diego New York Boston, pp 255–336.

37. Cohen, S.M., Wanibuchi, H., and Fukushima, S. (2002) Lower urinary tract, in *Handbook of toxicologic pathology*, Vol. 2, 2nd edition, (Haschek, W.M., Rousseaux, C.G., and Wallig, M.A., eds), Academic Press, San Diego New York Boston, pp 337–362.

38. Ferm, V.H. (1987) Embryology and comparative anatomy, Rodent reproductive tract, in *Monographs on pathology of laboratory animals. Genital system* (Jones, T.C., Mohr, U., and Hunt, R.D., eds), Springer, New York, pp 3–7.

39. Creasy, D.M., and Foster, P.M.D. Male reproductive system, in *Handbook of toxicologic pathology*, Vol. 2, 2nd edition, (Haschek, W.M., Rousseaux, C.G., and Wallig, M.A., eds), Academic Press, San Diego New York Boston, pp 785–846.

40. Lanning, L.L., Creasy, D.M., Chapin, R.E., Mann, P.C., Barlow, N.J., Regan, K.S., and Goodman, D.G. (2002) Recommended approaches for the evaluation of testicular and epididymal toxicity. *Toxicol. Pathol.* **30**, 507–520.

41. Boorman, G.A., Chapin, R.E., and Mitsumori, K. (1990) Testis and epididymis, in *Pathology of the Fischer rat. Reference and atlas* (Boorman, G.A., Eustis, S.L., Elwell, M.R., Montgomery, C.A., and MacKenzie, W.F., eds), Academic Press, San Diego New York, pp 405–418.

42. Lee, C.H., and Holland, J.M. (1987) Anatomy, histology, and ultrastructure (correlation with function), prostate, rat, in *Monographs on pathology of laboratory animals. Genital system* (Jones, T.C., Mohr, U., and Hunt, R.D., eds), Springer, Berlin Heidelberg New York, pp 239–251.

43. Boorman, G.A., Elwell, M.R., and Mitsumori, K. (1990) Male accessory sex glands, penis, and scrotum, in *Pathology of the Fischer rat. Reference and atlas* (Boorman, G.A., Eustis, S.L., Elwell, M.R., Montgomery, C.A., and MacKenzie, W.F., eds), Academic Press, San Diego New York, pp 419–428.

44. Heindel, J.J., and Chapin, R.E. (eds) (1993) *Methods in reproductive toxicology: female reproductive toxicology*, Vol. 3B. Academic Press, Orlando.

45. Yuan, Y.D., and Foley, G.L. (2002) Female reproductive system, in *Handbook of toxicologic pathology*, Vol. 2, 2nd edition (Haschek, W.M., Rousseaux, C.G., and Wallig, M.A., eds), Academic Press, San Diego New York Boston, pp 847–894.

46. Piper, R.C. (1981) Morphological evaluation of the heart in toxicologic studies, in *Cardiac toxicology*, Vol. 3 (Balazc, T., ed), CRC Press, Boca Raton, pp 111–136.

47. Van Vleet, J.F., Ferrans, V.J., and Herman, E. (2002) Cardiovascular and skeletal muscle system, in *Handbook of toxicologic pathology*, Vol. 2, 2nd edition (Haschek, W.M., Rousseaux, C.G., and Wallig, M.A., eds), Academic Press, San Diego New York Boston, pp 363–455.

48. Djikstra, C.D., and Sminia, T. (1990) Thymus. Structure and function. Normal anatomy, histology, immunohistology, ultrastructure, rat, in Monographs on pathology of laboratory animals. Hemopoietic system (Jones, T.C., Mohr, U., Hunt, R.D., Ward, J.M., and Burek, J.D., eds), Springer, New York, pp 249–256.

49. Kittel, B., Ernst, H., and Kamino, K. (1996) Anatomy, histology and ultrastructure, parathyroid, mouse, in *Monographs on pathology of laboratory animals. Endocrine system*, 2nd edition (Jones, T.C., Capen, C.C., and Mohr, U., eds), Springer, New York, pp 328–329.

50. Kittel, B., Ernst, H., and Kamino, K. (1996) Anatomy, histology and ultrastructure, parathyroid, rat, in *Monographs on pathology of laboratory animals. Endocrine system*, 2nd edition (Jones, T.C., Capen, C.C., and Mohr, U., eds), Springer, New York, pp 330–332.

51. Gopinath, C., Prentice, D.E., Lewis, D.J. (1987). The respiratory system, in *Atlas of experimental toxicological pathology*. MTP Press, Lancaster Boston The Hague, pp 22–42.

52. Plopper, C.G. (1996) Structure and function of the lung, in *Monographs on pathology of laboratory animals. Respiratory system*, 2nd edition (Jones, T.C., Dungworth, D.L., and Mohr, U., eds) Springer, New York, pp 135–150.

53. Cassella, J.P., Hay, J., and Lawson, S.J. (1997) *The rat nervous system*. John Wiley & Sons, Chichester.

54. Dorman, D.C., Brenneman, K.A., and Bolon, B. (2002) Nervous system, in *Handbook of toxicologic pathology*, Vol. 2, 2nd edition (Haschek, W.M., Rousseaux, C.G., and Wallig, M.A., eds), Academic Press, San Diego New York Boston, pp 509–537.

55. Mahler, J.F., and Elwell, M.R. (1999) Pituitary Gland, in *Pathology of the mouse. Reference and atlas* (Maronpot, R.R., Boorman, G.A., and Gaul, B.W. eds), Cache River Press, Vienna, pp 491–507.

56. Whiteley, H.E., and Peiffer, R.L. (2002) The eye, in Handbook of toxicologic pathology, Vol 2, 2nd edition (Haschek, W.M., Rousseaux, C.G., and Wallig,

57. Popp, J.A., and Monteiro-Riviere, N.A. (1985) Macroscopic, microscopic, and ultrastructural anatomy of the nasal cavity, rat, in *Monographs*

on pathology of laboratory animals. *Respiratory system*, 2nd edition (Jones, T.C., Dungworth, D.L., and Mohr, U., eds) Springer, Berlin Heidelberg New York Tokyo, pp 3–10.

58. Boorman, G.A., Morgan, K.T., and Uriah, L.C. (1990) Nose, larynx and trachea, in *Pathology of the Fischer rat. Reference and atlas* (Boorman, G.A., Eustis, S.L., Elwell, M.R., Montgomery, C.A., and MacKenzie, W.F., eds), Academic Press, San Diego New York, pp 315–337.

59. Copeland-Haines, D., and Eustis, S.L. Specialized sebaceous glands, in *Pathology of the Fischer rat. Reference and atlas* (Boorman, G.A., Eustis, S.L., Elwell, M.R., Montgomery, C.A., and MacKenzie, W.F., eds), Academic Press, San Diego New York, pp 279–294.

60. MCGavin, M.D. (1991) Procedures for morphological studies of skeletal muscle, rat, mouse, and hamster, in *Monographs on patholmusculoskeletal systems.* (Jones, T.C., Mohr, U., and Hunt, R.D., eds), Springer, New York, pp 101–108.

61. Valli, V.E., Villeneuve, D.C., Reed, B., et al. (1990) Evaluation of blood and bone marrow, rat, in *Monographs on pathology of laboratory animals. Hemopoietic system* (Jones, T.C., Mohr, U., Hunt, R.D., Ward, J.M., and Burek, J.D., eds), Springer, New York, pp 9–26.

62. Woodard, J.C., Burkhardt, J.E., and Lee, W. (2002) Bones and joints, in *Handbook of toxicologic pathology*, Vol. 2, 2nd edition (Haschek, W.M., Rousseaux, C.G., and Wallig, M.A., eds), Academic Press, San Diego New York Boston, pp 457–508.

63. Latendresse, J.R., Warbrittion, A.R., Jonassen, H., and Creasy, D.M. (2002) Fixation of testes and eyes using a modified Davidson's fluid: comparison with Bouin's fluid and conventional Davidson's fluid. *Toxicol. Pathol.* 30: 524–533.

64. Hoff, J. (2000) Methods of blood collection. *J. Lab. Anim.* **29(10)**, 47–53.

Chapter 4

Histopathology Procedures: From Tissue Sampling to Histopathological Evaluation

Mohamed Slaoui and Laurence Fiette

Abstract

Histological procedures aim to provide good quality sections that can be used for a light microscopic evaluation of human or animal tissue changes in either spontaneous or induced diseases. Routinely, tissues are fixed with neutral formalin 10%, embedded in paraffin, and then manually sectioned with a microtome to obtain 4–5 µm-thick paraffin sections. Dewaxed sections are then stained with hematoxylin and eosin (H&E) or can be used for other purposes (special stains, immunohistochemistry, *in situ* hybridization, etc.). During this process, many steps and procedures are critical to ensure standard and interpretable sections. Key recomendations are given here to achieve this objective.

Key words: Histology, Embedding, Sectioning, Staining, Histological slides

1. Introduction

Histopathology is the microscopic study of diseased tissue. It is an important investigative medical tool that is based on the study of human or animal histology (also called microscopic anatomy). It is performed by examining a thin tissue section under light microscopes. Histotechnique consists of a number of procedures that allow visualization of tissue and cell microscopic features and recognize specific microscopic structural changes of diseases.

Observation of tissues under a light microscope is an old concern for science and medicine. The earliest evidence of magnifying glass forming a magnified image dates back to 1021 when the physicist Ibn al-Haytham (965–1039) published the "Book of Optics." The name "microscope" was crafted by the German botanist Johann Faber (1574–1629). The light microscope used by Anton Van Leeuwenhoek's (1632–1723) was a small, single convex lens mounted on a plate. Nowadays, sophisticated light

Jean-Charles Gautier (ed.), *Drug Safety Evaluation: Methods and Protocols*, Methods in Molecular Biology, vol. 691,
DOI 10.1007/978-1-60761-849-2_4, © Springer Science+Business Media, LLC 2011

microscopes use multiple lenses and are widely used in research and in diagnostic.

Most histology techniques were described in the nineteenth century. They mostly use physicochemical reactions with tissue components that allow preservation, cutting or staining of tissues. It is only in the 1970s that the processing of tissue has become partially automated, but some critical steps such as embedding and sectioning are still manual. These steps are delicate and time and resource intensive.

Histopathology evaluation basically compares diseased or experimentally altered tissues with matching sample from healthy or control counterparts. Therefore, it is very important to rigorously standardize every histology process (i.e., specimen sampling, trimming, embedding, sectioning, and staining).

The purpose of this chapter is to describe some routine histological processing steps used for histopathological evaluation and, in particular, paraffin embedding, sectioning, and staining. Several other techniques are available and could be performed on tissues for specific purposes (special stains, immunohistochemistry, *in situ* hybridization, etc.) (1). Tissues can also be frozen or embedded in plastic, but these latter techniques are beyond the scope of this chapter. Many websites can be consulted to get further protocols in histological techniques (2, 3).

2. Materials

2.1. Fixation

1. Fixative solution (usually commercially available formalin).
2. Phosphate buffer (pH = 6.8).
3. Rubber or gloves (see Note 1).
4. Protective clothing.
5. Eyeglasses and mask.
6. Fume hood.
7. Containers with appropriate lids (volume is commensurate with sample size. Large neck plastic containers are preferable and can be reused).
8. Labels and permanent ink.

2.2. Trimming

1. Fume hood.
2. Rubber or gloves (see Note 1).
3. Protective clothing.
4. Eyeglasses and mask.
5. Dissecting board (plastic boards are preferred as they can be easily cleaned and autoclaved).

6. Blunt ended forceps (serrated forceps may damage small animal tissues).

7. Scalpels blades and handle.

8. Plastic bags and paper towels.

9. Containers for histological specimens, cassettes and permanent labels. Containers and cassettes, should be correctly labeled before starting tissue trimming.

2.3. Pre-embedding

1. Disposable plastic cassettes for histology (with appropriate lids). For small samples, disposable plastic cassettes for histology with subdivision (Microsette®).

2. Foam pads ($31 \times 25 \times 3$ mm) can be used to immobilize tissue samples inside the cassettes.

3. Commercial absolute ethyl alcohol and 96% ethanol solution.

4. 90% and 70% ethanol solutions.

5. Paraffin solvent/clearing agent: xylene or substitute (e.g., Histosol®, Neoclear®).

6. Paraffin wax for histology, melting point 56–57°C (e.g., Paraplast® Tissue Embedding Media).

7. Automated Tissue Processor (vacuum or carousel type).

2.4. Embedding

1. Tissue embedding station (a machine that integrates melted paraffin dispensers, heated and cooled plates).

2. Paraffin wax for histology, melting point 56–57°C (e.g. Paraplast® Tissue Embedding Media).

3. Histology stainless steel embedding molds. These are available in different sizes ($10 \times 10 \times 5$ mm; $15 \times 15 \times 5$ mm; $24 \times 24 \times 5$ mm; $24 \times 30 \times 5$ mm, etc.).

4. Small forceps.

2.5. Sectioning

1. Rotary microtome.

2. Tissue water bath with a thermometer. Alternatively a thermostatic warm plate can be used.

3. Disposable microtome blades (for routine paraffin sections use wedge-shaped blades).

4. Sharps container to discard used blades.

5. Fine paint brushes to remove paraffin debris.

6. Forceps to handle the ribbons of paraffin sections.

7. Clean standard 75×25 mm microscope glass slides (other dimension microscope glass slides are commercially available).

8. Laboratory oven (set at 37°C).

9. Coated glass slides (e.g., Superfrost® or Superfrost Plus®). This is especially recommended when slides are used for immunohistochemistry.

10. 0.1% gelatin in water (1 g of gelatin in 1 L of distilled water). This should not be used with Superfrost® or Superfrost Plus® slides and should be reserved for immunohistology sections.

2.6. Staining and Cover Slipping

1. Harris hematoxylin (commercial solution, ready to use).

2. Eosin Y solution.

3. Hydrochloric acid 37%.

4. Absolute ethanol.

5. Ethanol 96%.

6. Clearing agent (xylene or substitute e.g. Histosol®, Neoclear®).

7. Staining dishes and Coplin jars suitable for staining.

8. Permanent mounting medium (e.g. Eukitt®).

9. Glass cover slips (25 × 60 mm).

10. Filter paper.

11. Ethanol solutions:

    (a) Add 12.5 mL of water to 1 L of commercial 96% ethanol to obtain 95% ethanol.

    (b) Add 408 mL of water to 1 L of commercial 96% ethanol to obtain 70% ethanol.

2.7. Storage of Paraffin Blocks and Slides

1. Paraffin blocks storage cabinets.

2. Histological slides storage cabinets.

3. Methods

3.1. Fixation

Autolysis is a combination of postmortem changes due to rupture of cell homeostasis that leads to uncontrolled water and electrolytes dynamics in and out of the cell and of alteration of enzymatic activity. These changes are favorable conditions for bacterial and fungal growth and ultimately result in complete destruction of tissue structures. To halt autolysis, tissues should be preserved in an appropriate fixative that permanently cross-link its proteins and stabilize it.

The process of autolysis virtually begins immediately after death. Therefore, rapid and adequate fixation after sampling is essential. This can be achieved by immersion of the tissue sample in an adequate volume of fixative solution. There are several methods of fixation including aldehydes, mercurials, alcohols, oxidizing agents, and picric acid derivatives (4). Tissue immersion in aldehyde (formaldehyde or glutaraldehyde) is the most frequently used fixation method in biomedical research. Formalin (formaldehyde) is commercially available as 38–40% or 10% neutral phosphate-buffered solutions (see Note 2). It is generally accepted that a volume ratio of tissue to fixative of 1:10 to 1:20 is necessary for optimal fixation. Small tissue samples are usually fixed at room temperature after 12–48 h. Larger specimen may require more fixation time as formalin slowly penetrates tissues (see Note 3).

1. Place the fixative container under a fume hood.
2. Plunge tissue samples in the fixative solution.
3. Stir gently the fixative container for a few seconds to make sure the tissue sample does not stick to the container surface.
4. Replace cap over the container after each tissue (one container can be used for several tissue samples).
5. Add identification label on each container.

3.2. Trimming

After fixation, tissue samples need to be properly trimmed to reach the adequate size and orientation of the tissue. This step is also important to reach a sample size that is compatible with subsequent histology procedures such as embedding and sectioning.

Hard tissues (such as bones and teeth) must be decalcified before trimming.

1. Under a fume hood, remove tissue samples from the fixative container or jar.
2. Trim one or more small pieces of tissues and organs and fit them into cassettes.
3. Place a lid on the cassette.
4. Label each cassette with a permanent ink.
5. Store cassettes in a fixative container.

There are specific rules that should be followed for trimming of each tissue and organ. These depend on the goal of the histopathology evaluation. Standardized methods for toxicology studies in drug safety evaluation are available online (5). These are also described in the comprehensive papers from the RITA group (Registry of Industrial Toxicology Animal data) (6–8). Specific methods have been proposed for many organs: gut (9, 10), heart (11), male reproductive system (12–14), female reproductive system (15), or muscle (16).

3.3. Pre-embedding

The goal of pre-embedding is to infiltrate tissue samples with paraffin and replace water content of tissue by this wax material (17). Paraffin is used as a supporting material before sectioning. Histology grade paraffin wax has a melting point around 56 or 57°C, a temperature that does not alter the structures and key morphologic characteristics of tissues, thus allowing adequate microscopic evaluation by the pathologist. At room temperature, paraffin wax offers enough rigidity to allow very thin sections just a few micrometers thick (usually 4 or 5 μm).

Pre-embedding is a sequential process that consists of dehydration of tissues in increased concentrations of alcohol solutions, then gradual replacement of alcohol by a paraffin solvent. Xylene (or its substitutes; e.g., Histosol®, Neoclear®, and Histoclear®) has the advantage to be miscible in both alcohol and paraffin. As a result, the tissue sample is dehydrated and fully infiltrated by paraffin. This step is generally automated using a variety of vacuum or carousel type tissue processors (see Note 4).

When using a tissue processor, the following steps should be followed:

1. Check if the baskets and metal cassettes are clean and free of wax.
2. Do not pack the tissues too tightly to allow fluid exchange.
3. Check if the processor is free of spilt fluids and wax.
4. Check if the fluids levels are higher than the specimen containers.
5. Select the appropriate protocol and check the clock.
6. Prepare 95% and 70% ethanol solutions.
7. Dehydrate in a graded series of ethanol:
   (a) Wash in 70% ethanol for 1 h.
   (b) Wash in 95% ethanol for 1 h (two times).
   (c) Wash in 100% ethanol for 1 h (two times).
8. Clear with a paraffin solvent (xylene) for 1 h (two times).
9. Infiltrate with paraffin for 1 h (two times).
10. Tissue sampled are retrieved at the end of the processing program (automates are usually run overnight to start the embedding process in the next morning).

The following is a list of rescue procedures that can be helpful to consider in case the pre-embedding procedure is not completed normally:

1. Recovery of tissues that have air-dried because of mechanical or electrical failure of the processor:
   (a) Rehydrate the tissue in Sandison's solution (absolute alcohol 30 mL, formaldehyde 37% 0.5 mL, and sodium carbonate 0.2 g water up to 100 mL) or Van Cleve and Ross' solution (trisodium phosphate 0.25 g in 100 mL of water).
   (b) Immerse the tissues in one of these two solutions for 24–72 h (actually most of tissues rehydrate and soften within 4–6 h).

(c) Process to dehydration and pre-embedding as usual, starting in 70% ethanol.

2. Recovery of tissues accidentally returned to fixative following wax infiltration. Discard all contaminated fluids:

   (a) Rinse in 70% ethanol followed by 95% ethanol.

   (b) Rinse in absolute ethanol (two to three times).

   (c) Rinse in xylene (or substitute).

   (d) Carry out the paraffin infiltration three times, 30–60 min each.

3. Recovery of tissues accidentally returned to ethanol 70% following wax infiltration:

   (a) Discard all contaminated fluids.

   (b) Rinse in ethanol 95%.

   (c) Rinse in absolute ethanol (two changes).

   (d) Rinse in xylene (or substitute).

   (e) Carry out the paraffin infiltration two to three times, 30–60 min each.

The same steps can be used for manual tissue processing. Melt the paraffin in an oven at 60°C in glass containers. Immerse the specimens into the melted paraffin.

3.4. Embedding

Once tissue samples are infiltrated by paraffin, they are removed from the cassettes and carefully positioned inside a metal base mold.

This step is critical as correct orientation of the tissue is essential for accurate microscopic evaluation. The mold is filled with melted paraffin and then immediately placed on a cooling surface. To trace each tissue specimen, the cassette with permanent tissue and study identification is placed on top of the metal base mold and incorporated in the paraffin block before cooling. In this manner, the cassette will be used as a base of the paraffin block for microtome sectioning (once the metal base mold is removed) (see Note 5).

1. Check that the different compartments of the station have the appropriate temperature. Paraffin should be liquid in the paraffin reservoir, work surface should be warm, and cool plate should be cold. Stainless steel molds should be kept warm.

2. Remove the cassettes from the last tissue processor bath (normally melted paraffin) and transfer to the warm compartment of the embedding station.

3. Transfer one cassette onto the hot plate.

4. Snap off the cassette lid and discard it.

5. Select a preheated stainless steel mold of the appropriate size. The specimen must not come into contact with the edge of the mold.

6. Transfer the mold onto the hot plate.

7. Pour melted paraffin from the paraffin dispenser.

8. Transfer the paraffin-infiltrated tissues into the mold.

9. Using heated forceps, orientate the tissue inside the mold to obtain the desired position in relation with the cutting axis; the specimen surface in contact with the base of the mold being the one that will be on the slide after sectioning.

10. Center the specimen in the mold ensuring that paraffin entirely surrounds the edge of the tissue.

11. Carefully transfer the mold onto the cool plate. Allow a few seconds to paraffin to turn white (this means that paraffin returned to solid phase). During cooling, the paraffin will shrink (up to 15% of its initial volume); this compression will be fully recovered later after sectioning.

12. Make sure that the specimen does not move during this step and still keep its desired orientation. If not, put the mold back onto the warm work surface until the whole paraffin liquefies then start again from step 9.

    Immediately place the base of the original cassette on top of the mold. Incorporation of the cassette in the paraffin block before cooling allows tracing the specimen identification and uses the cassette as a holder during sectioning.

13. Carefully fill the mold with paraffin to above the upper edge of the cassette.

14. Carefully transfer the mold and cassette onto the cool plate and allow time (at least 15 min) until the paraffin has hardened.

15. Snap off the mold.

16. Bring the paraffin blocks together.

17. Store the paraffin blocks at room temperature until sectioning.

3.5. Sectioning

The objective of this step is to cut 4–5 µm-thick sections from paraffin blocks. This is achieved using precision knives (microtomes) (18). To obtain constant high quality and extremely thin tissue sections, disposable blades should be used and changed after a limited number of blocks.

The paraffin block is mounted on the microtome holder. Sections are cut as a ribbon and are floated on a water bath maintained at 45°C to stretch the paraffin section. A standard microscope glass slide is placed under the selected tissue section and removed from the water bath. Tissue sections are then allowed to dry, preferably in a thermostatic laboratory oven at 37°C.

Tissue sectioning and floating steps are delicate operations that should be performed by trained personnel.

1. Heat the tissue water bath to 45°C and fill it with water. To avoid microorganisms growth, the bath should be carefully cleaned every day and the water flotation bath discarded.

2. Put the paraffin blocks on a cold surface (e.g., refrigerated cold plate or ice) to harden the cut surface. Avoid prolonged cooling and very cold surfaces as they may lead to cracking in the block surface.

3. Install a disposable blade in the microtome.

4. Set angle between the blade edge bevel and the block to 2–5 degrees (clearance angle). A correct angle should be set to avoid compression in cut sections and to reduce friction as the knife passes through the block. Angles in the above mentioned range are recommended for paraffin sections, but the exact angle is generally found by trial and error.

5. Lock the blade in place.

6. Lock the microtome hand-wheel.

7. Trim the edges of one block with a sharp razor blade so that the upper and lower edges of the block are parallel to the edges of the knife. Otherwise a ribbon cannot be cut. Keep 2–3 mm of paraffin wax around the tissue.

8. Fit the cassette paraffin block onto the cassette holder of the microtome. Orientate the block so that its greater axis is perpendicular to the edge of the knife, and also that the edge offers the least resistance (e.g., the smallest edge will be cut first).

9. Unlock the hand-wheel.

10. Advance the block until it is in contact with the edge of the knife. Paraffin block edges must be parallel to the knife. If not, adjust the block orientation.

11. Set the section thickness around 15 microns.

12. Coarse cut the block at 15 microns until the whole surface of the embedded tissue can be cut.

13. Lock the microtome hand-wheel.

14. Return the trimmed block to cold plate for 1–2 min.

15. Set the section thickness to 4–5 μm.

16. Remove wax debris from the knife with alcohol. Avoid use of xylene to clean the paraffin debris as it often leaves an oily remnant on the knife and following sections will stick (not mentioning the xylene hazards for the operator).

17. Move to an unused area on the blade or install a new disposable blade.

18. Install the cassette paraffin block onto the cassette holder again.

19. Cut a series of paraffin sections. If sectioning is doing well, you will obtain a ribbon of serial sections.

20. Gently breath upon the sections to eliminate static electricity, to flatten the sections, and to facilitate the removal of the ribbon from the blade.

21. Separate the ribbon (including four to five sections) from the knife edge with a paint brush.

22. Transfer the piece of ribbon onto a glass slide coated with a drop of gelatin-water, or to the surface of the water bath.

23. Gently separate the floating sections on the water bath with pressure from the tips of forceps.

24. Collect sections on a clean glass slides. Hold the slide vertically beneath the section and lift carefully the slide up to enable tissue adherence.

25. Label slides with a histo-pen or pencil. Avoid pens with non-alcohol-resistant ink (ballpoint or felt-tipped pens).

26. Allow the slides to dry horizontally on a warm plate for 10 min to ensure that the section firmly adheres to the glass slide. Alternatively slides can be dried vertically in an oven for 20 min at 56°C.

27. Transfer the slides (vertically placed) to a laboratory oven overnight at 37°C.

28. Store the slides in dry boxes at room temperature. For immunohistochemistry, slides should be stored at 4°C to minimize antigen loss.

29. Empty the water bath and wipe it with a damp cloth at the end of each day.

3.6. Staining and Mounting

Unstained paraffin sections offer very low contrast and therefore cannot be evaluated microscopically in routine histopathology. It is necessary to apply coloring reagents (mostly chemicals) to stain tissue structures. There are many histochemistry staining techniques that can be applied to examine specific tissue or cell structures. As most of these dyes are water soluble, tissue sections should be rehydrated to remove paraffin (using xylene, alcohol solutions ending in water). Hematoxylin and Eosin (H&E) is the routine staining used to study histopathology changes in tissues and organs from animals in toxicity studies. Hematoxylin is a basic dye that has affinity for acid structures of the cell (mostly nucleic acids of the cell nucleus), and eosin is an acidic dye that binds to cytoplasmic structures of the cell. As a result, H&E stains nuclei in blue and cytoplasms in orange-red. A variant to this staining method is the Hematoxylin–Eosin and Saffron (HE&S) stain. As compared to the H&E method, HE&S stains collagen in yellow-orange, allowing a better highlight of interstitial conjunctive tissue (see Note 6).

The following protocol describes manual H&E staining technique. It is suitable for small series of slides. This operation is usually automated to allow high-throughput staining of slides.

1. Prepare the Harris hematoxylin working solution. Filter the commercial solution through filter paper to remove the metallic precipitant that forms in the solution upon standing.

2. Prepare 0.1% aqueous eosin Y working solution. Dissolve 1 g of eosin Y in 1 L of deionised water. Add four drops of HCl to obtain a pH between 4 and 5.

3. Add a thymol crystal to prevent molds growth.

4. Label and date the solutions. Aqueous eosin solution is stable for at least 2 months at room temperature.

5. Prepare the differentiation solution (acid alcohol). Add 1 mL of 37% HCl to 100 mL of 70% ethanol.

6. Dewax the paraffin sections in xylene 2×5 min each.

7. Rehydrate in 100% ethanol 2×5 min each.

8. Rehydrate in 95% ethanol 2×5 min each.

9. Wash in running tap water for 3 min.

10. Stain for 3–5 min in Harris hematoxylin.

11. Wash in running tap water for 3 min.

12. Decolorize briefly in acid alcohol for 2 s.

13. Wash and blue the sections in running tap water for 3 min.

14. Stain for 2–5 min in 0.1% aqueous eosin Y.

15. Rinse in tap water for 30 s.

16. Dehydrate in 95% ethanol two times for 2 min each.

17. Dehydrate in 100% ethanol two times for 2 min each.

18. Clear sections in clearing agent two times for 2 min each.

19. The slides may remain in clean clearing agent until cover slipping.

20. The nuclei will be stained in blue, the cytoplasms and other tissue components in pink-orange. Decreased staining intensity of the sections (after approximately 500 slides) indicates that the staining solutions should be renewed.

After staining, a very thin glass should be placed over the tissue section to protect it and to enhance the optical evaluation of the tissue. This also allows tissue section storage for several years. Cover slipping process consists of gluing the cover slip glass over the tissue section on the microscope slide glass. The mounting medium is usually insoluble in water. Therefore, the tissue should be dehydrated again using solutions of increasing concentrations of alcohol and xylene.

The following protocol describes manual cover slip mounting technique. It is suitable for small series of slides:

1. Wipe the surface under the slide while keeping the tissue section covered with the clearing agent.

2. Apply two or three drops of the mounting medium (e.g., Eukitt®).

3. Place a cover slip on the slide and avoid the formation of bubbles. Press gently with forceps to remove any bubble.

4. Dry the slides overnight at room temperature on a flat surface within the fume hood.

To allow high-throughput slide preparation, this operation is usually automated. These automated machines are commercially available from many suppliers.

3.7. Storage of Paraffin Blocks and Slides

1. After sectioning, store paraffin block at room temperature.

2. Store stained slides in appropriate boxes (avoid prolonged exposure to light).

4. Notes

1. Vinyl gloves are preferable as latex gloves may be allergenic.

2. Formaldehyde is an eye, nose, respiratory tract, and skin irritant. It is a strong skin sensitizer and can cause cancer in humans (19, 20). Therefore, it should not be handled without gloves or outside a fume hood. As a result, a variety of alternative fixatives, mostly compound fixatives containing chemicals with differing fixation characteristics, have been investigated (21). However, as of today, there is no unique formalin successor.

3. The best fixation is achieved by intracardial perfusion of the body with formaldehyde or glutaraldehyde. However, this technique needs specific training and is time consuming and therefore only used on a case by case basis.

4. The following is a non-exhaustive list of hazards associated with some of the above mentioned chemicals used during pre-embedding (*22*).

    (a) *Absolute ethanol* is inflammable and irritant to the eye. It should never be handled close to a naked flame or heat. The vapor is heavier than air and can travel a considerable distance to a source of ignition.

    (b) *Paraffin* is not hazardous for health when pure, but wax additives can be potential carcinogen as, e.g., dimethyl sulfoxide (DMSO). Molten wax should not be inhaled, as it produces small lipid droplets that can lead to lipid pneumonia. Prefer paraffin wax without DMSO.

(c) *Xylene* is an aromatic compound that contains benzene. It is moderately inflammable, a mild eye and mucous membrane irritant, a primary skin irritant that may causes dermatitis. It might cause central nervous system depression. Overexposure can lead to respiratory failure. Avoid contact with skin. Xylene substitutes are preferred, but if hazards of xylene are well documented, its substitutes have not been so thoroughly evaluated.

5. Alternative techniques of paraffin embedding exist; they use plastic or resin polymers that should be considered when paraffin embedding is not appropriate (i.e., methyl methacrylate to section nondecalcified bone, Epon to obtain very thin sections in the range of 1 μm or for electron microscopy, etc.) (23). These embedding media require specific reagents and equipment. These techniques will not be described in this chapter as they are not used in routine histology in the drug safety evaluation environment.

6. The following is a non-exhaustive list of hazards associated with some of the chemicals used during staining/cover slip mounting (20):

(a) *Harris hematoxylin*: irritant to eyes, skin, and mucous membranes. Toxic by inhalation and ingestion. Handle with care.

(b) *Eosin Y*: bromofluorescein dye and other dyes of this group are highly toxic. They are skin and eye irritant and reported as being carcinogens.

(c) *Mounting medium*: this is usually xylene or a xylene-based solvent. *See* xylene.

References

1. Paget, E.G., and Thompson, R. (1979) Standard operating procedures, in *Pathology*, MTP Press, Lancaster, pp 134–139.

2. European Course on the Pathology & Embryology of Genetically Engineered Animals (2005). At URL http://www.eurogems-2005.com/links.php.

3. Histology Procedure Manuals (1994). At URL http://library.med.utah.edu/WebPath/HISTHTML/MANUALS/MANUALS.html.

4. Leong, A.S.-Y. (1994) Fixation and fixatives, in *Laboratory histopathology, a complete reference* (Woods, A.E., and Ellis, R.C., eds), Churchill Livingstone, New York, Vol. 1, pp 4.1-1/4.2-26.

5. Revised Guides for Organ Sampling and Trimming in Rats and Mice (2003). At URL http://reni.item.fraunhofer.de/reni/trimming/index.php.

6. Ruehl-Fehlert, C., Kittel, B., Morawietz, G., Deslex, P., Keenan, C., Mahrt, C.R., Nolte, T., Robinson, M., Stuart, B.P., and Deschl, U. (2003) Revised guides for organ sampling and trimming in rats and mice – Part 1. *Exp. Toxic. Pathol.* **55**, 91–106.

7. Kittel, B., Ruehl-Fehlert, C., Morawietz, G., Klapwijk, J., Elwell, M.R., Lenz, B., O'Sullivan, M.G., Roth, D.R., and Wadsworth, P.F. (2004) Revised guides for organ sampling and trimming in rats and mice – Part 2. *Exp. Toxic. Pathol.* **55**, 413–431.

8. Morawietz, G., Ruehl-Fehlert, C., Kittel, B., Bube, A., Keane, K., Halm, S., Heuser, A., and Hellman, J. (2004) Revised guides for organ sampling and trimming in rats and mice – Part 3. *Exp. Toxic. Pathol.* **55**, 433–449.

9. Soul, N.W. (1987) Gut rolls: a better technique for GI tumor assessment. *Toxicol. Pathol.* **15**, 374.

10. Moolenbeek, C., and Ruitenberg, E.J. (1981) The "Swiss roll": a simple technique for histological studies of the rodent intestine. *Lab. Anim.* **15**, 57–59.

11. Piper, R.C. (1981) Morphological evaluation of the heart in toxicologic studies, in *Cardiac toxicology* (Balazc, T., ed), Vol. 3, CRC Press, Boca Raton, pp 111–136.

12. Latendresse, J.R., Warbrittion, A.R., Jonassen, H., and Creasy, D.M. (2002) Fixation of testes and eyes using a modified Davidson's fluid: Comparison with Bouin's fluid and conventional Davidson's fluid. *Toxicol. Pathol.* **30**, 524–533.

13. Lanning, L.L., Creasy, D.M., Chapin, R.E., Mann, P.C., Barlow, N.J., Regan, K.S., and Goodman, D.G. (2002) Recommended approaches for the evaluation of testicular and epididymal toxicity. *Toxicol. Pathol.* **30**, 507–520.

14. Creasy, D.M., and Foster, P.M.D. (2002) Male reproductive system, in *Handbook of toxicologic pathology* (Haschek, W.M., Rousseaux, C.G., and Wallig, M.A., eds), Vol. 2. Academic Press, San Diego New York Boston, pp 785–846.

15. Heindel, J.J., and Chapin, R.E. (1993) Female reproductive toxicology, in *Methods in reproductive toxicology* (Heindel, J.J., and Chapin, R.E., eds), Vol. 3B, Academic Press, Orlando.

16. McGavin, M.D. (1991) Procedures for morphological studies of skeletal muscle, rat, mouse, and hamster, in *Cardiovascular and musculoskeletal systems,* Monographs on pathology of laboratory animals (Jones, T.C., Mohr U., and Hunt, R.D., eds), Springer, New York, pp 101–108.

17. Windsor, L. (1994) Tissue processing, in *Laboratory histopathology, a complete reference* (Woods, A.E., and Ellis, R.C., eds), Churchill Livingstone, New York, Vol. 1, pp 4.2-1/4.2-42.

18. Ellis, C.R. (1994) The microtome function and design, in *Laboratory histopathology, a complete reference* (Woods, A.E., and Ellis, R.C., eds), Churchill Livingstone, New York, Vol. 1, pp 4.4-1/4.4-23.

19. TOXNET – Databases on Toxicology, Hazardous Chemicals, Environmental Health, and Toxic Releases (2008). At URL http://toxnet.nlm.nih.gov/cgi-bin/sis/htmlgen?HSDB.

20. IARC Monographs on the Evaluation of Carcinogenic Risks to Humans (2009). At URL http://monographs.iarc.fr/ENG/Monographs/vol88/index.php.

21. Titford, M., and Horenstein, M. (2005) Histomorphologic assessment of formalin substitute fixatives for diagnostic surgical pathology. *Arch. Pathol. Lab. Med.* **129**, (4), 502–506.

22. http://www2.hazard.com/msds/index.php (safety data).

23. Gormley, B., and Ellis, R.C. (1994) Resin embedding for light microscopy, in *Laboratory histopathology, a complete reference* (Woods, A.E., and Ellis, R.C., eds), Churchill Livingstone, New York, Vol. 1, pp 4.3-1/4.3-13.

Chapter 5

Principles and Methods of Immunohistochemistry

José A. Ramos-Vara

Abstract

Immunohistochemical techniques detect antigens in tissue sections by means of immunological and chemical reactions. This technique is highly sensitive and specific and can detect a wide variety of antigens in multiple animal species. This chapter reviews common immunohistochemical methods used in the characterization of normal and pathologic tissue and the reagents used. Pretreatments such as blocking steps for endogenous activities and antigen retrieval are included. Standard procedures on formalin-fixed, paraffin-embedded tissues as well as method standardization for new antibodies and troubleshooting are emphasized.

Key words: Antigen retrieval, Detection methods, Fixation, Immunohistochemistry, Standardization, Troubleshooting

1. Introduction

Immunohistochemistry (IHC) is the detection of antigens in tissue sections by means of specific antibodies. The unique advantage of IHC over other protein detection methods is the ability to correlate the presence of an antigen with its location in a tissue or cell. This is very important for the study of cell function in normal and pathological tissues. Since its introduction six decades ago, IHC has been applied extensively to multiple areas of biology including cell function and characterization of lesions (1). As its name indicates, IHC bridges three major disciplines: immunology, histology, and chemistry. This chapter will focus on the materials and methods used in immunohistochemistry. In addition, a strategy for standardization of immunohistochemical tests and troubleshooting in immunohistochemistry will be discussed.

Jean-Charles Gautier (ed.), *Drug Safety Evaluation: Methods and Protocols*, Methods in Molecular Biology, vol. 691,
DOI 10.1007/978-1-60761-849-2_5, © Springer Science+Business Media, LLC 2011

2. Materials

2.1. Buffers, Diluents, and Antigen Retrieval Solutions

1. Rinse buffer: corresponds to tris buffer normal saline (TBS) (0.05 M Tris, 0.15 M NaCl, 0.05% Tween 20, pH 7.6). Use TBS concentrate (Dako, Carpinteria, CA) and mix 100 ml of concentrate buffer and 900 ml of distilled water (working buffer) (see Notes 1 and 2).

2. Antibody diluent, background reducing from Dako.

3. Target retrieval solution citrate, pH 6, from Dako. Add 900 ml of distilled water to 100 ml of target retrieval solution to prepare a working dilution.

4. Target retrieval solution EDTA, pH 9.0 from Dako. To prepare a working dilution, add 900 ml of distilled water to 100 ml target retrieval solution.

5. Target retrieval solution, high pH Tris, pH 10.0 from Dako. To prepare a working dilution, add 900 ml of distilled water to 100 ml target retrieval solution (see Note 3).

6. Proteinase K (Dako).

2.2. Substrates, Chromogens, and Counterstain Solutions

1. Hydrogen peroxide-DAB Solution (Dako, Carpinteria, CA). This substrate is intended for peroxidase-based immunohistochemical methods (see Notes 4 and 5).

2. Permanent red substrate-chromogen from Dako.

3. Mayer's hematoxylin from Dako (see Note 6).

2.3. Endogenous Activities Blocking Solutions

1. Peroxidase and alkaline phosphatase blocking reagent (Dako) (see Notes 7 and 8).

2. Protein block, serum free, from Dako (see Note 9).

3. Biotin blocking system from Dako (see Note 10).

3. Methods

3.1. Tissue Fixation and Processing

Tissue fixation will depend in some ways on the type of antigen to be detected (e.g., some antigens will be destroyed during fixation in formaldehyde and tissues have to be frozen or fixed in a different fixative). Regardless of the antigen examined, collect and process samples before tissues undergo autolysis. Formaldehyde is the gold standard fixative for routine histology and immunohistochemistry. Formalin fixation is a progressive time- and temperature-dependent process. Overfixation has been considered deleterious for antigen detection. However, current antigen retrieval methods (see Subheading 3.2) are able to retrieve antigenic loss due to fixation, and overfixation is not a critical issue for many antigens. There is no universal optimal standard fixation time. Minimal fixation of 12–24 h is recommended (see Note 11).

1. Samples need to be <4 mm thick.

2. Immerse immediately the sample to be fixed in 10% neutral buffered formalin for 1–2 days.

3. Trim samples.

4. Embed samples in paraffin.

5. Cut 3–5 μm-thick sections with a microtome.

6. Place sections on silanized slides (see Note 12).

7. Dry sections in a 55–60°C oven for 30–60 min (see Note 13).

8. Stain the sections after deparaffinizing.

3.2. Antigen Retrieval Methods

Fixation with cross-linking agents modifies the tertiary and quaternary structure of many antigens making them undetectable by antibodies. Antigen retrieval (AR) methods are intended to retrieve the loss of antigenicity, theoretically returning proteins to their pre-fixation conformation. Approximately 85% of antigens fixed in formalin require some type of AR to optimize the immunoreactions (2). The need for AR depends not only on the antigen examined but also on the antibody used.

3.2.1. Detergents in Antigen Retrieval

Detergents solubilize membrane proteins by mimicking the lipid-bilayer environment, forming mixed micelles consisting of lipids and detergents and detergent micelles containing proteins (usually one protein molecule per micelle). The more common detergents used in IHC are of non-ionic type (e.g., Triton R-X 100, Tween 20, saponin, BRIJR, and Nonidet P40). These are usually added to rinsing buffers (e.g., 0.05% for Tween 20).

3.2.2. Enzymatic Antigen Retrieval

Protease-induced epitope retrieval (PIER) was the most commonly used antigen retrieval method before the advent of heat-based antigen retrieval methods. Many enzymes have been used for this purpose with the most common being trypsin, proteinase K, pronase, and pepsin. In this chapter, we advocate the use of proteinase K because it is active at room temperature. The mechanism of PIER is most likely digestion of protein cross-linkages introduced during formalin fixation, but this cleavage is nonspecific and some antigens may be negatively affected by this treatment. The effect of PIER depends on the concentration and type of enzyme, incubation parameters (time, temperature, and pH), as well as on the duration of fixation. The enzyme digestion time is directly proportional to the fixation time.

3.2.3. Heat-Induced Epitope Retrieval

Heat-Induced Epitope Retrieval (HIER) is based on a concept developed by Fraenklen-Conrat and collaborators who documented that the chemical reactions between proteins and formalin may be reversed, at least in part, by high temperature or strong alkaline hydrolysis (3). The mechanism involved in HIER is unknown, but its final effect is to revert conformational changes produced during fixation. The degree of fixation can dramatically modify the response of antigens to antigen retrieval. Unfixed proteins are denatured at temperatures of 70–90°C, whereas such proteins do not exhibit denaturation at the same temperatures when they have been fixed in formaldehyde. Caution must be taken when testing new antibodies using different AR protocols. The possibility of unexpected immunostaining should always be considered when using HIER, particularly with buffers at low pH. Regardless of the HIER method used, do not let the slides dry out at any time after being dewaxed and rehydrated.

3.2.3.1. HIER in a Microwave Oven

1. Using a microwave with revolving plate, timer and choice of watt settings, heat 500 ml of target retrieval solution (either citrate pH 6.0 or EDTA pH 9.0 or Tris pH 10.0) in a plastic jar that will hold the slides and a plastic beaker with 200 ml of water for 2 min at 750 W. At the end of this time, remove the beaker of water.

2. Immerse the dewaxed slides completely in the warm buffer. Cover the container loosely with its lid.

3. Microwave at 750 W for 5 min (the solution needs to boil).

4. Check the level of the solution and fill to the original volume with the warm water.

5. Repeat steps 3 and 4 for the required length of time (usually 15–20 min).

6. Remove the container from the microwave oven and place it in cold tap water for 15 min.

7. Rinse the slides in distilled water and transfer to rinse buffer.

3.2.3.2. HIER in a Pressure Cooker

1. Plug in the unit and place the pan into the decloaker's body.

2. Fill the pan of the decloaker (Biocare Medical) with 500 ml of deionized water and turn the unit on.

3. Place slides into Tissue Tek™ containers filled with 250 ml of target retrieval solution (either citrate pH 6.0 or EDTA pH 9.0 or Tris pH 10.0). Alternatively, plastic Coplin jars may be used and filled with 50 ml of target retrieval solution.

4. Place containers with slides into center of pan.

5. Place the heat shield in the center of the pan.

6. Place the monitor steam strip on top of the staining dish, put the lid on and secure.

7. Put the weight on the vent nozzle.

8. Push the display set and check each of the displayed parameters.

9. Set the SP1 function (heating time) between 30 s and 5 min, depending on the antigen.

10. Push the display set button to SP1 and push start.

11. When the timer goes off, push the start/stop button.

12. When the temperature reaches 90°C, the timer will sound off again.

13. Push the start/stop button to end the program. The pressure should read 0.

14. Open the lid and let the slides cool for several minutes.

15. Remove slide container and slowly rinse the slides in running tap water.

16. Transfer slides to rinse buffer.

3.2.3.3. HIER in a Steamer

1. Fill bottom of steam container with water.

2. Place Tissue Tek™ containers filled with 250 ml of retrieval buffer into steamer basket. Alternatively, plastic Coplin jars may be used and filled with 50 ml of target retrieval solution (either citrate pH 6.0 or EDTA pH 9.0 or Tris pH 10.0).

3. Turn steamer on and preheat the AR buffer in the Tissue Tek™ containers/Coplin jars. Place thermometer through steam holes in the lid of the steamer suspended in the AR buffer. Bring the buffer up to 95°C.

4. When the temperature reads 95°C, quickly place the slides in the AR buffer (avoid touching it with bare hands) and increase the temperature of the buffer back to 95°C.

5. Steam for 20 min or the required time for antigen retrieval only after the temperature reaches 95°C.

6. Remove the beaker with the slides from the steamer and let it cool at room temperature for 20 min.

7. Wash in tap water for 10 min.

8. Put the slides in rinse buffer and continue with immunohistochemical staining.

3.3. Immunoenzyme Techniques

The final aim of any immunohistochemical method is to detect the maximum amount of antigen with the least possible background (maximum signal-to-noise ratio). As a rule, with some exceptions, the more complex the technique, the more sensitive it is. The choice of method will depend on the amount of antigen present, the level of sensitivity required, and the technical capabilities of the laboratory. There are numerous commercially available detection kits. The methods included in this chapter use some of these commercial kits in an automatic stainer, but manual staining following these procedures is also possible. The number of steps that can be done in the automatic stainer depends on the model.

3.3.1 Direct Methods

1. Dewax sections in three changes of xylene or substitute, 5 min each.

2. Hydrate sections using 100% ethanol (two changes, 5 min each) and 95% ethanol (three changes, 2 min each). Rinse slides in water to adequately remove alcohol.

3. HIER or antigen retrieval with enzymes at 37°C, if needed (see Note 3).

4. Place the slides in rinse buffer for 5 min and transfer to the autostainer.

5. Block endogenous peroxidase with peroxidase and alkaline phosphatase-blocking reagent and block endogenous biotin with biotin-blocking system.

6. Rinse in buffer.

7. Antigen retrieval with proteinase K at RT (if needed), 5 min.

8. Incubate sections with serum free nonspecific binding blocking solution for 10–20 min.

9. WITHOUT rinsing, blow (blot if done manually) the fluid off the slide.

10. Incubate with primary labeled antibody for 30 min (see Note 14).

11. Rinse with rinsing buffer three times.

12. Incubate sections in the DAB solution for 5–10 min.

13. Rinse sections in distilled water.

14. Counterstain with Mayer's hematoxylin.

15. Rinse sections in distilled water. Blue sections using diluted ammonium hydroxide solution.

16. Dehydrate using 95% ethanol (two changes, 3–5 min), 100% ethanol (two changes, 3–5 min), and xylene or substitute (three changes, 3–5 min).

17. Mount in synthetic mounting medium.

3.3.2. Indirect Methods

3.3.2.1. Two-Step Method

1. Follow steps 1–11 as in Subheading 3.3.1.

2. Incubate with labeled secondary antibody for 30 min.

3. Follow steps 11–17 as in Subheading 3.3.1.

3.3.2.2. Polymer-Based Immunoenzyme Method

This method is more sensitive than the indirect method. It is based on the capability of binding many molecules of label (e.g., peroxidase) to an inert backbone of polymer (e.g., dextran) to which molecules of immunoglobulin (e.g., goat anti-rabbit immunoglobulins) recognizing the primary antibody (in this case, rabbit immunoglobulins) are also bound. Another advantage of this method is the lack of avidin or biotin molecules involved in the reaction and therefore the lack of endogenous avidin–biotin activity (EABA) background. A second generation of polymer-based immunoenzyme methods uses a second (link) unlabeled antibody between the primary and the polymer incubations. This method is more sensitive than the one-step polymer-based method.

1. Follow steps 1–11 as in Subheading 3.3.1.
2. Incubate with polymer–immunoglobulin–enzyme complex for 30 min.
3. Follow steps 11–17 as in Subheading 3.3.1.

3.3.3. Multiple-Step Methods

Multiple-step methods are more laborious than indirect methods but usually are more sensitive. Most commonly used multiple-step methods are based on the high affinity of avidin (glycoprotein found in egg white) or streptavidin (glycoprotein from *Streptomyces avidinii*) for biotin (glycoprotein present in egg yolk). Streptavidin produces less background due to its lack of oligosaccharide residues and its neutral isoelectric point. Avidin–biotin methods are highly sensitive and are currently the most widely used IHC methods.

3.3.3.1. Streptavidin–Biotin Complex (ABC) Method

1. Follow steps 1–11 as in Subheading 3.3.1.
2. Incubate with biotinylated secondary antibody for 30 min.
3. Rinse with rinsing buffer three times.
4. Incubate with tertiary reagent (preformed avidin/streptavidin-peroxidase complex) for 30 min.
5. Follow steps 11–17 as in Subheading 3.3.1.

3.3.3.2. Tyramide-Based Methods

Tyramide-based methods amplify the immune reaction 100–1,000-fold when compared with a conventional ABC method. Also the dilution of the primary antibody can be increased several hundred-fold. These methods are based on the deposition of molecules of labeled (biotin, fluorescein) tyramide followed by a secondary reaction with peroxidase conjugated to streptavidin- or peroxidase-conjugated anti-fluorescein.

1. Follow steps 1–11 as in Subheading 3.3.1.
2. Incubate with $F(ab')_2$ biotinylated secondary antibody (avidin–biotin method) or peroxidase–IgG secondary antibody (fluorescein method), 15 min.

3. Rinse with rinsing buffer three times.

4. Incubate with primary peroxidase–streptavidin–biotin complex (avidin–biotin method) or fluorescyl-tyramide amplification reagent (fluorescein method), 15 min.

5. Rinse with rinsing buffer three times.

6. Incubate with biotinyl–tyramide amplification reagent (avidin–biotin method), 15 min or anti-fluorescein-peroxidase (fluorescein method), 15 min.

7. Rinse with rinsing buffer three times.

8. Incubate with peroxidase–streptavidin complex (avidin–biotin method), 15 min.

9. Follow steps 11–17 as in Subheading 3.3.1. For fluorescein method, follow steps 12–17 as in Subheading 3.3.1.

3.3.4. Immunohistochemical Detection of Multiple Antigens

Currently, there are detection kits that allow the detection of at least two antigens using two different enzymes as labels (e.g., peroxidase and alkaline phosphatase). These detection kits are highly effective but also very expensive. The key issue in multiple detection of antigens is their location (different or same tissues, cells, or cellular compartments). A careful selection of the chromogen for each antigen is also necessary to achieve the best distinction between antigens. Examples of enzyme substrate combinations in double immunostaining are included in Vector Laboratories catalog (http://www.vectorlabs.com). The chance of good visualization of both antigens is reduced if they are anatomically close to each other (e.g., both antigens are within the nucleus of the same cell type). Double immunodetection is also complicated by the variety of AR methods used for different antigens. In other words, an AR necessary for one antigen might have deleterious effects for the second antigen to be detected. For a comprehensive review of multiple immunostaining, read van der Loos' monograph (4) on multiple immunoenzymatic staining. The method included can be used for primary antibodies from same or different species.

3.3.4.1. Sequential Double Immunoenzymatic Staining Using Primary Antibodies from Same or Different Species (Modified from Van der Loos) (4) (see Note 15)

1. Follow steps 1–11 as in Subheading 3.3.1.

2. Incubate with ENVISION™/peroxidase reagent, 30 min.

3. Rinse with rinsing buffer three times.

4. Develop peroxidase activity with DAB-chromogen reagent, 5 min.

5. Elution step with DAKO double staining block or alternatively, 5 min boiling in citrate pH 6.0.

6. Rinse with rinsing buffer three times.

7. Incubate sections with nonspecific binding blocking solution for 10 min.

8. WITHOUT rinsing, blow (blot if done manually) the fluid of the slide.

9. Incubate with second primary unlabeled antibody, 30–90 min.

10. Rinse with rinsing buffer three times.

11. Incubate with ENVISION™/alkaline phosphatase reagent, 30 min.

12. Rinse with rinsing buffer three times.

13. Develop alkaline phosphatase activity with Fast Red, 5–30 min.

14. Rinse with distilled water.

15. Light counterstain with Mayer's hematoxylin.

16. Mount in aqueous mounting medium.

3.4. Standardization of a New Immunohistochemical Test

The standardization of a new IHC test is a challenging process in which many factors affect the outcome. Most commercial antibodies have been tested in human tissues and rarely in other species. Information from the manufacturer of the antibody is essential to determine the suitability of the antibody for a particular species as well as the IHC detection of a particular antigen in frozen sections and/or by western blot. However, many times this information is unavailable, and the researcher needs to develop a standard protocol to test new antibodies. The following protocol assumes that tissues have been fixed in formalin and embedded in paraffin.

1. Select the tissue that is most likely to be used as a positive control. Ideally, it should have areas known to lack the antigen of interest.

2. Processing (e.g., fixation, embedding) of the control tissue should be done in the same manner as for test tissues. Control tissue should be from the same species as test tissues (an additional control tissue from a species known to react with that antibody, if available, is also recommended).

3. Prepare dilutions of the primary antibody (usually four twofold dilutions will suffice).

4. Prepare three sets of slides: one without AR; another with enzymatic AR (e.g., proteinase K); the third set of slides with heat-induced epitope retrieval (HIER) with citrate buffer at pH 6.0.

5. Run the IHC test following a standard procedure. Incubation of the primary antibody (time, temperature) will depend on the antigen in question. Default incubation time, 30–60 min.

6. After the IHC test is done, examine the slides to determine staining quality (see Note 16).

3.5. Troubleshooting

*3.5.1. Excessive
Background Staining*

1. *Pre-staining problems*

    (a) Inadequate fixation, necrosis, and autolysis.

    (b) Tissue sections allowed to dry out. Reduce incubation time; incubate in a humidified chamber.

    (c) Sections not completely deparaffinized. Use fresh dewaxing solutions.

    (d) Slide adhesive inappropriate or too thick. Use adhesives specific for IHC or positive charged slides.

    (e) Tissue section too thick. Prepare thinner sections.

    (f) Inappropriate antigen retrieval used. Re-evaluate antigen retrieval conditions.

    (g) Incubation temperature too high. Reduce temperature.

2. *Blocking problems*

    (a) Endogenous enzyme activity not suppressed. Increase concentration of blocking agent.

    (b) Inadequate protein blocking. Use a different blocking agent.

    (c) Inadequate blocking of endogenous avidin–binding activity. Use an avidin–biotin blocking step or use a nonavidin-biotin detection method.

    (d) Inadequate blocking of endogenous biotin. Use an avidin–biotin blocking step or a nonavidin–biotin detection method.

    (e) Blocking serum from improper species. Use blocking serum from same species as the link (secondary) antibody.

3. *Primary antibody problems*

    (a) Primary antibody too concentrated. Re-titrate the primary antibody.

    (b) Primary antibody incubation time too long. Reduce incubation time.

    (c) Primary antibody is from a similar or identical species as the test tissue (mouse on mouse, rat on mouse, etc.). Use specific protocols (i.e. MOM or ARK commercial kits) or additional blocking steps.

    (d) Inadequate buffer washes (inappropriate buffer ion concentration). Modify ionic strength of the buffer solution.

4. *Secondary antibody problems*

    (a) Secondary antibody and label concentration too high.

    (b) Secondary antibody and label incubation time too long.

    (c) Buffer washes insufficient.

    (d) Secondary antibody recognizes endogenous (tissue) immunoglobulins.

5. *Chromogen and counterstains problems*

   (a) Chromogen concentration too high. Reduce concentration of chromogen.

   (b) Chromogen allowed to react too long. Reduce incubation time with chromogen.

   (c) Buffer washes insufficient. Prolong buffer washes.

   (d) Counterstain obscures the IHC reaction. Use a different counterstain that does not interfere with immunohistochemical staining.

3.5.2. Inadequate or No Staining of the Test Slide and Adequate Staining of the Positive Control Slide

1. The antigen in question is not present in the test tissue.

2. The antigen is present in the test tissue, but in a concentration below the method's detection limits. Consider using an amplification procedure, or increasing the primary antibody concentration, incubation time or temperature, or a combination thereof.

3. The test tissue is over- or under-fixed. Modify antigen retrieval protocol.

4. The test tissue is from a different species than the control tissue and has different reactivity with the primary antibody. Validate the IHC test with same species control and test tissues.

3.5.3. Weak or No Staining of Positive Control and Weak or No Staining of Test Slides

1. All slides from some of the primary antibodies used in the run are affected. Check for inadequacy of the primary antibody, method incompatibility, primary and link antibody incompatibility, or inadequate antigen retrieval.

2. The whole run is affected. Check assay log and adequacy of reagent volumes and sequence of reagent delivery to the slide. Determine whether reagents were delivered to all slides (e.g. buffer, chromogen).

3. If it is hit-and-miss throughout the run, consider technical problems or problems with the tissues. Check for inadequate sequence of reagents, unbalanced autostainer, and inadequate drop zone.

3.5.4. No Staining of Positive Control Slide and Adequate Staining of the Test Slide

1. Technical error in the staining or handling of the positive control slide. The log or check list should be reviewed; if everything is in order, the assay should be repeated. For control blocks for infectious diseases, the antigen to be tested may not be present through the entire block.

2. Tissue section aging (5–7). This is probably the result of tissue photo-oxidation and dehydration during prolonged storage of tissue control sections (8). Test the tissue control section with a known positive case by IHC or test a fresh cut tissue control section.

4. Notes

1. The average shelf life of TBS working solution at room temperature is 4 days and at 4°C is 7 days.

2. Do not add sodium azide as preservative to enzyme-labeled reagents because it inhibits enzyme activity.

3. When using heat-induced epitope retrieval (antigen retrieval), use the target retrieval solution more appropriate to detect that particular antigen of the three included in Materials. Several antigen retrieval methods may need to be tested to achieve optimal immunohistochemical reaction.

4. The incubation time depends on the amount of antigen. Longer incubation times tend to increase background.

5. Disposal of DAB. DAB is considered toxic or potentially carcinogenic, so proper disposal is necessary. Each institution has its own regulations. Contact your waste hazard office. In general, to inactivate DAB, add several drops of household bleach or sodium hypochlorite. The solution will turn black (due to oxidation of DAB) and can be washed down the sink with plenty of water. An FDA-approved alternative method consists of preparing a solution containing 15 ml of concentrated sulfuric acid added slowly to 85 ml of water. Add 4 g of potassium permanganate. Add this solution to the used DAB and leave overnight. Neutralize with sodium hydroxide, then discard.

6. It is critical to use a counterstain that is compatible with the color produced by the histochemical reaction. In this chapter we use hematoxylin as a counterstain for a histochemical reaction producing a brown or red color. However, other combinations of chromogen-counterstain are available. For a list of compatibility between counterstains and chromogens, look at the Vector Laboratories catalog or at http://www.vectorlabs.com.

7. Pretreatment of the sections for antigen retrieval can be done before or after the endogenous peroxidase blocking step.

8. For some antigens, particularly those in the cytoplasmic membrane, this treatment is deleterious and should be done after the incubation with the primary antibody.

9. Alternatively, a solution of bovine serum albumin (BSA) or normal serum can be used.

10. This solution should be added immediately before the incubation with the biotinylated antibody. This solution is only needed with endogenous biotin background is likely to occur (9).

11. Other fixatives. Many of the formalin substitutes are coagulating fixatives that precipitate proteins by breaking hydrogen

bonds in the absence of protein crosslinking. The typical noncrosslinking fixative is ethanol. Other fixatives used in IHC are glyoxal (dialdehyde), a mixture of glyoxal and alcohol, 4% paraformaldehyde (PFA), and zinc formalin. A trial-and-error approach starting with the recommendations on the manufacturer's antibody specification sheet should be used.

12. Other slide adhesives can be used (e.g., poly-L-lysine).

13. Drying paraffin sections at higher temperatures may destroy antigenicity (10).

14. All antibody incubations are at room temperature. However, incubation duration and incubation temperature (e.g., 37°C, 4°C) can be modified as necessary.

15. This method is laborious and needs an elution or blocking step between the primary and second immune reactions. There are commercially available kits based on polymer-based technology (e.g., ENVISION™). The concentrations of the primary antibodies should be at least double concentrated to those used in separate IHC methods. For sequential double immunostaining, it is recommended that peroxidase activity using DAB as chromogen is developed first (11). It is critical to choose the right color combination, which will depend greatly on the amount of antigen and its location in the tissue section. The counterstain should not mask the color of the immune reaction.

16. If specific staining is achieved, the concentration of the primary antibody, incubation times, and incubation temperature, as well as antigen retrieval procedures, may need to be optimized to obtain the best signal-to-noise ratio. If there is no staining, the concentration of the primary antibody, incubation and temperature time (including overnight or longer incubation at 4°C), and antigen retrieval procedures (use of other enzymes or buffers at different pH) may need to be modified. Keep in mind that the detection of the antigen may not be possible due to fixation, animal species lack of cross-reactivity of primary antibody, and lack or low amount of the epitope recognized by the antibody.

References

1. Ramos-Vara, J.A., Kiupel, M., Baszler, T., Bliven, L., Brodersen, B., Chelack, B., Czub, S., Del Piero, F., Dial, S., Ehrhart, E.J., Graham, T., Manning, L., Paulsen, D., Valli, V.E., and West, K. (2008) Suggested guidelines for immunohistochemical techniques in veterinary diagnostic laboratories. *J. Vet. Diagn. Invest.* **20**, 393–413.

2. Ramos-Vara, J.A., and Beissenherz, M.E. (2000) Optimization of immunohistochemical methods using two different antigen retrieval methods on formalin-fixed, paraffin-embedded tissues: experience with 63 markers. *J. Vet. Diagn. Invest.* **12**, 307–311.

3. Ramos-Vara, J.A. (2005) Technical aspects of immunohistochemistry. *Vet. Pathol.* **42**, 405–426.

4. Van der Loos, C.M. (1999) *Immunoenzyme Multiple Staining Methods*, Bios Scientific Publishers, Oxford, UK.

5. Atkins, D., Reiffen, K.-A., Tegtmeier, C.L., Winther, H., Bonato, M.S., and Störkel, S. (2004) Immunohistochemical detection of EGFR in paraffin-embedded tumor tissues: variation in staining intensity due to choice of fixative and storage time of tissue sections. *J. Histochem. Cytochem.* **52**, 893–901.

6. Fergenbaum, J.H., Gracia-Closas, M., Hewitt, S.M., Lissowska, J., Sakoda, L.C., and Sherman, M.E. (2004) Loss of antigenicity in stored sections of breast cancer tissue microarrays. *Cancer Epidemiol. Biomarkers Prev.* **13**, 667–672.

7. Mirlacher, M., Kasper, M., Storz, M., Knecht, Y., Durmuller, U., Simon, R., Mihatsch, M.J., and Sauter, G. (2004) Influence of slide aging on results of translational research studies using immunohistochemistry. *Mod. Pathol.* **17**, 1414–1420.

8. Blind, C., Koepenik, A., Pacyna-Gengelbach, M., Fernahl, G., Deutschmann, N., Dietel, M., Krenn, V., and Petersen, I. (2008) Antigenicity testing by immunohistochemistry after tissue oxidation. *J. Clin. Pathol.* **61**, 79–83.

9. Wood, G.S., and Warnke, R. (1981) Suppression of endogenous avidin-binding activity in tissues and its relevance to biotin-avidin detection systems. *J. Histochem. Cytochem.* **29**, 1196–1204.

10. Henwood, A.F. (2005) Effect of slide drying at 80°C on immunohistochemistry. *J. Histotechnol.* **28**, 45–46.

11. Malik, N.J., and Daymon, M.E. (1982) Improved double immunoenzyme labeling using alkaline phosphatase and horseradish peroxidase. *J. Clin. Pathol.* **35**, 1092–1094.

Chapter 6

Tissue Microarrays and Digital Image Analysis

Denise Ryan, Laoighse Mulrane, Elton Rexhepaj,
and William M. Gallagher

Abstract

Tissue microarrays (TMAs) have recently emerged as very valuable tools for high-throughput pathological assessment, especially in the cancer research arena. This important technology, however, has yet to fully penetrate into the area of toxicology. Here, we describe the creation of TMAs representative of samples produced from conventional toxicology studies within a large-scale, multi-institutional pan-European project, PredTox. PredTox, short for Predictive Toxicology, formed part of an EU FP6 Integrated Project, Innovative Medicines for Europe (InnoMed), and aimed to study pre-clinically 16 compounds of known liver and/or kidney toxicity. In more detail, TMAs were constructed from materials corresponding to the full face sections of liver and kidney from rats treated with different drug candidates by members of the consortium. We also describe the process of digital slide scanning of kidney and liver sections, in the context of creating an online resource of histopathological data.

Key words: Tissue microarrays, Immunohistochemistry, Digital image analysis, Predictive toxicology

1. Introduction

Tissue microarray (TMA) technology is a powerful technology originally described by Wan and colleagues in 1987 (1). The technique has gained extensive recognition, however, following a publication in *Nature Medicine* by Kononen and colleagues in the laboratory of Olli Kallioneimi in 1998 (2, 3). TMAs are created from multiple cores of tissue taken from histologic paraffin blocks arrayed onto one single master block. This allows one TMA to be subjected to a variety of tests, such as immunohistochemical/immunofluorescent staining or fluorescent *in situ* hybridisation (FISH) (2, 4, 5) (Fig. 1).

On average, between 50 and 100 slides may be created from a single TMA allowing for a large number of tests to be carried

Jean-Charles Gautier (ed.), *Drug Safety Evaluation: Methods and Protocols*, Methods in Molecular Biology, vol. 691,
DOI 10.1007/978-1-60761-849-2_6, © Springer Science+Business Media, LLC 2011

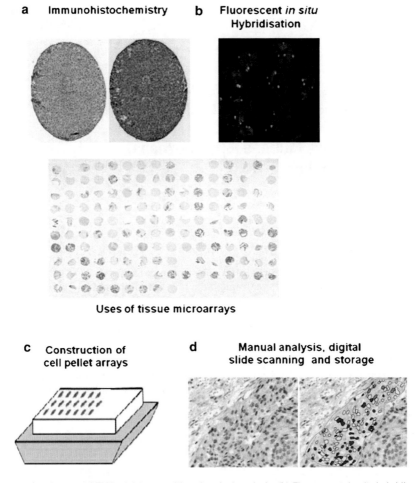

a   Immunohistochemistry   **b   Fluorescent *in situ* Hybridisation**

Uses of tissue microarrays

c   Construction of cell pellet arrays   **d   Manual analysis, digital slide scanning and storage**

Fig. 1. Summary of main uses of TMAs. (**a**) Immunohistochemical analysis. (**b**) Fluorescent *in situ* hybridisation. (**c**) Cell lines which are formalin-fixed, paraffin embedded and incorporated into a cell pellet array can be used for immunohistochemistry. (**d**) Manual analysis, digital slide scanning and storage.

out (6, 7). Moreover, due to the advent of digital slide technology, tissue specimens can now be scanned to create digital slide images, and these can then be analysed rapidly by computer software at full resolution. Quantitative image analysis has become increasingly important in aiding pathologists and automating tasks and, recently, there has been an increase in the development of automated imaging and assessment technologies (8, 9).

While TMAs have gained considerable prominence in the cancer research field, this is still a relatively new technology within the toxicological arena, although the use of TMAs constructed from animal tissue has been demonstrated for the quantitation of target distribution studies in drug discovery pathology (5). We have recently created a comprehensive series of TMAs from a large-scale pre-clinical toxicology study in the rat (10) and now describe in detail the workflow involved.

PredTox, short for Predictive Toxicology, formed part of the EU FP6 Integrated Project, Innovative Medicines for Europe (InnoMed), and aimed to study pre-clinically sixteen compounds of known liver and/or kidney toxicity. These include proprietary drug candidates which had failed during the development and reference compounds (gentamicin and troglitazone) known to have certain toxic effects. PredTox aimed to better understand mechanisms of toxicity and to identify biomarkers of toxicity by combining conventional toxicological data (histopathology, clinical pathology) and the newer technologies of proteomics, transcriptomics, and metabolomics. Our contribution to this project involved the process of digital slide scanning of kidney and liver slices from rats treated with different drug candidates by members of the consortium, as well as the construction of TMAs from materials corresponding to the full face sections of liver and kidney scanned (10). In this project, we utilised TMAs for immunohistochemical and *in situ* hybridisation studies.

2. Materials

2.1. Construction of TMAs

1. Leica EG1150H Paraffin Embedding Station (Leica Microsystems, Wetzlar, Germany).
2. Paraffin wax (Sigma-Aldrich, St Louis, MO).
3. Beecher MTA-1 Arrayer (Beecher Instruments; Wisconsin, USA).
4. TMA Punches 0.6/1/1.5 mm (Beecher Instruments Klisconsin, USA).
5. Leica RM2135 Microtome (Leica Microsystems).
6. SuperFrost® Plus Slides (Microm International, Walldorf, Germany).

2.2. Construction of Cell Pellet Arrays

1. Phosphate buffered saline (PBS) with 1 mM EDTA (Gibco).
2. Trypsin-EDTA (1×) Liquid 0.05% stored at −20°C (Gibco).
3. 4% v/v formalin is used to resuspend the pellet (Sigma-Aldrich).
4. 5% w/v agarose (Sigma-Aldrich).

2.3. Frozen Tumour TMA

1. Optimum cutting temperature (OCT) compound embedding medium (Miles, Inc. Diagnostic Division, Elkhart, IN).
2. Tissue-Tek standard cryomold (Miles, Inc.).
3. Plastic biopsy cassette (Simport Histosette II Biopsy Cassette from Fisher Scientific, with lid removed).

2.4. Immunohisto-chemistry

1. Lab Vision Autostainer XL (Thermo Fisher Scientific).

2. Leica Autostainer 360 (Leica Microsystems).

3. Lab Vision PT Module (Thermo Fisher Scientific).

4. Citrate buffer, pH 6 100× (Thermo Fisher Scientific). Dilute to 1× (0.01 M at the working dilution).

5. Tris–EDTA (Tris Base) pH 9 100× (Thermo Fisher Scientific). Dilute to 1× (0.01 Molar at the working dilution).

6. Tris–HCl (hydrochloric acid), pH 10 100× (Thermo Fisher Scientific). Dilute to 1× (0.01 M at the working dilution).

7. PBS, pH 7.3 (8 tablets in 1 L of distilled H_2O; Oxoid Ltd, Hampshire, UK) with 1 mL Tween®20 (Sigma-Aldrich). (PBS; sodium chloride 0.16 mol, potassium chloride 0.003 mol, disodium hydrogen phosphate 0.008 mol, potassium dihydrogen phosphate 0.001 mol).

8. Xylol (Sigma-Aldrich).

9. Ethanol (Sigma-Aldrich).

10. H_2O_2 30 wt. % solution in water (Sigma-Aldrich). Dilute by tenfold to 3%.

11. UltraVision LP Detection System (containing UV Block, Horse Radish Peroxidase, Polymer & Primary Antibody Enhancer; Thermo Fisher Scientific).

12. UltraVision Plus Detection System (Thermo Fisher Scientific). Add one drop of DAB Plus Chromagen to 2 mL DAB Plus Substrate.

13. Mayer's Haematoxylin (ClinTech Ltd.).

2.5. Fluorescent In Situ Hybridisation

1. LB agar (Sigma-Aldrich).

2. Chloroamphenicol (working conc.; 25 μg/mL) (Sigma-Aldrich).

3. LB broth (Sigma-Aldrich).

4. 0.1 mM dTTP (Abbott Laboratories. Abbott Park, Illinois, U.S.A.).

5. 0.1 mM dNTP (Abbott Laboratories).

6. Extracted P1, BAC, or YAC DNA (0.2–1 μg/μL solution of extracted DNA in Tris–EDTA (Tris Base) (10 mM Tris, 1 mM EDTA, pH 8.5) buffer.

7. COT-1 DNA (Gibco).

8. Human placental DNA/Salmon sperm DNA (Invitrogen).

9. 3 M sodium acetate (Sigma-Aldrich).

10. Centromeric control (Cepheid UK, UK).

11. Hybridisation buffer (Abbott Laboratories).

12. Xylene (Sigma-Aldrich).

13. 100% IMS (Sigma-Aldrich).

14. 0.2 M HCl (Abbott Laboratories).

15. 20× SSC (3 M sodium chloride, 0.3 M sodium citrate, pH 5.3) (Abbott Laboratories).

16. Protease buffer (Abbott Laboratories).

17. 10% formalin (Sigma-Aldrich).

18. Denaturing solution (70% formamide/2× SSC, pH 7.0–8.0) (Abbott Laboratories).

19. Ethanol solutions: Prepared v/v dilutions of 70%, 85%, and 100% using 100% ethanol and purified water.

20. Post-hybridisation wash buffer (2× SSC/0.3% NP-40) (Abbott Laboratories).

21. DAPI (4',6-diamidino-2-phenylindole) (Abbott Laboratories).

3. Methods

3.1. Construction of TMAs

1. These instructions assume the use of a Beecher MTA-1 Arrayer.

2. Prepare paraffin blocks as standard using metal moulds and plastic inserts.

3. Allow to cool for 2 min and place on cold tray/ice.

4. Tissue blocks are prepared as per standard procedure.

5. Before beginning construction, it is essential to design a map for each TMA. Ensure if it is to be evenly spaced (i.e. same number of cores in all rows/columns), that a reference core of a tissue unrelated to the rest of the material to be arrayed be placed in a prominent position e.g. (1, 1). This is to provide orientation should the TMA section be placed upside-down on the slide, as often happens.

6. Using the Beecher MTA-1 Arrayer, attach needles of chosen size (0.6, 1, 1.5, 2 mm). 0.6 mm cores are generally sufficient for most uses, although 1 mm cores may be needed to see specific toxicological effects, should this be required. The red needle is screwed in to the left, the blue to the right. These needles are of slightly different sizes to ensure that each core is fitted securely into the paraffin block.

7. The empty block is heated slightly to aid adhesion of cores to recipient block.

8. The punches are moved to the starting position and the arrayer is set to zero.

9. The empty paraffin block is screwed into the indent, ensuring that its position is fixed.

10. A blank core is taken from the empty paraffin block using the red punch and discarded.

11. The donor core may then be extracted from the tissue block using the blue punch. Twist lever back and forth to remove core and slowly dispense into hole in recipient block by pushing gently on the needle, taking care that the top of the core is level with the block. If a core is pushed too deep, it will move down towards the slide during the cutting preparation. However, if a core protrudes over the top of the TMA, this tissue will be wasted. This is important to note when arraying valuable samples of limited quantity (see Note 1).

12. Samples are usually arrayed in triplicate or quadruplicate. However, depending on the size of the cores, it may not be possible to fit all these samples into one block. In this case, multiple TMAs are constructed, although it is more desirable to have all cores within the one TMA to reduce staining variability.

13. The handle is moved across by a chosen distance. It is generally sufficient to leave 1–1.5 mm spacing between cores. The closer the cores, the more likely it is to lose samples or mix them up on a slide.

14. At the end of the row, the needles are moved down a chosen distance as above. Samples may now be arrayed from right to left although it is possible to have any arrangement of cores with a manual arrayer.

15. Continue as above until all samples are arrayed (Fig. 2).

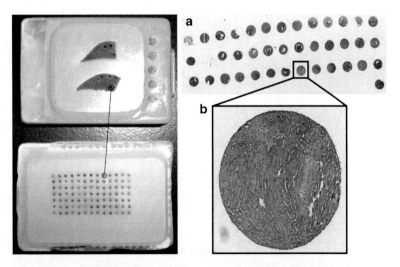

Fig. 2. TMA construction. The *left image* shows a representation of the construction of a TMA from individual blocks of rat liver. The newly constructed TMA consists of numerous samples from different blocks of rat liver. The *right image* depicts an immunohistochemically stained TMA made from FFPE rat kidney (**a**) at ×1 and (**b**) at ×5.

16. Once the TMA is fully constructed, sections may be cut using a microtome. Standard sections are usually 5–7 μm thick. Place sections on slides and dry at 60°C for 1 h. Heating the recipient block slightly before use can prevent cores from falling out and decrease the likelihood of cores being lost in the tissue section (see Note 1).

3.2. Construction of Cell Pellet Arrays

After the specificity of a particular antibody was determined via Western blot analysis, further work could be carried out such as using immunohistochemical methodologies on formalin-fixed paraffin-embedded tissue. It is often useful to construct some cell pellet arrays from the cell lines used in Western blot analysis before proceeding to TMA analysis. This allows one to determine cellular localisation and staining quality. Cell pellet arrays are useful as an early antibody optimisation step before moving to precious TMAs (7). The following protocol demonstrates the method of constructing a cell pellet from a cell line.

1. PBS with 1 mM EDTA is used to wash a T175 flask of adherent cells.

2. Trypsin is added and the flask is incubated for several minutes or until the cells have detached.

3. Once detached, cold culture media is added and the cells are centrifuged at $500 \times g$ for 10 min at 4°C.

4. The supernatant is removed and the pellet is resuspended in cold PBS.

5. The cells are centrifuged again at $500 \times g$ for 5 min at 4°C.

6. The supernatant is removed and the pellet is resuspended in 10 mL of 4% formalin for approximately 1 h at room temperature.

7. After fixation with formalin, the cells are centrifuged again, the supernatant is taken off and 750 μL of formalin is added.

8. A solution of 5% agarose in PBS is made and microwaved to dissolve fully; following this, it is then placed in a waterbath at 65°C.

9. The tube with the cells is placed into a waterbath and ~750 μL of agarose is added.

10. The suspension is mixed thoroughly and transferred to a 24-well plate. It is allowed to cool at 4°C for at least 30 min, but not more than 72 h.

11. The agarose block is removed and placed in a specimen bag in a cassette and carried through standard tissue processing.

12. Once tissue processing is complete, it can be embedded in paraffin and then used as a donor block for a cell pellet array.

3.3. Frozen Tumour TMA

Fejzo and Slamon (11) described the construction of a frozen tumour TMA in 2001. The technique involves the use of frozen tissue instead of FFPE tissue which eliminates the fixation and embedding processes where changes in the tissue sometimes occur and result in damage to or blocking of antigenic sites. One disadvantage of this approach is the greater expertise required to construct the TMA, and the storage of frozen tissue can be a problem.

1. Fresh tissue is taken and frozen at –70°C.

2. The tissue is embedded in OCT compound, and the frozen tissue is then arrayed into a recipient OCT block.

3. Tissue biopsies (diameter 0.6 and 1.0 mm; height 3–4 mm) can be punched from tumours in OCT and placed into an OCT array block using a tissue microarrayer (Beecher Instruments, Silver Spring, MD).

4. Tissue-Tek standard cryomold filled with OCT can be used to make the recipient OCT array block. The OCT filled mould is then mounted to the base of a plastic biopsy cassette (see Note 2).

5. Dry ice is important to keep the recipient block from melting. The same needle can be used for coring the recipient array block and collecting the core biopsy, rather than switching to a larger needle for the biopsies.

6. The dry ice is also used to keep the needle frozen before and after punching the tissue and also while dispensing the tissue core into the recipient block (see Note 2).

7. The recipient array was kept frozen by placing a piece of dry ice on its upper surface at all times except when punching and filling holes. Generally, a space of about 1 mm is kept between cores on the array.

8. The recipient block is sectioned, and the array is evaluated without fixation.

9. OCT arrays have been shown to work well for DNA, RNA, and protein analyses (11).

3.4. Immunohisto-chemistry

Immunohistochemistry (IHC) is a commonly used method of protein detection and localisation in frozen or FFPE tissue and has become a routine method of biomarker validation in both the cancer field and other areas of research. Although the discovery of IHC is credited to Coons and Jones who published their technique in 1941 (12), it did not become a standard pathological tool until the late 1970s. This technique has now been widely adopted in diagnostic laboratories owing primarily to the development of machines which automate the process, making it cheap and relatively quick to use. It is based on the premise that antigens in the tissue will be recognised by a specific antibody which can, in turn, be localised using a secondary antibody conjugated to an enzyme, such as a peroxidase or alkaline phosphatase. This enzyme catalyses a colourimetric substrate reaction (e.g. 3,3′-diaminobenzidine tetrahydrochloride (DAB) or 3-amino-9-ethylcarbazole (AEC)] allowing visualisation of the antibodies and thus proteins on the slide.

1. These instructions assume the use of the Lab Vision Autostainer XL and Leica Autostainer 360, and we discuss the use of the horseradish peroxidase (HRP)-DAB staining system. The slides are pre-treated in the Leica Autostainer XL using the following conditions:

   (a) Heat to 62°C for 10 min.

   (b) Treat with xylol for 10 min × 2.

   (c) Treat with 100% ethanol for 3 min × 2.

   (d) Treat with 70% alcohol for 3 min × 2. Wash with water.

2. Slides are then heated to 95°C for 15 min in the Lab Vision PT Module to enhance antigen retrieval. This can be done in a variety of buffers, including citrate, Tris–HCl, or Tris–EDTA and at a variety of pH levels. It is essential to optimise this treatment for each batch of slides as staining may be greatly affected.

3. Prepare the Lab Vision Autostainer 360 for staining and dispense correct amounts of diluted antibody, substrate, enzyme blocker, secondary reagent, and protein blocker into barcoded bottles.

4. Set up desired programme on dedicated desktop computer and run. An example of a typical programme using the HRP detection system runs as follows:

   (a) The number of slides is inputted into the programme and each slide is given a name.

   (b) Labels for slides and bottles are printed.

   (c) The machine can be set up to dispense between 100 and 600 µL. It is usually sufficient to dispense either 150–200 µL of each solution in the centre of the slide or 100 µL in the centre and each extreme of the slide, depending on the position and size of tissue on the slides.

   (d) Slides are rinsed with PBS-T (PBS, 0.01% Tween).

   (e) The enzyme block is added (for HRP, 3% H_2O_2) for 7 min.

   (f) Slides are rinsed with PBS-T.

   (g) The protein block (UV block) is added for 10 min.

   (h) Slides are dried briefly to remove excess liquid.

(i) A sufficient dilution of primary antibody is added for 30 min.

(j) Slides are rinsed with PBS-T and dried × 3.

(k) The secondary reagent (PAE – Primary Antibody Enhancer) is added for 20 min. This is a proprietary formulation containing both mouse and rabbit secondary antibodies.

(l) Slides are rinsed with PBS-T and dried × 3.

(m) The labelled polymer is added for 15 min.

(n) Slides are rinsed with PBS-T and dried × 3.

(o) The colourimetric substrate (DAB) is added for 10 min.

(p) Slides are rinsed with distilled water × 4.

5. Counterstain slides in the Leica Autostainer XL using Programme 6 and coverslip:

(a) Treat with haematoxylin for 45 s.

(b) Treat with spirit for 30 s × 2.

(c) Treat with 100% ethanol for 30 s × 2.

(d) Treat with xylol for 5 min × 2.

3.5. Fluorescent In Situ Hybridisation

TMA technology allows the analysis of numerous tissue specimens at a time, either at the DNA, RNA, or protein level. TMAs can be used for genomics-based diagnostics and drug target discovery. FISH is suitable for the analysis of genetic alterations on TMA slides. A single hybridisation allows visualisation of specific genetic changes in large numbers of tissue specimens (13). There is a huge need for image analysis algorithms for automatically scoring FISH to be developed further, as manual assessment is extremely tedious and labour-intensive.

1. Place a microcentrifuge tube on ice and allow the tube to cool.

2. Add the following components to a tube, briefly centrifuge and vortex the tube before adding the enzyme (last component): nuclease free water, 1 µg extracted DNA, 2.5 µL of fluorescently labelled DNA probes (spectrum red/green or orange), 0.1 mM dTTP, dNTP mix, 10× nick translation buffer, nick translation enzyme.

(a) Briefly centrifuge and vortex the tube.

(b) The tubes are incubated for 8–16 h at 15°C.

(c) The reaction is stopped by heating in a 70°C water bath for 10 min.

(d) Chill tubes on ice.

3. The probe size is determined by running an agarose gel.

4. The probe is then precipitated by dispensing ~100 ng from the nick translation reaction mixture into a microcentrifuge

tube and by adding 1 µg COT-1 DNA, 2 µg human placental DNA, and 4 µL purified water to the tube.

5. 1.2 µL (0.1 vol.) 3 M sodium acetate, then 30 µL (2.5 vol.) of 100% EtOH are added to precipitate the DNA.

6. The mixture is then vortexed briefly and placed on dry ice for 15 min.

7. Mixture is centrifuged at 12,000 × g for 30 min at 4°C to pellet the DNA.

8. The supernatant is removed and the pellet dried for about 10 min under a speed vacuum at ambient temperature for 5–10 min.

9. The pellet is resuspended in 2 µL centromeric control, 1 µL purified water and 7 µL Hybridisation Buffer (see Note 3).

10. The slides are dewaxed in xylene (2 × 5 min) at this stage and re-hydrated in 100% IMS (2 × 5 min) and air dried (no dH$_2$O needed) (see Note 5).

11. The slides are then immersed in 0.2 M HCL for 20 min, washed in distilled water for 2 min, and then washed in 2× SSC for 3 min × 2.

12. Following this, the slides are immersed in pre-treatment solution at 80°C for 30 min before being washed in 2× SSC for 3 min × 2 (see Note 6).

13. Protease treatment involves the removal of slides from 2× SSC, the removal of excess liquid and immersion in protease solution at 37°C for 48 min. If staggering after protease treatments, put first slide in 2× SSC and wait for other slide. Drying of slides before denaturation is not necessary (see Note 4).

14. Slides are then washed in 2× SSC for 3 min × 2 and immersed in 10% formalin for 10 min (see Note 7).

15. The slides are placed in a hybridiser and 100 µL of denaturing solution is applied for 5 min (see Note 8).

16. The probe is denatured by heating the probe mix for 5 min in a 73°C water bath.

17. Slides are dehydrated through 70%, 85%, and 100% alcohol for 1 min each and then air dried.

18. 10 µL of probe mix is added to each slide and covered with a coverslip, and the edges are sealed with rubber cement.

19. The slides are placed in the hybridiser at 37°C overnight.

20. On day two, the slides are placed in Post-hybridisation buffer (PHB) at room temperature to remove the rubber cement and float off the coverslip.

21. Following this, the slides are immersed in PHB in the 74°C water bath for 5 min before being removed and air dried in the dark in the incubator (37°C) for 1 h.

22. 10 µL DAPI counterstain is applied, covered with a glass coverslip and sealed.

23. Slides are stored in the dark before visualisation using a fluorescent microscope.

3.6. Manual Analysis

The stained TMA needs to be evaluated for the presence or absence and cellular localisation of the particular protein of interest. Manual analysis also involves determining the percentage and intensity of staining in the tissue of interest.

1. Intensity of staining on tissues can be scored by allocating a numerical value (e.g. 0, 1, 2, and 3) to the stain. As well as allocating a score on the basis of staining intensity, percentage of cells stained can also be recorded.

2. An intensity of 0 indicates negative staining, 1 indicates mild staining, 2 indicates moderate staining, and 3 indicates strong staining.

3. Staining results can also be reported as positive or negative.

4. Once a scoring system is decided upon, the cores are then scored in a blinded manner by two independent pathologists. Document staining in all compartments and percentage of cells staining during the first analysis (see Note 9).

5. If the scoring is discordant for a core, it is reviewed again and a consensus is reached and a score allocated.

6. The TMAs are usually analysed at 20× for the percentage of stained tumour cells at each level of staining intensity; however, 40× or higher resolution maybe be required for some tissues such as kidney.

7. The scoring results are recorded in an Excel database and then are transferred into the TMA database containing the clinical information on the TMA.

8. When samples are arrayed in duplicate, the mean of scoring results is often taken for statistical analysis. When samples are arrayed in quadruplicate, the median value is often taken.

9. Problems of inter- and intra-variability should be considered when manually scoring a TMA. Manual scoring produces only a limited amount of data and is difficult to duplicate due to its subjective nature. Hence, there is a need for automated analysis which can distinguish stain patterns and quantify staining (14).

3.7. Digital Slide Scanning and Storage

For this part, we assume the use of an Aperio XT scanner. This system is composed of three parts, namely, the glass slide scanner, the light source box, and a working station that provides the necessary software to use the scanner and manage the digital slides.

1. Preparation of glass slides for scanning involves cleaning of slides with alcohol and tissue to remove dust and chemical residues from the staining process.

2. Preparation of scanner

    (a) Switch on the light to warm up the light box. The bulb inside the light box might need to be changed if the intensity of the light is too weak.

    (b) Switch on the working station beside the scanner and open the ScanScope Console program needed to operate the scanner. Wait until the LCD screen on the top of the scanner displays the message "*Scanscope ready*".

    (c) Leave the whole system for 25 min in order to let the light source box reach the optimum temperature.

3. Scanning

    (a) The XT scanner operates in both manual and batch automatic mode. In manual mode, one slide can be scanned per run; in batch automatic mode, it is possible to scan up to 120 slides. For the purpose of this chapter, we would refer to the manual mode. Please refer to the XT manual for the batch mode.

    (b) Click on manual load on the ScanScope Console.

    (c) If you want to scan at 20×, move the doubler (black knob) backwards towards the front of the machine or at 40× move the doubler inwards.

    (d) The glass slide holder is automatically brought outside the right-side of the scanning box.

    (e) Put the glass slide on the slide holder on the top right-side of the scanner. The slide label should be on the top and faced towards the back side of the scanner.

    (f) A snapshot of the glass slide is automatically displayed in the ScanScope Console.

    (g) In the Scanscope Console window, go to the "Scan Area" tab. Click on "Find Tissue" and a green box is overlayed on the slide snapshot demarcating the area where the tissue is being scanned. If the green box is too small or too big you can change the size by stretching it.

    (h) A blue diamond appears over the snapshot. This indicates the focus area for scanning and needs to be moved to the area with no tissue by left clicking on it and moving to another position.

    (i) If scanning a full face section, go to the menu bar at the top of the screen and select "Tools" and then "Configure". Select the "Scan*scope Properties*" tab and inside select as "*Parameter set*", "*Coverslip*".

(j) If scanning a TMA, go to the menu bar at the top of the screen select "Tools" and then "Configure". Select the "Scanscope Properties" tab and inside select as "Parameter set", "TMA".

(k) Close the window and go back to the main window of ScanScope console. Go to the "Focus points" tab and click on the "Auto Select" button. This will automatically select the scanning focus points.

(l) Move along to the next tab "Prescan". Click on the "Prescan" button. If the prescanning image displayed in the middle of the window is not clear grey in colour, move the position of the prescanning focus point and repeat the prescan. There should be no tissue/dirt visible in this prescanned image.

(m) Move to the next tab "Scan" and click on "Scan". When finished, the "View *slide*" button is activated. By clicking on "*View slide*", the Aperio ScanScope viewer will be opened to look at the digital glass slide at different resolutions.

3.8. Management of Digital Slides

1. Local storage of glass slides: By default, slides are stored locally in the hard drive of the desktop connected to the scanner. The images are stored in a folder in C:\Images named using the date on which the image were scanned. The file extension for the digital slides is ".svs".

2. Accessing the digital slides: Digital slides can be directly open by clicking on them. This brings up the Aperio ScanScope viewer.

3. Slides can also be opened by using Spectrum, the digital slide management programme developed by Aperio.

4. Notes

1. Punching and coring should be done slowly with minimal pressure to prevent needle breakage.

2. Heating the recipient block slightly before use can prevent cores from falling out and decrease the likelihood of cores being lost in the cut section.

3. The recipient OCT block has the same size base as the paraffin recipient block that the tissue microarrayer was made to accommodate, and therefore it is easily mounted in the tissue microarrayer (Beecher Instruments).

4. If staggering after protease treatments, put first slide in 2× SSC and wait for other slide. Drying of slides before denaturation is not necessary.

5. Two water baths are set up at this stage; one for pre-treatment and the other for protease treatment at 80°C and 37°C,

respectively, and the pre-treatment solutions and protease buffers are removed from the fridge.

6. Protease is added to protease buffer and mixed well at this point.

7. If staggering after protease treatments, put first slide in 2× SSC and wait for other slide. Drying of slides before denaturation is not necessary.

8. Check denaturing solution is at pH 7–8.

9. When scoring a TMA where hundreds of cores are to be evaluated, it is advisable to document staining in all compartments and percentage of cells staining during the first analysis, as this will prevent the need to come back again at a future date and repeat what can be a very tedious process.

Acknowledgments

Funding is acknowledged under the EU FP6 Integrated Project, InnoMed, and the Health Research Board of Ireland. The UCD Conway Institute and the Proteome Research Centre is funded by the Programme for Research in Third Level Institutions (PRTLI), as administered by the Higher Education Authority (HEA) of Ireland from the Health Research Board of Ireland. The UCD Conway Institute is funded by the PRTLI, as administered by the HEA of Ireland.

References

1. Wan, W.H., Fortuna, M.B., and Furmanski, P. (1987) A rapid and efficient method for testing immunohistochemical reactivity of monoclonal antibodies against multiple tissue samples simultaneously. *J. Immunol. Methods* **103**(1), 121–129.

2. Kallioniemi, O.P., Wagner, U., Kononen, J., and Sauter, G. (2001) Tissue microarray technology for high-throughput molecular profiling of cancer. *Hum. Mol. Genet.* **10**(7), 657–662.

3. Kononen, J., Bubendorf, L., Kallioniemi, A., Barlund, M., Schraml, P., Leighton, S., Torhorst, J., Mihatsch, M.J., Sauter, G., and Kallioniemi, O.P. (1998) Tissue microarrays for high-throughput molecular profiling of tumor specimens. *Nat. Med.* **4**(7), 844–847.

4. Bubendorf, L., Nocito, A., Moch, H., and Sauter, G. (2001) Tissue microarray (TMA) technology: miniaturized pathology archives

for high-throughput *in situ* studies. *J. Pathol.* **195**(1), 72–79.

5. McKay, J.S., Bigley, A., Bell, A., Jenkins, R., Somers, R., Brocklehurst, S., White, A., and Goodwin, L. (2006) A pilot evaluation of the use of tissue microarrays for quantitation of target distribution in drug discovery pathology. *Exp. Toxicol. Pathol.* **57**(3), 181–193.

6. Englert, C.R., Baibakov, G.V., and Emmert-Buck, M.R. (2000) Layered expression scanning: rapid molecular profiling of tumor samples. *Cancer Res.* **60**(6), 1526–1530.

7. Chung, J.Y., Braunschweig, T., Baibakov, G., Galperin, M., Ramesh, A., Skacel, M., Gannot, G., Knezevic, V., and Hewitt, S.M. (2006) Transfer and multiplex immunoblotting of a paraffin embedded tissue. *Proteomics* **6**(3), 767–774.

8. Hassan, S., Ferrario, C., Mamo, A., and Basik, M. (2008) Tissue microarrays: emerging

standard for biomarker validation. *Curr. Opin. Biotechnol.* **19(1)**, 19–25.

9. Taranger-Charpin, C., Andrac-Meyer, L., Dales, J.P., Carpentier-Meunier, S., Andonian, C., Lavaut, M.N., Allasia, C., and Bonnier, P. (2007) High-throughput quantification of tissue microarrays: identification of candidate target proteins in inflammatory breast cancer. *Bull. Acad. Natl. Med.* **191(2)**, 361–374; discussion 374–376.

10. Mulrane, L., Rexhepaj, E., Smart, V., Callanan, J.J., Orhan, D., Eldem, T., Mally, A., Schroeder, S., Meyer, K., Wendt, M., *et al.* (2008) Creation of a digital slide and tissue microarray resource from a multi-institutional predictive toxicology study in the rat: an initial report from the PredTox group. *Exp. Toxicol. Pathol.* **60(4–5)**, 235–245.

11. Schoenberg Fejzo, M., and Slamon, D.J. (2001) Frozen tumor tissue microarray technology for analysis of tumor RNA, DNA, and proteins. *Am. J. Pathol.* **159(5)**, 1645–1650.

12. Coons, A.H., and Jones, R.N. (1941) Immunological properties of an antibody containing a fluorescent group. *Proc. Soc. Exp. Biol. Med.* **47**, 200–202.

13. Summersgill, B., Clark, J., and Shipley, J. (2008) Fluorescence and chromogenic *in situ* hybridization to detect genetic aberrations in formalin-fixed paraffin embedded material, including tissue microarrays. *Nat. Protoc.* **3(2)**, 220–234.

14. Murlane, L., Rexhepaj, E., Penney, S., and Gallagher, W.M. (2008) Automated image analysis in histopathology: a valuable tool in medical diagnosis. *Expert Rev. Mol. Diagn,* **8(6)**, 707–725

Part III

Genetic Toxicology

Chapter 7

Micronucleus Assay and Labeling of Centromeres with FISH Technique

Ilse Decordier, Raluca Mateuca, and Micheline Kirsch-Volders

Abstract

The cytokinesis-block micronucleus (CBMN) assay has since many years been applied for *in vitro* genotoxicity testing and biomonitoring of human populations. The standard *in vitro/ex vivo* micronucleus test is usually performed on human lymphocytes and has become a comprehensive method to assess genetic damage, cytostasis, and cytotoxicity. The predictive association between the frequency of micronuclei (MN) in cytokinesis-blocked lymphocytes and cancer risk has recently been demonstrated. MN frequencies can be influenced by inherited (or acquired) genetic polymorphisms (or mutations) in genes responsible for the metabolic activation, detoxification of clastogens, and for the fidelity of DNA replication. An important advantage of the CBMN assay is its ability to detect both clastogenic and aneugenic events by centromere and kinetochore identification and contributes to the high sensitivity of the method. The objective of the present chapter is to review the mechanisms of induction of micronuclei, the method of the micronucleus assay and its combination with centromeric labeling in the FISH technique. Furthermore, an overview is given of recent results obtained by our laboratory by the application of the micronucleus assay.

Key words: Micronuclei, Fluorescence *in situ* hybridization, Aneugens, Clastogens, Biomonitoring, Genetic polymorphisms

1. Introduction

In the late 1800s and early 1900s, micronuclei (MN) were described for the first time by Howell and Jolly as Feulgen-positive nuclear bodies in human reticulocytes, known as Howell–Jolly bodies, and representing chromosomes separated from the mitotic spindle. In the following decades, many cytogeneticists described MN formed by the presence of acentric fragments and the exclusion of these fragments from the daughter nuclei at telophase following *in vitro* irradiation of cells (1, 2). Boller and Schmidt (3) and Heddle (4) suggested the term micronucleus test for the first

Jean-Charles Gautier (ed.), *Drug Safety Evaluation: Methods and Protocols*, Methods in Molecular Biology, vol. 691,
DOI 10.1007/978-1-60761-849-2_7, © Springer Science+Business Media, LLC 2011

time in the early 1970s and showed that this assay provided a simple method to detect the genotoxic potential of mutagens after *in vivo* exposure of animals using bone marrow erythrocytes. A few years later, it was shown that also peripheral blood lymphocytes could be used for the micronucleus approach, and MN were recommended as a biomarker in testing schemes (5). In the recent years, the *in vitro* micronucleus test has become an attractive tool for *in vitro* genotoxicity testing because of its simplicity of scoring and wide applicability in different cell types and has been applied successfully for biomonitoring of *in vivo* genotoxic exposure.

In this chapter, we aim at reviewing the mechanisms of induction of MN, the method of the micronucleus assay and its combination with centromeric labeling in the fluorescence *in situ* hybridization (FISH) technique. Furthermore, an overview is given of recent results obtained by our laboratory by the application of the micronucleus assay.

2. Micronucleus Formation

MN can be found in dividing cells as small, extranuclear bodies resulting from chromosome breaks (leading to acentric fragments) and/or whole chromosomes that did not reach the spindle poles during cell division. At telophase, when the nuclear envelope is reconstituted around the two daughter cells, these lagging chromosomes or fragments are not incorporated into the main nucleus but encapsulated into a separate, smaller nucleus, a micronucleus. MN represent therefore a measure of both chromosome breakage and chromosome loss.

MN containing whole chromosomes/chromatids may be formed from defects in the chromosome segregation machinery, such as failure of the mitotic spindle, kinetochore, or other parts of the mitotic apparatus, or by damage to chromosomal substructures. Other phenomena giving rise to MN are deficiencies in cell cycle controlling genes, mechanical disruption (6), and hypomethylation of centromeric DNA (7). MN harboring chromosomal fragments can arise by direct double-strand DNA breakage (DSB), conversion of single-strand breaks (SSB) into DSB after cell replication, or inhibition of DNA synthesis. Furthermore, MN may have their origin in fragments derived from broken anaphase bridges formed due to chromosome rearrangements, such as dicentric chromatids, intermingled ring chromosomes, or union of sister chromatids (8). MN may also result from gene amplification via breakage-fusion-bridge (BFB) cycles when amplified DNA is selectively localized to specific sites at the periphery of the nucleus and eliminated via nuclear budding (NBUD) during the S-phase of the cell cycle (reviewed in (9)). Figure 1 gives an overview of the possible mechanisms leading to MN formation (reviewed in (9)).

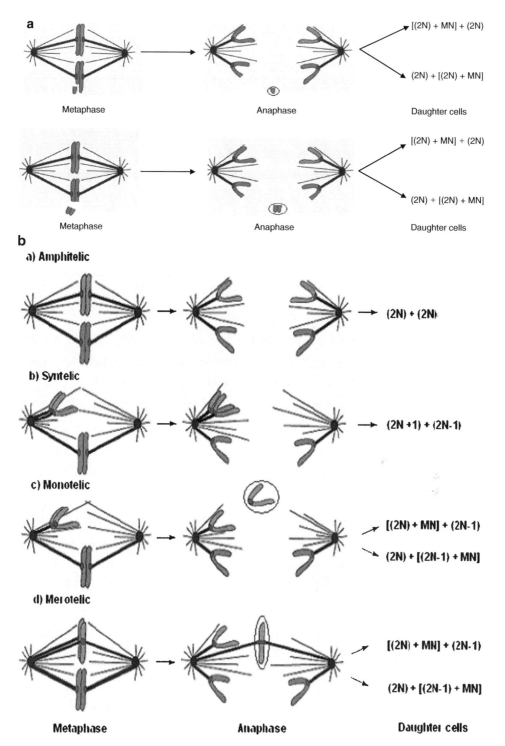

Fig. 1. Mechanisms of micronuclei (MN) formation. MN can mainly arise from: acentric chromosome/chromatid fragments resulting from DNA breakage events (**a**) and whole chromosomes/chromatids that lag behind in anaphase due to: misattachment of tubulin fibers on kinetochore (**b**); tubulin depolymerization.

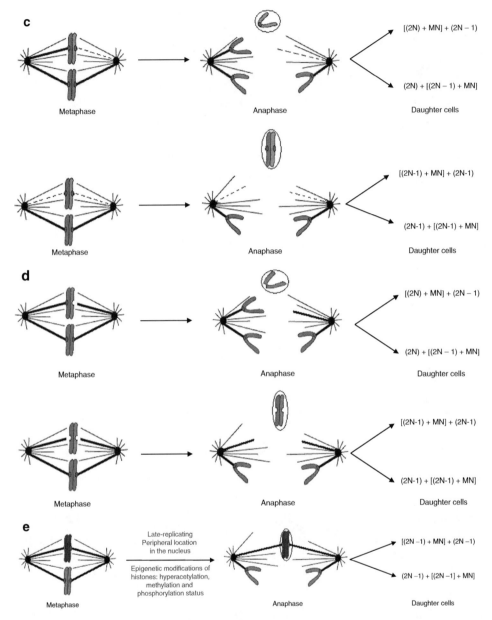

Fig. 1. (continued) (**c**); defects in centromeric DNA, in kinetochore proteins or in kinetochore assembly (**d**); late replication, peripheral location in the nucleus, and epigenetic modifications of histones (**e**). MN can also arise as a result of NPB formation/breakage **f**(1) and **f**(2). Misrepair of two chromosome breaks **f**(1) may lead to an asymmetrical chromosome rearrangement producing a dicentric chromosome and an acentric fragment; alternatively, dicentric chromosomes may also arise by telomere end fusions **f**(2). Centromeres of the dicentric chromosomes are pulled to opposite poles of the cells at anaphase resulting in the formation of a NPB between the daughter nuclei [**f**(1) and **f**(2)]. In the first case **f**(1), the lagging acentric fragment accompanying the dicentric chromosome will form MN. In both of the above cases, MN could also arise by breakage of the NPB [**f**(1) and **f**(2)].

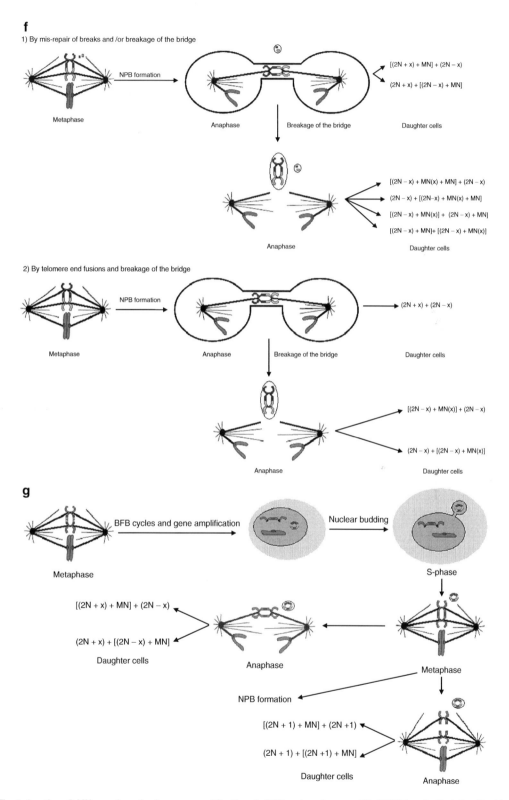

Fig. 1. (continued) MN can also arise by gene amplification via BFB cycles when amplified DNA is selectively localized to specific sites at the periphery of the nucleus and eliminated via NBUD during the S-phase of the cell cycle (**g**) (reviewed in ref. 9).

3. The Micronucleus Assay

The scoring of MN has become an important assay for *in vitro* genotoxicity testing and as a reliable biomarker assay for human genotoxic exposure and effect. The standard *in vitro/ex vivo* micronucleus test is usually performed on human lymphocytes but has also been adapted to other cell lines of different origin and other cell types relevant for human biomonitoring, such as fibroblasts and exfoliated epithelial cells. The *in vivo* micronucleus test generally involves assessing the induction of MN in bone marrow erythrocytes of mice or rats. Additional methods have been developed to detect MN in other, more relevant target tissues, such as the gut (10) or lung (11).

Since the formation of MN requires a nuclear division, it is necessary to be able to distinguish dividing cells from resting cells. Fenech and Morley (12) developed a simple method, the cytokinesis-block micronucleus assay (CBMN), to identify cells that have divided by adding cytochalasin B to the cells. Cytochalasin B is a metabolite of the mold *Helminthosporium dematioideum* and acts as an inhibitor of actin polymerization required for the formation of the microfilament ring that constricts the cytoplasm between the daughter nuclei during cytokinesis (13) (Fig. 2). The CBMN methodology allows distinction between a binucleated cell that has divided once, and a mononucleated cell, that did not divide. MN present in mononucleated cells (MNMONO) may provide an indication of the genome instability accumulated *in vivo*, while MN in binucleated cells (MNCB) indicate the chromosome/genome mutations accumulated before cultivation plus lesions expressed during *in vitro* culture (Fig.3). Other mechanisms accounting for the origin of MNMONO are: (1) mononucleated

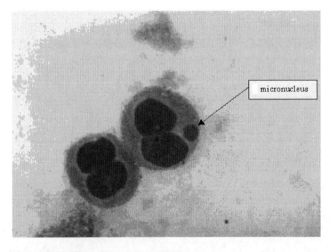

Fig. 2. A binucleated PBMC with a micronucleus.

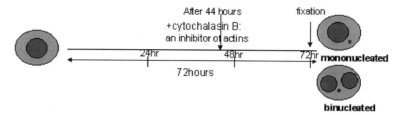

Fig. 3. *In vitro* cytochalasin-B micronucleus assay: methodology. The standard *in vitro* cytochalasin-B micronucleus assay is usually performed on human lymphocytes but has also been adapted to various cell lines of different origin. In a classical test, human lymphocytes are cultured in the presence of phytohemagglutinin to stimulate mitosis. After 44 h, cytochalasin-B is added to the culture. The use of this inhibitor of actin polymerization will block cytokinesis allowing the distinction between binucleated cells (cells that have divided once in culture) and mononucleated cells (cells that did not divide or escaped the cytokinesis-block). At 72 h, the cells are harvested onto microscopic slides, fixed and stained.

cells are cells remaining in first interphase as a result of cell cycle delay, (2) mononucleated cells containing MN are cells that underwent normal cell division, being insensitive to cytochalasin B, resulting in two mononucleated cells instead of the expected binucleated cells, (3) cells with a deficient mitotic spindle can escape mitotic arrest and undergo mitotic slippage in the presence of microtubule inhibitors after mitotic arrest (14). These cells do not undergo cytokinesis and give rise to tetraploid mononucleated cells with or without micronuclei. This is important to take into account when testing the aneugenic potential of chemicals. Therefore, it was suggested by Kirsch-Volders and Fenech (15) that MNMONO should also be scored when performing the CBMN assay.

Furthermore, the assessment of cell proliferation and cytotoxicity in the CBMN assay was recommended for a more comprehensive assessment of the genetic damage (15–18). Many agents can induce multiple effects at molecular, chromosomal, or cellular level at the same time. Analysis of the genotoxic events without information on apoptosis or necrosis can be confounding because increases in genotoxic damage can be the result of indirect events, such as inhibition of apoptosis or disturbed cell cycle checkpoints leading to shorter cell cycle times and higher rates of chromosome malsegregation (18). In addition, in cytogenetic assays, such as the CBMN assay, requiring cell division in culture for the expression of the measured endpoint (MN), not all damaged cells may be observed because they may undergo apoptosis or necrosis instead of completing nuclear division. These additional biomarkers can relatively easily be integrated in the CBMN assay, as they can be distinguished by means of morphological criteria and scored alongside the micronucleated cells. The assessment of proliferation is important for evaluating potential cytostatic effects of a compound and allows the identification of molecules that can stimulate cell division (17). In human peripheral blood mononuclear cells (PBMC), the proliferation index is also a measure of mitogen response, a useful biomarker of immune response in nutrition studies which can also be related to genotoxic exposure (19–21).

The International Collaborative Project on Micronucleus Frequency in Human Populations (the HUMN project, http://www.humn.org) established scoring criteria for MN using isolated human lymphocyte cultures and used combined databases to assess intra- and interlaboratory variation in MN scoring, background MN frequencies, and the influence of age, gender, and smoking on MN frequencies (22–27).

As a result of two International Workshop on Genotoxicity Test Procedures (IWGTP) workshops an internationally harmonized protocol was designed for both human primary lymphocytes and cell lines (17, 28, 29). Recently, the *in vitro* micronucleus test has been recognized as a scientifically valid alternative for the *in vitro* chromosome aberration assay for genotoxicity testing by ECVAM and a new guideline 487 for the protocol for the *In Vitro* Mammalian Cell Micronucleus Test (Mnvit) has been proposed by OECD. The protocol for the CBMN cytome assay has been recently described by Fenech (18).

Combined with FISH with probes for centromeric, pericentromeric, or telomeric regions (see below) micronucleus scoring in the cytokinesis-block method also allows the identification of the major mechanisms responsible for micronucleus induction: chromosome breakage leading to MN with acentric fragments and failure of the mitotic apparatus resulting in MN with entire chromosomes. The CBMN assay is now also used for the assessment of nucleoplasmic bridges (NPBs), a biomarker of dicentric chromosomes resulting from telomere end-fusions or DNA misrepair, and of NBUDs, a biomarker of gene amplification.

Since the CBMN assay not only does provide information on the chromosome breakage and loss, but also on additional measures of genotoxicity and cytotoxicity, such as apoptosis, necrosis, cell division inhibition (by estimation of the proliferation index), NBUDs, and NPBs, the concept of the CBMN assay as a "cytome" assay has been introduced by Fenech (18). This concept of "cytome" indicates that every cell is scored cytologically for its viability status (apoptosis or necrosis), its mitotic status (mono-, bi-, or polynucleated), and its chromosomal damage or instability status (the presence of MN, NPB, NBUD, number of centromeric signals if combined with FISH). However, it is known that MN frequency measured by the CBMN method may not identify all chromosome damage events, e.g., aberrations, such as symmetrical reciprocal translocations, are not expressed as MN but asymmetrical translocations, such as dicentric chromosomes, and

Table 1
Advantages and disadvantages of the CBMN assay

Advantages	Disadvantages
• End point = chromosome + genome mutations • + FISH: discrimination between clastogen/aneugen and chromosome loss/non-disjunction • Estimation of nuclear division index • Possible codetection of NPB, NBUD, apoptosis/necrosis • Sensitive • Simple, fast, cheap, automation possible • Statistical power	• Does not detect all chromosomal damage events (e.g., symmetrical reciprocal translocations) • Requires cell division for expression of MN • Effect of cytochalasin B on MN frequency

their associated acentric fragments may be observed as NPBs and MN, respectively (23).

In comparison with the scoring of chromosomal aberrations (CAs), the scoring of MN is simpler, requires shorter training and is less time consuming (8). Moreover, the statistical power obtained from scoring larger numbers of cells (thousands) than are typically used for metaphase analysis (a hundred or a few hundred) is a major advantage of the CBMN assay. These large numbers of binucleated cells can be achieved because it is possible to cytokinesis block cultures for 24–48 h; on the contrary, colchicine blocking for metaphase analysis can only be performed for 1–4 h as longer times cause chromosome condensation making metaphases unscorable. Automated scoring of MN will further increase the statistical power of the assay by eliminating interindividual variation in assessing this type of chromosomal damage. The advantages and disadvantages of the CBMN assay are presented in Table 1.

4. Micronuclei and Predictivity for Cancer

Recently, a prospective study was performed in the framework of the HUMN project in which 6,718 subjects from ten countries, screened for MN frequencies between 1980 and 2002 and followed-up for cancer incidence and mortality. This multinational collaborative study demonstrated a significantly higher prospective cancer risk (RR 1.67, $P=0.002$) in those diagnosed with MN frequencies in the medium or high tertile as compared to those in the low MN frequency tertile (30). These evidences that baseline frequency of MN in peripheral blood lymphocytes is a predictive biomarker of cancer risk was confirmed by a study of Murgia et al. (31) who validated the frequency of MN in peripheral blood lymphocytes as an early cancer risk biomarker in a nested case-control study performed 14 years after the original recruitment. Rajagopalan et al. (32) observed that cells from human colorectal cancers and adenomas, deficient in G1-S checkpoint control as a result of hCDC4 mutations, showed an increased genome instability corresponding to a high frequency of micronuclei, thereby demonstrating a functional link between MN and cancer.

5. Micronucleus Assay and Labeling of Centromeres with FISH Technique

As already mentioned, the *in vitro* cytochalasin-B block methodology allows discrimination between mutagens inducing DNA breakage (clastogens) or chromosome loss (aneugens).

MN arising from lagging chromosomes can be identified with immunochemical labeling of kinetochores proteins that are assembled on centromeres (CREST) or by the presence of centromere-specific DNA using FISH. MN that do not contain kinetochore proteins or centromeric DNA sequences are interpreted as harboring acentric chromosomal fragments (6). However, the use of antikinetochore antibodies does not distinguish between unique chromosomes and MN formed from entire chromosomes with disrupted or detached kinetochore which may result in MN with no kinetochore signal. Furthermore, chemicals can interact with the synthesis of kinetochore proteins. Therefore, the preferred method is to use FISH with pancentromeric probes to identify MN containing whole chromosomes (Fig. 4). In addition, centromeric chromosome-specific probes also allow an accurate analysis of non-disjunction (unequal distribution of unique homologous chromosome pairs in the daughter nuclei) (Fig. 3). This is very helpful to perform risk assessment of compounds with threshold type of dose-responses. Our laboratory used the MN assay in combination with FISH for the *in vitro* demonstration of thresholds for microtubule inhibitors aneugenic compounds binding specifically to β-tubulin and inhibiting tubulin polymerization, such as nocodazole, a chemotherapeutic drug or carbendazim, a pesticide (33, 34). The two endpoints reflecting aneuploidy were studied *in vitro* in human lymphocytes: chromosome loss and non-disjunction. To assess chromosome loss the detection of centromere-positive versus centromere-negative MN by FISH with a general alphoid centromeric probe was performed on cytochalasin-B blocked binucleates resulting from cultures exposed to the spindle poisons. For chromosome nondisjunction, the same compounds were investigated on cytokinesis-blocked binucleated lymphocytes in combination with FISH using chromosome-specific centromeric probes for chromosome 1 and

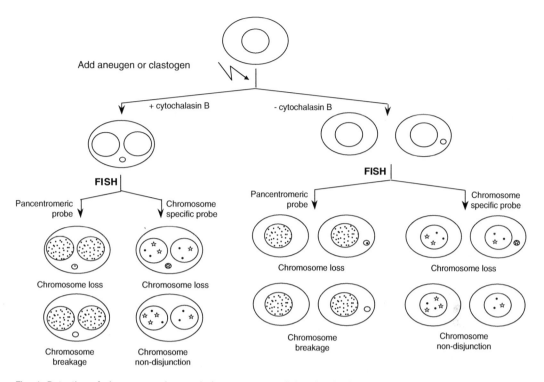

Fig. 4. Detection of chromosome loss and chromosome nondisjunction in the cytokinesis-block micronucleus assay combined with FISH.

chromosome 17. This allowed the accurate evaluation of non-disjunction since artifacts were excluded from the analysis as only binucleates with the correct number of hybridization signals were taken into account. We demonstrated dose dependency of the aneugenic effects and the existence of thresholds for the induction of chromosome non-disjunction and chromosome loss by these spindle inhibitors (lower for non-disjunction than for chromosome loss) (Fig. 5).

6. Micronuclei and Apoptosis

From a mechanistic point of view, one can expect that apoptosis contributes to the elimination of cells with premutagenic/mutagenic lesions. Therefore, we evaluated whether aneuploid cells, i.e., cells bearing non-disjunctions and MN formed after chromosome loss, cells were selectively eliminated by apoptosis (35). For this purpose, apoptotic and viable cells were separated by magnetic microbead cell sorting combined with annexin-V staining. In the two collected populations micronuclei, chromosome loss and chromosome non-disjunction were scored in binucleated cells

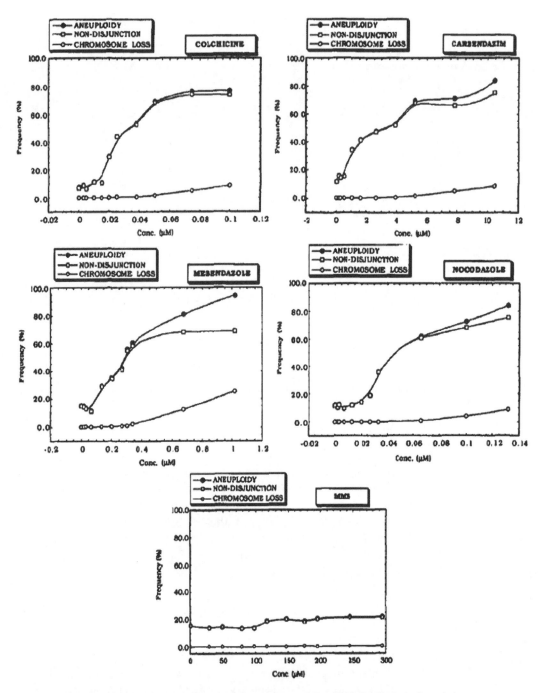

Fig. 5. Dose dependency of aneugenic effects and the existence of thresholds for the induction of chromosome non-disjunction and chromosome loss by spindle inhibitors.

(MNCB) obtained in the *in vitro* cytokinesis-block MN assay, using FISH. This methodology, combining cell sorting and FISH identification of chromosomes, seemed to be adequate to analyze whether chromosome loss or non-disjunction themselves trigger

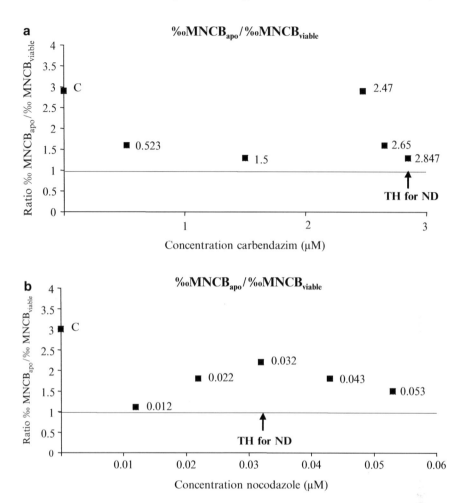

Fig. 6. Induction of micronucleated cytokinesis-blocked lymphocytes (‰MNCB) in the apoptotic versus viable cells, induced by carbendazim (**a**) and nocodazole (**b**). 500–1,000 cytokinesis-blocked lymphocytes were scored. The ratio between frequencies of micronucleated cytokinesis-blocked lymphocytes (‰MNCB) in the apoptotic fraction versus the viable fraction was calculated for each studied concentration. A ratio equal to one expresses the same probability of finding that class of cells among viable and apoptotic cells. A higher ratio value indicates that those cells preferentially undergo apoptosis. The threshold value for non-disjunction (TH for ND) is indicated by the *arrow*. 2.847 μM for carbendazim and 0.032 μM for nocodazole. The actual tested concentrations are reported close to each experimental point.

apoptosis. The results suggest that the elimination of aneuploid cells, i.e., micronucleated cells or cells with chromosome non-disjunction, does occur, even below the threshold concentrations for chromosome loss and non-disjunction (Figs. 6 and 7). However, apoptosis provoked by micronucleated cells is much stronger than for cells presenting chromosome non-disjunction. Therefore, micronucleated cells constitute a strong apoptotic signal (35).

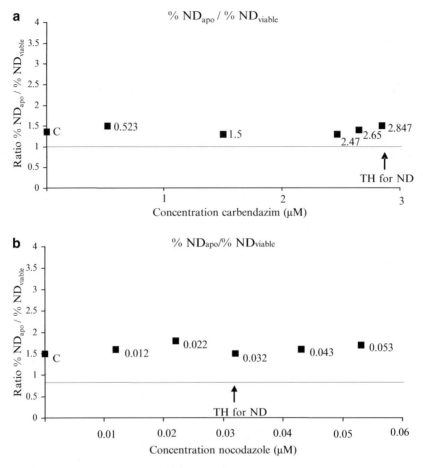

Fig. 7. Induction of chromosomal non-disjunction for the total genome (% Tot. ND) cytokinesis-blocked lymphocytes in the apoptotic versus viable cells, by carbendazim (**a**) and nocodazole (**b**). 500–1,000 cytokinesis-blocked lymphocytes were scored. The ratio between frequencies of chromosomal non-disjunction (% Tot. ND) in the apoptotic fraction versus the viable fraction was calculated for each concentration. A ratio equal to one expresses the same probability of finding that class of cells among viable and apoptotic cells. A higher ratio value indicates that those cells preferentially undergo apoptosis. The threshold value for non-disjunction (TH for ND) is indicated by the *arrow*. The actual tested concentrations are reported close to each experimental point.

Our findings that MN can be eliminated by apoptosis were confirmed by the use of specific caspase inhibitors (36). Our rationale for this was that, if micronucleated cells can be eliminated by apoptosis, inhibition of apoptosis would result in an increased frequency of micronucleated cells. An increase of micronucleated cells was observed with inhibitors of the two main initiator caspase-8 and -9, confirming that micronucleated cells can be eliminated by apoptosis (Fig. 8).

Some other studies investigated the elimination of MN from cells. Schriever-Schwemmer et al. (37) demonstrated the extrusion of MN induced by colchicine and acrylamide during the

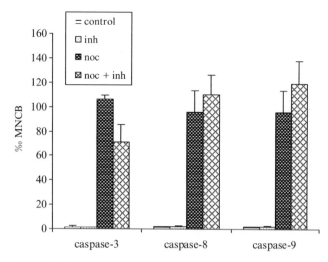

Fig. 8. Frequencies of nocodazole-induced MNCB in the presence of caspase-9 inhibitor Ac-LEHD-CMK, the caspase-8 inhibitor Boc-AEVD-CHO and the caspase-3 inhibitor Ac-DEVD-CHO in PBMC. *Each bar* represents the mean of two donors, per donor two parallel cultures and per culture 1,000 binucleates were scored for the incidence of MN. Statistical analysis was performed using Mann-Whitney *U*-test to determine significant differences in lymphocytes treated with different experimental conditions (SPSS 12.0), *$P < 0.05$, presence of the caspase inhibitor versus absence of the caspase inhibitor.

maturation of erythrocytes. This phenomenon was observed for MN containing lagging chromosomes as well as for MN containing acentric fragments. Furthermore, MN containing amplified DNA (double minutes) have been reported to be selectively eliminated from the cell (38). Results obtained by Schwartz and Jordan (39) suggested that apoptosis contributes to the selective removal of cells bearing unstable types of aberrations, such as dicentrics, rings and chromosome fragments, in a p53-dependent manner. This was not the case for stable aberrations like balanced translocations. These observations were confirmed in another study by Bassi et al. (40) who showed that the preferential elimination of cells containing unstable aberrations occurs via p53/survivin-dependent apoptosis. Moreover, Taga et al. (41) demonstrated that also during early development apoptosis contributes to the elimination of cells carrying a damaged or unstable genome (42).

How the presence of a micronucleus in a cell can lead to apoptosis has still to be elucidated. A question that remains unanswered is whether it is the micronucleus itself or its content, i.e., a whole chromosome/chromatid or a chromosome fragment resulting from a non-repaired DSB, which is responsible for the death signal. The experiments carried out in our studies were only performed with nocodazole, which is an aneugen. We observed that high concentrations of nocodazole do not induce double-strand DNA breaks using the alkaline comet assay and analysis of centromere-positive and -negative MN demonstrated only an increase of centromere-positive MN in the presence of high concentrations of nocodazole (43). However, one cannot exclude that some of these MN originated from an indirect clastogenic effect of nocodazole (e.g., decrease of trafficking enzymes for repair of endogenous DNA damage) may also constitute an apoptotic trigger (reviewed in (42)).

7. Role of Caspase-3 in the Formation of Micronuclei

On the contrary to what was observed with caspase-8 and -9 inhibitors, our results showed a decrease of the frequencies of nocodazole-induced MN in PBMC in the presence of a caspase-3 inhibitor (Fig. 8). These observations suggested that caspase-3 is not involved in the elimination of micronucleated cell, but rather in the formation of MN. Therefore, we attempted to investigate the possible role of caspase-3 in the formation of MN more in detail by using the paired human breast carcinoma cell lines MCF-7, which is caspase-3 deficient, and the MCF-7 stably transfected with functional caspase-3 gene (MCF-7casp3+). The results obtained showed that, in every condition where caspase-3 was not working properly, i.e., in the caspase-3 deficient or in the MCF-7casp3+ cell treated with the caspase-3 inhibitor, a lower frequency of MN was observed (Fig. 9). These results suggested that caspase-3, in addition to its function in apoptosis, is also involved in the formation of MN. Since the same phenomenon was observed in the presence of the clastogen MMS, the contribution of caspase-3 to the formation of MN seemed to be irrespective of the content of the micronucleus (a whole chromosome or a chromosome fragment) (36). It remains to be elucidated how caspase-3 exhibits its function in the formation of MN. One could hypothesize that components of the nuclear envelope could be potential targets of caspase-3, and that their cleavage is involved in the formation of MN. The nuclear lamina is composed of lamins and lamin-associated proteins. Lamins are type-V intermediate-filament proteins and are grouped in A- and B-types according to their biochemical properties and behavior during mitosis (44). Nuclear reassembly occurs at the end of mitosis and follows the following regulated sequence of molecular interactions, in a temporal order: (a) targeting of individual nucleoskeletal proteins to the chromosomal surface, (b) membrane recruitment and fusion, (c) assembly of the nuclear pore complexes (NPCs), (d) transport of lamins into the nucleus through newly formed NPCs, and (e) formation of the nuclear lamina (45). One can hypothesize that a similar sequence of events occurs when a micronucleus is formed. Since lamin B (46, 47) and the nuclear

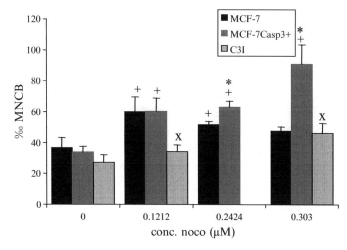

Fig. 9. Nocodazole-induced micronuclei after 48 h treatment in the MCF-7 cell line, the MCF-7$^{casp-3+}$ cell line and in the MCF-7$^{casp-3+}$ cell line in the presence 300 μM of the caspase-3 inhibitor Ac-DEVD-CHO (C-3I). Parallel cultures were analyzed for each treatment and 1,000 binucleated cells per culture were scored. Statistical analysis was performed using Student's t-test (since the data were normally distributed) to compare between pairs of groups for each dose in the two cell lines [Statistical Package for the Social Sciences (SPSS) 12.0], +, $P < 0.05$ as compared to the control; *, $P < 0.05$ MCF-7^{casp3+} as compared to MCF-7; ×, $P < 0.05$ with inhibitor as compared without. The experiment with the caspase-3 inhibitor Ac-DEVD-CHO was not performed with 0.2424 μM nocodazole.

pore complex protein Nup153 (48) have been shown to be substrates of caspase-3, one cannot exclude that the interaction between caspase-3 and these components of the nuclear envelope contributes to the formation of a micronucleus. However, the exact mechanisms still need to be clarified (reviewed in (42)).

8. Influence of Genetic Polymorphisms on Micronuclei

MN frequencies can be influenced by inherited (or acquired) genetic polymorphisms (or mutations) in genes responsible for the metabolic activation and detoxification of clastogens, for the fidelity of DNA replication (mismatch repair), DNA repair and/ or chromosome segregation. The relationship between MN frequencies and genetic polymorphisms provides insight on how genetic variants can modulate the effect of genotoxic exposure, host factors, such as age and gender, lifestyle characteristics, such as smoking and folate and diseases such as cancer. In the last four years, our laboratory has performed several human population studies addressing the influence of genetic polymorphisms on MN frequencies (49–53).

The influence of GSTM1 and GSTT1 polymorphisms on micronucleus frequencies in peripheral blood lymphocytes of the general population and of groups exposed to known or suspected genotoxic substances was recently assessed by a pooled analysis of eight biomonitoring studies using the *in vivo* CBMN assay (54). The results of the pooled analysis indicated that the *GSTT1* null subjects had lower micronucleus frequencies than their positive counterparts in the total population. A significant overall increase in micronucleus frequency with age and gender was observed, females having higher micronucleus frequencies than males, when occupationally exposed. Nonoccupationally exposed smokers had lower micronucleus frequencies than nonsmokers, whereas no significant difference in micronucleus level was observed between smokers and nonsmokers in the occupationally exposed group.

The pooled approach was also used to study the influence of polymorphisms in genes involved in DNA repair on the micronucleus frequencies in human lymphocytes *in vivo* (55). Three polymorphic genes *hOGG1*, *XRCC1*, and *XRCC3*, involved in the repair of oxidized bases, SSBs and DSBs, respectively, were studied. The results of that study provided evidence that single DNA repair gene polymorphisms are not likely to have a major impact on MN frequencies but rather combinations of different DNA repair genes. In addition, the results indicated that complex interplay between *hOGG1*[326], *XRCC1*[399], *XRCC3*[241] genotypes, and environmental factors modulates MN levels.

Several studies have also addressed the relationship between genetic polymorphisms and MN frequencies (56–58). Crott et al. (57) demonstrated that the methylenetetrahydrofolate reductase (MTHFR) C677T polymorphism did not influence the levels of chromosome damage as assessed by the CBMN assay in human lymphocytes. Kimura et al. (56) on the other hand, found higher MN frequencies in the lymphocytes of variant MTHFR TT genotypes as compared with the wild type MTHFR CC genotypes, and a lower NBUD level in TT homozygotes relative to CC homozygotes for the MTHFR C677T mutation. A significant association between the methionine synthase reductase (MTRR) 66GG variant genotype and higher micronucleus levels was observed by Zijno et al. (58) after correction for age, gender, and GSTM1 genotype. Ishikawa et al. (59) investigated the relationships between MN frequency, smoking habits and five folate metabolic enzyme gene polymorphisms (*MTHFR* C677T and A1298C, *MTR* A2756G, *MTRR* A66G and *TYMS* 3'UTR) in 132 healthy Japanese men. The results of this study indicated that the MTRR AA genotype acts to increase the MN frequency resulting from cigarette smoking.

9. Conclusion

Due to its simplicity, accuracy, multipotentiality, potential to detect early effects of mutagens/carcinogens, capacity to identify inheritable changes, its predictivity for cancer and large tissue applicability the *ex vivo/in vitro* micronucleus assay has become an important cytogenetic biomarker to assess genetic damage. The assay has applications in many research areas: *in vitro* genotoxicity testing, biomonitoring of human populations for *in vivo* genotoxic exposure, nutrigenomics, pharmacogenomics, preventive medicine, ecotoxicology, and as predictor of normal tissue and tumor radiation sensitivity and cancer. Its importance is also demonstrated by the high level of international validation.

A next step in the MN technology is the automation of MN scoring and its combination with FISH. Validation of automated MN scoring is currently in progress. This would allow high throughput applicability and a faster and more reliable nonsubjective analysis for the prescreening of new chemicals for genotoxic effects and primary prevention through risk assessment of human populations exposed to environmental and/or occupational mutagens.

Acknowledgments

This work was supported by the EU research programs "The Detection and Hazard Evaluation of Aneugenic Chemicals (ENV4-CT97-0471)," Protection of the European Population from Aneugenic Chemicals (PEPFAC) (QLK4-CT-2000-00058), ChildrenGenoNetwork (QLRT-2001-02198), Cancer Risk Biomarkers (QLK4-2000-00628), ECNIS (FOOD-CT-2005-513943), NewGeneris (FOOD-CT-2005-016320-2) and by the Belgian Offices for Scientific, Technical and Cultural Affairs of the Prime Minister's Office (contract PS/03/35).

References

1. Thoday, J.M. (1951) The effect of ionizing radiation on the broad bean root. Part IX. Chromosome breakage and the lethality of ionizing radiations to the root meristem. *Br. J. Radiol.* **24**, 276–572.

2. Evans, H.J., Neary, G.J., and Williamson, F.S. (1959) The relative biological efficiency of single doses of fast neutrons and gamma rays in Vicia faba roots and the effect of oxygen. Part II. Chromosome damage; the production of micronuclei. *Int. J. Rad. Biol.* **1**, 230–240.

3. Boller, K., and Schmid, W. (1970) Chemical mutagenesis in mammals. The Chinese hamster bone marrow as an *in vivo* test system. Hematological findings after treatment with trenimon. *Humangenetik* **11**, 35–54.

4. Heddle, J.A. (1970) A rapid *in vivo* test for chromosome damage. *Mutat. Res.* **18**, 187–190.

5. Countryman, P.I., and Heddle, J.A. (1976). The production of micronuclei from chromosome aberrations in irradiated cultures of

human lymphocytes. *Mutat. Res.* **41**, 321–332.

6. Albertini, R.J., Anderson, D., Douglas, G.R., Hagmar, L., Hemminki, K., Merlo, F., Natarajan, A.T., Norppa, H., Shuker, D.E., Tice, R., Waters, M.D., and Aitio, A. (2000) IPCS guidelines for the monitoring of genotoxic effects of carcinogens in humans. International Programme on Chemical Safety. *Mutat. Res.* **463**, 111–172.

7. Fenech, M., Baghurst, P., Luderer, W., Turner, J., Record, S., Ceppi, M., and Bonassi, S. (2005) Low intake of calcium, folate, nicotinic acid, vitamin E, retinol, beta-carotene and high intake of pantothenic acid, biotin and riboflavin are significantly associated with increased genome instability – results from a dietary intake and micronucleus index survey in South Australia. *Carcinogenesis* **26**, 991–999.

8. Norppa, H., and Falck, G.C. (2003) What do human micronuclei contain? *Mutagenesis* **18**, 221–233.

9. Mateuca, R., Lombaert, N., Aka, P.V., Decordier, I., and Kirsch-Volders, M. (2006) Chromosomal changes: induction, detection methods and applicability in human biomonitoring. *Biochimie* **88**, 1515–1531.

10. Vanhauwaert, A., Vanparys, P., and Kirsch-Volders, M. (2001) The *in vivo* gut micronucleus test detects clastogens and aneugens given by gavage. *Mutagenesis* **16**, 39–50.

11. De Boeck, M., Hoet, P., Lombaert, N., Nemery, B., Kirsch-Volders, M., and Lison, D. (2003) *In vivo* genotoxicity of hard metal dust: induction of micronuclei in rat type II epithelial lung cells. *Carcinogenesis* **24**, 1793–1800.

12. Fenech, M., and Morley, A.A. (1985) Measurement of micronuclei in lymphocytes. *Mutat. Res.* **147**, 29–36.

13. Carter, S.B. (1976) Effects of cytochalasins on mammalian cells. *Nature* **213**, 261–264.

14. Elhajouji, A., Cunha, M., and Kirsch-Volders, M. (1998) Spindle poisons can induce polyploidy by mitotic slippage and micronucleate mononucleates in the cytokinesis-block assay. *Mutagenesis* **13**, 193–198.

15. Kirsch-Volders, M., and Fenech, M. (2001) Inclusion of micronuclei in non-divided mononuclear lymphocytes and necrosis/apoptosis may provide a more comprehensive cytokinesis block micronucleus assay for biomonitoring purposes. *Mutagenesis* **16**, 51–58.

16. Fenech, M. (1999) Micronucleus frequency in human lymphocytes is related to plasma vitamin B12 and homocysteine. *Mutat. Res.* **428**, 299–304.

17. Kirsch-Volders, M., Sofuni, T., Aardema, M., Albertini, S., Eastmond, D., Fenech, M., Ishidate, M. Jr., Lorge, E., Norppa, H., Surralles, J., von der Hude, W., and Wakata, A. (2004) Corrigendum to "Report from the *in vitro* micronucleus assay working group" [*Mutat. Res.* 2003, **540**, 153–163]. *Mutat. Res.* **564**, 97–100.

18. Fenech, M. (2007) Cytokinesis-block micronucleus cytome assay. *Nat. Protoc.* **2**, 1084–1104.

19. Fenech, M. (2000) The *in vitro* micronucleus technique. *Mutat. Res.* **455**, 81–95.

20. Umegaki, K., and Fenech, M. (2000) Cytokinesis-block micronucleus assay in WIL2-NS cells: a sensitive system to detect chromosomal damage induced by reactive oxygen species and activated human neutrophils. *Mutagenesis* **15**, 261–269.

21. Wu, D., Han, S.N., Meydani, M., and Meydani, S.N. (2006) Effect of concomitant consumption of fish oil and vitamin E on T cell mediated function in the elderly: a randomized double-blind trial. *J. Am. Coll. Nutr.* **25**, 300–306.

22. Fenech, M. (1998) Chromosomal damage rate, aging, and diet. *Ann. N. Y. Acad. Sci.* **854**, 23–36.

23. Fenech, M., Holland, N., Chang, W.P., Zeiger, E., and Bonassi, S. (1999) The Human MicroNucleus Project – an international collaborative study on the use of the micronucleus technique for measuring DNA damage in humans. *Mutat. Res.* **428**, 271–283.

24. Bonsái, S., Fenech, M., Lando, C., Lin, Y.P., Ceppi, M., Chang, W.P., Holland, N., Kirsch-Volders, M., Zeiger, E., Ban, S., Barale, R., Bigatti, M.P., Bolognesi, C., Jia, C., Di Giorgio, M., Ferguson, L.R., Fucic, A., Lima, O.G., Rehíla, P., Krishnaja, A.P., Lee, T.K., Migliore, L., Mikhalevich, L., Mirkova, E., Mosesso, P., Müller, W.U., Odagiri, Y., Scarffi, M.R., Szabova, E., Vorobtsova, I., *et al.* (2001) Human MicroNucleus Project: international database comparison for results with the cytokinesis-block micronucleus assay in human lymphocytes: I. Effect of laboratory protocol, scoring criteria, and host factors on the frequency of micronuclei. *Environ. Mol. Mutagen.* **37**, 31–45.

25. Bonassi, S., Neri, M., Lando, C., Ceppi, M., Lin, Y.P., Chang, W.P., Holland, N., Kirsch-Volders, M., Zeiger, E., and Fenech, M. (2003) HUMN collaborative group. Effect of smoking habit on the frequency of micronuclei in human lymphocytes: results from the Human MicroNucleus project. *Mutat. Res.* **543**, 155–166.

26. Fenech, M., Bonassi, S., Turner, J., Lando, C., Ceppi, M., Chang, W.P., Holland, N.,

Kirsch-Volders, M., Zeiger, E., Bigatti, M.P., Bolognesi, C., Cao, J., De Luca, G., Di Giorgio, M., Ferguson, L.R., Fucic, A., Lima, O.G., Hadjidekova, V.V., Hrelia, P., Jaworska, A., Joksic, G., Krishnaja, A.P., Lee, T.K., Martelli, A., McKay, M.J., Migliore, L., Mirkova, E., Müller, W.U., Odagiri, Y., Orsiere, T., Scarfi, M.R., Silva, M.J., Sofuni, T., Surralles, J., Trenta, G., Vorobtsova, I., Vral, A., and Zijno, A. (2003) HUman MicroNucleus project. Intra- and inter-laboratory variation in the scoring of micronuclei and nucleoplasmic bridges in binucleated human lymphocytes. Results of an international slide-scoring exercise by the HUMN project. *Mutat. Res.* **534**, 45–64.

27. Fenech, M., Chang, W.P., Kirsch-Volders, M., Holland, N., Bonassi, S., and Zeiger, E. (2003). HUman MicronNucleus project. HUMN project: detailed description of the scoring criteria for the cytokinesis-block micronucleus assay using isolated human lymphocyte cultures. *Mutat. Res.* **534**, 65–75.

28. Kirsch-Volders, M., Sofuni, T., Aardema, M., Albertini, S., Eastmond, D., Fenech, M., Ishidate, M. Jr., Lorge, E., Norppa, H., Surralles, J., von der Hude, W., and Wakata, A. (2001) Report from the *In vitro* Micronucleus Assay Working Group. *Environ. Mol. Mutagen.* **35**, 167–172.

29. Kirsch-Volders, M., Sofuni, T., Aardema, M., Albertini, S., Eastmond, D., Fenech, M., Ishidate, M. Jr., Kirchner, S., Lorge, E., Morita, T., Norppa, H., Surralles, J., Vanhauwaert, A., and Wakata, A. (2003) Report from the *in vitro* micronucleus assay working Group. *Mutat. Res.* **540**, 153–163.

30. Bonassi, S., Znaor, A., Ceppi, M., Lando, C., Chang, W.P., Holland, N., Kirsch-Volders, M., Zeiger, E., Ban, S., Barale, R., Bigatti, M.P., Bolognesi, C., Cebulska-Wasilewska, A., Fabianova, E., Fucic, A., Hagmar, L., Joksic, G., Martelli, A., Migliore, L., Mirkova, E., Scarfi, M.R., Zijno, A., Norppa, H., Fenech, M. (2007) An increased micronucleus frequency in peripheral blood lymphocytes predicts the risk of cancer in humans. *Carcinogenesis* **28**, 625–631.

31. Murgia, E., Ballardin, M., Bonassi, S., Rossi, A.M., and Barale, R. (2008) Validation of micronuclei frequency in peripheral blood lymphocytes as early cancer risk biomarker in a nested case-control study. *Mutat. Res.* **39**, 27–34.

32. Rajagopalan, H., Jallepalli, P.V., Rago, C., Velculescu, V.E., Kinzler, K.W., Vogelstein, B., and Lengauer, C. (2004) Inactivation of hCDC4 can cause chromosomal instability. *Nature* **428**, 77–81.

33. Elhajouji, A., Van Hummelen, P., and Kirsch-Volders, M. (1995) Indications for a threshold of chemically-induced aneuploidy *in vitro* in human lymphocytes. *Environ. Mol. Mutagen.* **26**, 292–304.

34. Elhajouji, A., Tibaldi, F., and Kirsch-Volders, M. (1997) Indication for thresholds of chromosome non-disjunction versus chromosome lagging induced by spindle inhibitors *in vitro* in human lymphocytes. *Mutagenesis* **12**, 133–140.

35. Decordier, I., Dillen, L., Cundari, E., and Kirsch-Volders, M. (2002) Elimination of micronucleated cells by apoptosis after treatment with inhibitors of microtubules. *Mutagenesis* **17**, 337–344.

36. Decordier, I., Cundari, E., and Kirsch-Volders, M. (2005) Influence of caspase activity on micronuclei detection: a possible role for caspase-3 in micronucleation. *Mutagenesis* **20**, 173–179.

37. Schriever-Schwemmer, G., Kliesch, U., and Adler, I.D. (1997) Extruded micronuclei induced by colchicine or acrylamide contain mostly lagging chromosomes identified in paintbrush smears by minor and major mouse DNA probes. *Mutagenesis* **12**, 201–207.

38. Shimizu, N., Shimura, T., and Tanaka, T. (2000) Selective elimination of acentric double minutes from cancer cells through the extrusion of micronuclei. *Mutat. Res.* **448**, 81–90.

39. Schwartz, J.L., and Jordan, R. (1997) Selective elimination of human lymphoid cells with unstable chromosome aberrations by p53-dependent apoptosis. *Carcinogenesis* **18**, 201–205.

40. Bassi, L., Carloni, M., Meschini, R., Fonti, E., and Palitti, F. (2003) X-irradiated human lymphocytes with unstable aberrations and their preferential elimination by p53/survivin-dependent apoptosis. *Int. J. Radiat. Biol.* **79**, 943–954.

41. Taga, M., Shiraishi, K., Shimura, T., Uematsu, N., Oshimura, M., and Niwa, O. (2000) Increased frequencies of gene and chromosome mutations after X-irradiation in mouse embryonal carcinoma cells transfected with the bcl-2 gene. *Jpn. J. Cancer Res.* **91**, 994–1000.

42. Decordier, I., Cundari, E., and Kirsch-Volders, M. (2008) Survival of aneuploidy, micronucleated and/or polyploid cells: crosstalk between ploidy control and apoptosis. *Mutat. Res.* **651**, 30–39.

43. Decordier, I. (2006) Crosstalk between ploidy control and apoptosis in human cells. VUB, Brussels, 237 pp. 229–230.

44. Gruenbaum, Y., Margalit, A., Goldma, R.D., Shumaker, D.K., and Wilson, K.L. (2005) The nuclear lamina comes of age. *Nat. Rev. Mol. Cell. Biol.* **6**, 21–31.

45. Margalit, A., Vlcek, S., Gruenbaum, Y., and Foisner, R. (2005) Breaking and making of the nuclear envelope. *J. Cell. Biochem.* **95**, 454–465.

46. Slee, E.A., Adrain, C., and Martin, S.J. (2001) Executioner caspase-3, -6, and -7 perform distinct, non-redundant roles during the demolition phase of apoptosis. *J. Biol. Chem.* **276**, 7320–7326.

47. Kottke, T.J., Blajeski, A.L., Meng, X.W., Svingen, P.A., Ruchaud, S., Mesner, P.W., Boerner, S.A., Samejima, K., Henriquez, N.V., Chilcote, T.J., Lord, J., Salmon, M., Earnshaw, W.C., and Kaufmann, S.H. (2002) Lack of correlation between caspase activation and caspase activity assays in paclitaxel-treated MCF-7 breast cancer cells. *J. Biol. Chem.* **277**, 804–815.

48. Buendia, B., Santa-Maria, A., and Courvalin, J.C. (1999) Caspase-dependent proteolysis of integral and peripheral proteins of nuclear membranes and nuclear pore complex proteins during apoptosis. *J. Cell. Sci.* **112**, 1743–1753.

49. Aka, P., Mateuca, R., Buchet, J.P., Thierens, H., and Kirsch-Volders, M. (2004) Are genetic polymorphisms in OGG1, XRCC1 and XRCC3 genes predictive for the DNA strand break repair phenotype and genotoxicity in workers exposed to low dose ionising radiations? *Mutat. Res.* **556**, 169–181.

50. Mateuca, R., Aka, P.V., De Boeck, M., Hauspie, R., Kirsch-Volders, M., and Lison, D. (2005) Influence of hOGG1, XRCC1 and XRCC3 genotypes on biomarkers of genotoxicity in workers exposed to cobalt or hard metal dusts. *Toxicol. Lett.* **156**, 277–288.

51. Godderis, L., De Boeck, M., Haufroid, V., Emmery, M., Mateuca, R., Gardinal, S., Kirsch-Volders, M., Veulemans, H., and Lison, D. (2004) Influence of genetic polymorphisms on biomarkers of exposure and genotoxic effects in styrene-exposed workers. *Environ. Mol. Mutagen.* **44**, 293–303.

52. Godderis, L., Aka, P., Mateuca, R., Kirsch-Volders, M., Lison, D., and Veulemans, H. (2006) Dose-dependent influence of genetic polymorphisms on DNA damage induced by styrene oxide, ethylene oxide and gamma-radiation. *Toxicology* **219**, 220–229.

53. Decordier, I., De Bont, K., De Bock, K., Mateuca, R., Roelants, M., Ciardelli, R., Haumont, D., Knudsen, L.E., and Kirsch-Volders, M. (2007) Genetic susceptibility of newborn daughters to oxidative stress. *Toxicol. Lett.* **172**, 68–84.

54. Kirsch-Volders, M., Mateuca, R.A., Roelants, M., Tremp, A., Zeiger, E., Bonassi, S., Holland, N., Chang, W.P., Aka, P.V., Deboeck, M., Godderis, L., Haufroid, V., Ishikawa, H., Laffon. B., Marcos, R., Migliore, L., Norppa, H., Teixeira, J.P., Zijno, A., and Fenech, M. (2006) The effects of GSTM1 and GSTT1 polymorphisms on micronucleus frequencies in human lymphocytes *in vivo*. *Cancer Epidemiol. Biomarkers Prev.* **15**, 1038–1042.

55. Mateuca, R.A., Roelants, M., Iarmarcovai, G., Aka, P.V., Godderis, L., Tremp, A., Bonassi, S., Fenech, M., Bergé-Lefranc, J.L., and Kirsch-Volders, M. (2008) hOGG1326, XRCC1399 and XRCC3241 polymorphisms influence micronucleus frequencies in human lymphocytes *in vivo*. *Mutagenesis* **23**, 35–41.

56. Kimura, M., Umegaki, K., Higuchi, M., Thomas, P., and Fenech, M. (2004) Methylenetetrahydrofolate reductase C677T polymorphism, folic acid and riboflavin are important determinants of genome stability in cultured human lymphocytes. *J. Nutr.* **134**, 48–56.

57. Crott, J.W., Mashiyama, S.T., Ames, B.N., and Fenech, M. (2001) The effect of folic acid deficiency and MTHFR C677T polymorphism on chromosome damage in human lymphocytes *in vitro*. *Cancer Epidemiol. Biomarkers Prev.* **10**, 1089–1096.

58. Zijno, A., Andreoli, C., Leopardi, P., Marcon, F., Rossi, S., Caiola, S., Verdin, A., Galati, R., Cafolla, A., and Crebelli, R. (2003) Folate status, metabolic genotype, and biomarkers of genotoxicity in healthy subjects. *Carcinogenesis* **24**, 1097–1103.

59. Ishikawa, H., Ishikawa, T., Miyatsu, Y., Kurihara, K., Fukao, A., and Yokoyama, K. (2006) A polymorphism of the methionine synthase reductase gene increases chromosomal damage in peripheral lymphocytes in smokers. *Mutat. Res.* **599**, 135–143.

Chapter 8

The Use of Bacterial Repair Endonucleases in the Comet Assay

Andrew R. Collins

Abstract

The comet assay is a sensitive electrophoretic method for measuring DNA breaks at the level of single cells, used widely in genotoxicity experiments, biomonitoring, and in fundamental research. Its sensitivity and range of application are increased by the incorporation of an extra step, after lysis of agarose-embedded cells, in which the DNA is digested with lesion-specific endonucleases (DNA repair enzymes of bacterial or phage origin). Enzymes with specificity for oxidised purines, oxidised pyrimidines, alkylated bases, UV-induced cyclobutane pyrimidine dimers, and misincorporated uracil have been employed. The additional enzyme-sensitive sites, over and above the strand breaks detected in the standard comet assay, give a quantitative estimate of the number of specific lesions present in the cells.

Key words: Comet assay, DNA damage, Altered bases, Electrophoresis, Repair endonucleases

1. Introduction

The comet assay (single cell gel electrophoresis) is widely used in genetic toxicology for measuring DNA damage in the form of strand breaks (SBs). It can be applied to cells from animal tissues after *in vivo* testing or to cultured cells used in *in vitro* experiments. Cells are embedded in agarose on a microscope slide, and lysed with 2.5 M NaCl and non-ionic detergent; this removes membranes and soluble cell components, including most of the histones, leaving the DNA still attached to the nuclear matrix in a structure known as a nucleoid. Although the nucleosomes (round which the DNA is wound in the living cell) are disrupted by the removal of histones, the turns of the DNA around the histone–nucleosome core are retained in the form of (negative) supercoils. The DNA is not free to rotate, being constrained as a series of loops attached at their bases to the matrix.

Jean-Charles Gautier (ed.), *Drug Safety Evaluation: Methods and Protocols*, Methods in Molecular Biology, vol. 691, DOI 10.1007/978-1-60761-849-2_8, © Springer Science+Business Media, LLC 2011

After lysis, the gel-embedded nucleoids are incubated in an alkaline solution and then electrophoresed at high pH. DNA is attracted to the anode, but little migration occurs unless there are breaks present in the DNA. A single break in a DNA loop relaxes supercoiling in the loop, and it is then free to extend. After electrophoresis, gels are neutralised and "comets" visualised by fluorescence microscopy with a suitable stain. The relative intensity of fluorescence in the comet tail, reflecting the number of relaxed DNA loops, is thus a quantitative measure of DNA break frequency.

SBs are just one form of DNA damage. Most chemical genotoxic agents induce other kinds of damage, such as small base changes (oxidation or alkylation), base loss, cross-links, or addition of large chemical groups (bulky adducts). Enzymes with specific endonucleolytic activity against some of these DNA lesions have been employed in conjunction with the comet assay to enhance its sensitivity and selectivity. The gels containing nucleoids are incubated with enzyme following the lysis step, in parallel with control gels incubated with enzyme buffer alone. Thus, endonuclease III or Nth (EC 4.2.99.18) is used to detect oxidised pyrimidines (1); formamidopyrimidine DNA glycosylase (FPG: EC 3.2.2.23) recognises oxidised guanines (2); and 3-methyladenine DNA glycosylase or AlkA (EC 3.2.2.21) has activity against alkylated bases (3). T4 endonuclease V, also known as DenV endonuclease V (EC 3.1.25.1), repairs UV-damaged DNA, and has been used to detect cyclobutane pyrimidime dimers in the comet assay (4). Uracil DNA glycosylase (UDG: EC 3.2.2.3) detects uracil that has been misincorporated in DNA (5). UvrABC, which recognises bulky adducts, unfortunately has not yet been used successfully in the comet assay. Net enzyme-sensitive sites are calculated by subtracting the comet score for the enzyme buffer control from the comet score for digestion with enzyme.

This article describes the use of specific endonucleolytic enzymes in this way. A general knowledge of the comet assay is assumed, or the reader is referred to a review article such as (6). However, sufficient information is included to enable the assay for specific DNA damage to be set up without prior comet assay experience.

2. Materials

2.1. Equipment

Standard comet assay equipment (electrophoresis tank, power supply, fluorescence microscope).

Staining jars, vertical or horizontal (depending on how many slides are to be incubated).

Enzyme incubation box: this can be a plastic food-storage box with lid, with water in the bottom to maintain humidity, and a platform above the water for the slides to be placed on. The box should be kept at 37°C (pre-warmed so that the enzyme reaction is optimal).

2.2. Solutions

Prepare solutions from appropriate stocks, such as 0.5 M Na_2EDTA, 1 M Tris base, 10 M NaOH, 1 M KCl, etc. Keep solutions at 4°C. It is also useful to keep a stock of distilled water at 4°C for rapid preparation of cold solutions.

1. Lysis solution: 2.5 M NaCl, 0.1 M EDTA, 10 mM Tris base. Prepare 1 l. Set pH to 10 with either solid NaOH or preferably concentrated (10 M) NaOH solution. Add 35 ml of NaOH straight away to ensure that EDTA dissolves, and then add dropwise to pH 10. Add 1 ml Triton X-100 per 100 ml immediately before use.

2. Enzyme reaction buffer (see Notes 1 and 2): 40 mM HEPES, 0.1 M KCl, 0.5 mM EDTA, 0.2 mg/ml bovine serum albumin, pH 8.0 with KOH. This buffer can be made as 10× stock, adjusted to pH 8.0 and frozen at −20°C.

3. Electrophoresis solution: 0.3 M NaOH, 1 mM EDTA.

4. Neutralising buffer: Phosphate-buffered saline (PBS) (see Note 3).

5. 4′6-diamidine-2-phenylindol dihydrochloride (DAPI) 1 μg/ml in distilled H_2O (stored at −20°C)

6. Agarose: Normal melting point, electrophoresis grade and low melting point (LMP) (necessary for embedding cells at 37°C).

7. Enzymes: the repair enzymes endonuclease III, FPG (see Note 4), T4 endonuclease V, AlkA, and UDG may be obtained commercially in purified form, in which case the supplier's instructions for use should be followed. An alternative source is the various researchers who produce their own enzyme from bacteria containing overproducing plasmids. Crude extract is generally satisfactory because the enzyme represents such a high proportion of the protein in the extract, and there is unlikely to be significant non-specific nuclease activity.

The final working dilution of the enzyme will vary from batch to batch (see Note 5). To illustrate the best way to handle the enzymes (avoiding repeated freezing and thawing and minimising wastage), we refer here to FPG as an example, with a recommended final dilution of 3,000×. On receipt, the enzyme (which should have been frozen in transit) should be dispensed into small aliquots (say, 5 μl) and stored at −80°C (this minimises repeated freezing and thawing). Take one of these aliquots and dilute to 0.5 ml using the regular enzyme reaction buffer – with the addition of 10% glycerol. Dispense this into 10 μl aliquots (label as "100× diluted") and freeze at –80°C. For use, dilute one of these 10 μl aliquots to 300 μl with buffer (no glycerol) and keep on ice until you add it to the gels: do not refreeze this working solution.

3. Methods

3.1. Preparing Agarose

1. Normal melting point agarose is used for precoating slides. Prepare a 1% solution in water, heating in a microwave oven to near boiling point, shaking occasionally; the agarose should form a transparent gel. It can then be cooled, stored at 4°C, and melted in the microwave oven whenever needed for precoating slides.

2. LMP agarose is used for the gel containing cells. Prepare a 1% solution in PBS, dissolving the agarose by heating, as above. Make no more than 10 or 20 ml (enough for several experiments). If a larger quantity is made, and repeatedly melted, evaporation occurs and the concentration is then significantly higher than 1%.

3.2. Slide Preparation

Early versions of the comet assay used fully frosted slides, which give good anchorage for agarose, but can only be used a few times before agarose layers begin to detach. The use of ordinary clear glass slides with frosted end, precoated with agarose, is now recommended. The use of plain slides (as well as being cheaper) has the advantage that, if slides are dried down after electrophoresis for storage and later examination, the comets (now very close to the glass surface) do not suffer from the high background of reflection from the frosted surface. Another advantage is that the comets, after drying, are in the same plane, obviating the need for constant refocusing.

1. Dip each slide in a beaker of melted 1% standard agarose in H$_2$O.

2. Drain off excess agarose, wiping the back clean with tissue.

3. Leave the slides, coated side up, on a clean surface at 37°C overnight to dry.

4. Mark one corner of the frosted end to indicate which side of the slide is coated.

5. Slides can then be returned to a slide box for storage at room temperature until needed.

6. (The slides for precoating should be grease-free; clean if necessary by soaking in alcohol and then wiping dry with a clean tissue.)

3.3. Embedding Cells in Agarose

1. Suspend cells in PBS at approximately 10^6/ml.

2. For each slide, take an aliquot of 40 µl in a microcentrifuge tube.

3. Quickly add 140 µl of 1% LMP agarose in PBS at 37°C and mix by tapping the tube and then pipet once up and down.

4. Using a 70 µl pipettor, quickly place two separate drops on one slide, and cover each with an 18 × 18 mm coverslip. Work quickly as the agarose sets quickly at room temperature.

5. Leave the slides on a cold metal plate at 4°C for 5 min. Cells maintain metabolic activity even after embedding, and can be treated in the gel with DNA-damaging agents, and then incubated in medium to monitor DNA repair (7) (see Note 6).

3.4. Lysis

1. Add 1 ml Triton X-100 to 100 ml of lysis solution (4°C). Use a pipettor tip with the end cut off, as Triton is viscous.

2. Mix thoroughly.

3. Remove cover slips from slides and place in this solution in a staining jar.

4. Leave at 4°C for 1 h (see Note 6).

3.5. Enzyme Incubation

1. Prepare 300 ml of enzyme reaction buffer. Put aside a few ml for enzyme dilutions.

2. Wash slides in three changes of this buffer (4°C) in a staining jar, for 5 min each in order to equilibrate with enzyme buffer.

3. Dilute an aliquot of enzyme with enzyme buffer. The final dilution of the working solution will vary from batch to batch.

4. Remove slides from last wash, and dab off excess liquid with tissue.

5. Place 50 µl of enzyme solution (or buffer alone, as control) onto each gel, and cover with 22 × 22 mm cover slip. As an alternative, you can cover the gel with a square cut from Parafilm (see Note 7).

6. Put slides into moist box (to prevent desiccation) and incubate at 37°C for 45 min.

3.6. Alkaline Treatment and Electrophoresis

1. Ensure that electrophoresis solution is cold before use, e.g. by pouring into the electrophoresis tank in the cold room an hour or so before it is needed.

2. Gently place slides (minus cover slips) on platform in tank, forming one or two complete rows (gaps should be filled with blank slides). Gels must be (just) covered with electrophoresis solution.

3. Leave for 40 min.

4. For most tanks (i.e. of standard size), run at 25 V (constant voltage setting) for 30 min (see Note 8). If there is too much

electrolyte covering the slides, the current may be so high that it exceeds the maximum – so set this at a high level. If necessary, i.e. if 25 V is not reached, remove some solution. Normally, the current is around 300 mA.

3.7. Neutralisation and Staining

1. Wash 5 min with neutralising buffer in staining jar at 4°C, followed by 5 min in water; then dry (room temperature) for storage (or proceed to stain immediately).

2. Stain with DAPI: place 20 µl of a 1 µg/ml solution DAPI in distilled H_2O (stored at –20°C) onto each slide and cover with a 22×22 mm cover slip.

3. Keep slides in a dark, moist chamber until they are viewed. They may be left overnight before viewing, either stained or unstained (however, if stained, some fluorescence is lost) (see Note 9).

3.8. Image Analysis and Calculation

1. Image analysis. Generally, 50 or 100 comets are analysed per gel. There are numerous commercially available comet image analysis software packages, linked to a charge-coupled device (CCD) camera, or visual scoring can be used (see (6) for details). Visual scoring depends on sorting comets into one of the five classes with "values" from 0, no visible tail, to 4, almost all DNA in tail, and adding the individual values for 100 comets to give a score of between 0 and 400 arbitrary units. The computer-based systems offer a selection of parameters, some more useful than others. Comet tail length is only useful at very low damage levels; once the tail is established its length hardly changes as the damage level increases (as expected if the tail is a collection of relaxed DNA loops). % Tail DNA is the most useful parameter, being proportional to DNA break frequency over a relatively wide range of damage levels before saturation is reached. Tail moment combines tail length and intensity (% tail DNA), and is unaccountably popular. It does not show a linear relation to break frequency, since it includes the tail length factor which saturates at low dose. Furthermore, it deprives us of valuable information: it has no generally recognised units, and so there is no way of visualising a comet of a particular tail moment value. In contrast, given a value of % tail DNA, it is immediately clear what kind of comet is being described.

2. Calculation. The control gels (no enzyme treatment) provide an estimate of the background level of SBs (strictly speaking, strand breaks plus alkali-labile sites) in the DNA. The enzyme-treated gels reveal strand breaks plus base damage (SBs + BD). Assuming a linear dose response, whether working in % DNA in tail or in arbitrary units, subtraction of SBs from (SBs + BD) gives net enzyme-sensitive sites as a measure of damaged bases (see Note 10).

3. Calibration. Ionising radiation produces SBs in DNA with known efficiency. If the breaks introduced in cells by different doses of X-rays are detected with the comet assay, a standard curve can be drawn, with break frequency expressed as Gray-equivalents, or as breaks per unit length of DNA (8).

3.9. Storage and Re-Examination

1. Place slides in a warm oven, or leave on bench, until the gel has dried.

2. Slides can then be stored at room temperature.

3. For re-examination, stain as above.

3.10. Quality Control

1. Reference standards: It is important to include cells containing DNA damage as a positive control in experiments to assess genotoxicity. When the lesion-specific enzymes are being used in the comet assay, the reference cells should be treated with an appropriate agent, i.e. an alkylating agent for AlkA, UV(C) for T4 endonuclease V, a reactive oxygen generating agent for FPG or endonuclease III. (H_2O_2 is often used, but as it produces many SBs as well as oxidised bases, it is important to incubate the cells to allow repair of these breaks (see Note 5).

   When measuring DNA damage in human lymphocytes, as part of a population study, standard lymphocyte samples should be included in every batch of samples (e.g. on one day each week). The standard lymphocytes are prepared from 50 ml of blood from one or more donors; after isolation the lymphocytes are pooled, counted, and aliquoted at about 10^6/ml in ice-cold freezing medium (cell culture medium, e.g. MEM or RPMI, with 10% foetal calf serum and 10% DMSO), each tube containing enough cells for several gels. Freeze slowly to $-80°C$ and store until needed. Results from the standard lymphocytes should not show variation from week to week; if they do, there is a problem with the procedure which should be sorted out. If the variation is large, then the samples may need to be re-analysed.

2. Visual scoring and image analysis: If using visual scoring, each operator should be "calibrated" against the computer image analysis system at regular intervals. This simply involves scoring comets on a slide showing a range of damage levels, visually (classes 0–4) and then by computer image analysis (% DNA in tail), until there are 20 of each class. For all class 0 comets, calculate the mean % DNA in tail, and similarly for all comets of the other classes. Then, plot *mean % DNA in tail* against *comet class*. The resulting line is unlikely to be perfectly straight, but should show a near-linear relationship. More important than the exact relationship is the point that individual operators should be trained (if necessary) to give a similar "calibration curve" when plotted in this way.

3.11. Interpretation of Results

In comet assay experiments with enzymes, there should always be a "buffer control", incubated alongside the enzyme-treated gels but without enzyme. After alkaline treatment and electrophoresis, this gives the level of SBs plus alkali-labile sites. Subtracting the buffer control value from the value obtained with enzyme gives "net enzyme-sensitive sites" (but see Note 10), and this is the preferred way to express results – rather than the combined total of SBs plus enzyme-sensitive sites.

Careful use of lesion-specific endonucleases in the comet assay can give valuable information about the different kinds of DNA damage that may be present, either as "natural" background, or induced by a particular genotoxic agent. However, it is important to be aware that the enzyme specificities are not absolute. FPG-sensitive sites are often equated with 8-oxoguanine (9), but FPG also recognises purine breakdown products, formamidopyrimidines (fapy). Speit et al. (10) reported the recognition by FPG of alkylation damage. Endonuclease III recognises a range of oxidised pyrimidines. AlkA has as its main substrate 3-methyladenine, but will also attack other alkylated bases and even, at high enough concentration, undamaged DNA (11). In addition, many of the enzymes have a hydrolytic activity against AP sites (apurinic/apyrimidinic sites), which occur in DNA spontaneously. This should not be a problem, since AP sites are alkali-labile, and therefore should appear as SBs and be included in the enzyme buffer control score – but it has not been definitively established that the comet assay conditions are sufficiently alkaline to break all AP sites.

4. Notes

1. The HEPES buffer is used for FPG, endonuclease III, AlkA, and T4 endonuclease V. The recommended buffer for UDG is: 60 mM Tris–HCl, 1 mM EDTA, pH 8.0.

2. The buffer in which the enzyme is prepared and stored normally contains β-mercaptoethanol or dithiothreitol to preserve the enzyme. However, inclusion of sulphydryl reagents in the reaction buffer significantly increases background DNA breakage. It is therefore recommended to omit this reagent from the reaction buffer.

3. Three washes in 0.4 M neutral Tris buffer were originally recommended for neutralising gels after electrophoresis. One wash in standard, cheaper buffer, such as PBS is adequate. Even water will bring the pH down to a level at which DNA no longer unwinds, which is all that is required.

4. OGG1, the mammalian analogue of FPG, has been used in the comet assay (12). It has a rather narrower specificity, detecting 8-oxoguanine and methyl fapy guanine but is as yet

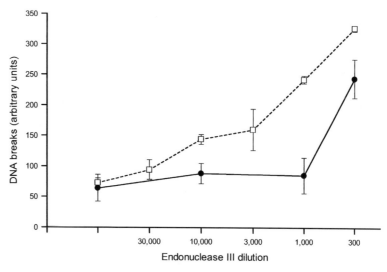

Fig. 1. Titration of endonuclease III. HeLa cells were incubated with 0.6 mM H_2O_2 for 5 min on ice, to induce strand breaks and oxidised bases. During subsequent incubation at 37°C for 45 min, the strand breaks were repaired, leaving oxidised bases. Slides were prepared for the comet assay, and after lysis, gels were incubated with endonuclease III at different dilutions from the stock (and without enzyme – data on far left), and breaks measured by visual scoring (range 0–400). *Solid symbols* (*filled circle*): control cells, not treated with H_2O_2. *Open symbols* (*square*): after H_2O_2 and incubation. *Bars* indicate range, in duplicate experiments. At high enzyme concentrations, non-specific DNA breakage occurs (as is seen from the steep rise in breaks in the DNA from the untreated cells). The working range of the endonuclease III is therefore a dilution of 10,000- to 3,000-fold.

not routinely used if only because it is not available in large quantities from an overproducing plasmid.

5. Suppliers of enzyme will normally recommend a working concentration and incubation time. However, you are recommended to carry out a titration experiment, varying both incubation period and enzyme concentration, to be sure that damage detection is optimised. To do this, cells containing the specific damage are required. HeLa cells (or another common transformed cell line) can be treated with H_2O_2, and incubated for 1 h so that virtually all SBs are repaired, leaving oxidised bases, which are much more slowly repaired by the cell (see Fig. 1). Incubation of cells with a photosensitiser, Ro19-8022 (supplied by F. Hoffmann-La Roche), followed by irradiation with visible light, induces 8-oxoguanine and provides a good substrate for titrating FPG. Alkylation damage can be induced by treating cells with methylmethanesulphonate. UV(C) irradiation induces cyclobutane pyrimidine dimers that can be used to titrate UV endonuclease.

6. Sometimes, cells are treated with a genotoxic chemical after embedding in the gel. If this is the case, it is advisable to dip the slides in water before lysis, and to keep treated and control slides in separate lysis vessels to avoid cross-contamination.

7. If dealing with a large number of slides, carry out this step (addition of enzyme) with the slides on a cold plate before transferring to the moist box, to ensure that they all have the same period of incubation at 37°C.

8. It is the voltage drop across the gels that causes the movement of DNA into the tail. The current is not critical (8).

9. Propidium iodide (2.5 μg/ml), Hoechst 33258 (0.5 μg/ml), ethidium bromide (20 μg/ml), or SybrGold (10–25,000 diluted with respect to manufacturer's stock) are often used in place of DAPI for the visualisation of comet DNA.

10. Subtraction of the comet score for enzyme buffer control from the score for enzyme digestion gives an accurate estimate of net enzyme-sensitive sites – if the response curve for the relative tail intensity against DNA break frequency is linear. This is the case at relatively low damage levels, but at higher levels the assay tends towards saturation, and the curve is distinctly non-linear. In that case, it is necessary to calibrate the assay, for example, using ionising radiation as a standard DNA-damaging agent so that results can be expressed as, e.g. Gray equivalents or DNA breaks per 10^9 Da (since the DNA breakage efficiency of radiation is known).

Acknowledgments

I thank Katja Lange and Anna Tirado for excellent technical support.

References

1. Collins, A.R., Duthie, S.J., and Dobson, V.L. (1993) Direct enzymic detection of endogenous oxidative base damage in human lymphocyte DNA. *Carcinogenesis* **14**, 1733–1735.

2. Dusinska, M., and Collins, A. (1996) Detection of oxidised purines and UV-induced photoproducts in DNA of single cells, by inclusion of lesion-specific enzymes in the comet assay. *Alternatives to Laboratory Animals* **24**, 405–411.

3. Collins, A.R., Dusinska, M., and Horska, A. (2001) Detection of alkylation damage in human lymphocyte DNA with the comet assay. *Acta Biochimica Polonica* **48**, 611–614.

4. Collins, A.R., Mitchell, D.L., Zunino, A., de Wit, J., and Busch, D. (1997) UV-sensitive rodent mutant cell lines of complementation groups 6 and 8 differ phenotypically from their human counterparts. *Environmental and Molecular Mutagenesis* **29**, 152–160.

5. Duthie, S.J., and McMillan, P. (1997) Uracil misincorporation in human DNA detected using single cell gel electrophoresis. *Carcinogenesis* **18**, 1709–1714.

6. Collins, A.R. (2004) The comet assay for DNA damage and repair. *Molecular Biotechnology* **26**, 249–261.

7. Collins, A.R., and Horvathova, E. (2001) Oxidative DNA damage, antioxidants and DNA repair; applications of the comet assay. *Biochemical Society Transactions* **29**, 337–341.

8. Collins, A.R., Azqueta Oscoz, A., Brunborg, G. et al. (2008) The comet assay: topical issues. *Mutagenesis* **23**, 143–151.

9. Collins, A.R., Cadet, J., Moller, L., Poulsen, H.E., and Vina, J. (2004) Are we sure we know how to measure 8-oxo-7,8-dihydroguanine in DNA from human cells? *Archives of Biochemistry and Biophysics* **423**, 57–65.

10. Speit, G., Schütz, P., Bonzheim, I., Trenz, K., and Hoffmann, H. (2004) Sensitivity of the FPG protein towards alkylation damage in the comet assay. *Toxicology Letters* **146**, 151–158.

11. Berdal, K.G., Johansen, R.F., and Seeberg, E. (1998) Release of normal bases from intact DNA by a native DNA repair enzyme. *EMBO Journal* **17**, 363–367.

12. Smith, C.C., O'Donovan, M.R., and Martin, E.A. (2006) hOGG1 recognizes oxidative damage using the comet assay with greater specificity than FPG or ENDOIII. *Mutagenesis* **21(3)**, 185–190.

Part IV

Safety Pharmacology

Chapter 9

Manual Whole-Cell Patch-Clamping of the HERG Cardiac K⁺ Channel

Xiao-Liang Chen, Jiesheng Kang, and David Rampe

Abstract

Delayed ventricular repolarization, as measured by a prolongation of the QT interval on the electrocardiogram, is a major safety issue in the drug development process. It is now recognized that most cases of drug-induced QT prolongation arise from direct pharmacological inhibition of the human *ether-a-go-go*-related gene (HERG) cardiac K⁺ channel. It is standard practice to test a drug's ability to interact with the HERG channel prior to entry into clinical trials. This testing is used, as part of a larger battery of tests, to help predict the cardiac safety profile of a drug. Manual whole-cell patch-clamping provides the most sensitive and accurate way to examine the biophysical and pharmacological properties of the HERG cardiac K⁺ channel.

Key words: HERG, Patch-clamp, Potassium channels, Arrhythmia, *Torsades de pointes*, QT interval

1. Introduction

Voltage-dependent ion channels are membrane-spanning proteins that control electrical activity in the human heart. During the heartbeat, the opening of voltage-dependent Na⁺ and Ca⁺⁺ channels produces excitation and contraction of the myocardium while the reversal of this process, known as repolarization, is primarily carried out by the opening of voltage-dependent K⁺ channels. Several distinct types of voltage-dependent K⁺ channels are known to exist in human cardiac myocytes. The human *ether-a-go-go*-related gene (HERG) encodes one of these K⁺ channels (1). The HERG cardiac K⁺ channel contributes to repolarization in the human heart, and its activity helps to determine the length of the QT interval measured on the electrocardiogram (ECG).

A major safety concern in the drug development process is a phenomenon known as acquired long QT syndrome. Acquired

Jean-Charles Gautier (ed.), *Drug Safety Evaluation: Methods and Protocols*, Methods in Molecular Biology, vol. 691,
DOI 10.1007/978-1-60761-849-2_9, © Springer Science+Business Media, LLC 2011

long QT syndrome occurs when a drug, often as an unintended side effect, delays the repolarization process of the heart. This effect is measured as a prolongation of the QT interval on the ECG. Prolongation of cardiac repolarization can result in the sometimes fatal ventricular arrhythmia known as *torsades de pointes*. Over the past decade, a number of marketed drugs have been withdrawn, or their use severely restricted, because they produced QT prolongation and *torsades de pointes* arrhythmia. These include drugs from many pharmacological classes, including antipsychotics (pimozide, sertindole, and thioridazine), antihistamines (terfenadine and astemizole), antibiotics (grepafloxacin), and gastric prokinetics (cisapride). Furthermore, it has been revealed that virtually all cases of acquired long QT syndrome result from drugs specifically inhibiting the HERG cardiac K^+ channel (2). This appears to be due to the unique architecture of the channel that allows it to bind, and to be inhibited by, a wide range of structurally distinct molecules (3, 4). For this reason, elimination of drug/HERG interactions has become a major focus of the pharmaceutical industry and has led to the creation of a branch of safety pharmacology that specifically studies HERG and the consequences of its inhibition.

As is the case with most ion channels, a variety of assays have been developed to measure the interactions of drugs with HERG. These include radioligand binding, Rb^+ efflux, and newer "high-throughput" electrophysiological assays (5, 6). All of these assays can provide information on drug/HERG interactions and are used to varying degrees in the drug development process. However, it is generally accepted that none of these assays provides the degree of reliability and accuracy that is obtained with the "classical" manual patch-clamp technique. By "classical" we mean the measurement of HERG channel currents in single cells stably expressing the channel protein, using the whole-cell configuration of the patch-clamp technique (7). A description of the set-up and basic principles of patch clamp electrophysiology is far beyond the scope of this paper, and so it must be assumed that the reader has some background in this technique. Instead, the intent of this manuscript is to provide the reader with some basic insights and common problems associated with measuring HERG channel currents using standard whole-cell electrophysiology. Nevertheless, we have also made an effort to describe in some detail the equipment that we use in an effort to make this paper as complete as possible. Likewise, this paper is not intended to describe the molecular biology techniques involved in the cloning and stable expression of the cDNA encoding HERG. Cell lines stably expressing the channel are available from a variety of commercial and academic sources or can be produced "from scratch" by those familiar with molecular cloning techniques. The method described here uses Chinese hamster ovary (CHO) cells stably transfected with HERG. With these caveats in mind, this paper describes the materials and methods necessary to conduct whole-cell patch-clamping of the HERG channel stably expressed in CHO cells.

2. Materials

2.1. Cell Preparation

1. F-12 nutrient mixture (Ham, Gibco/Invitrogen, Grand Island, NY).
2. Fetal bovine serum (FBS, Gibco/Invitrogen) stored in aliquots of 50 mL at –20°C.
3. Geneticin (50 mg/mL, Gibco/Invitrogen).
4. Penicillin/Streptomycin mixture (5,000 units/mL of penicillin and 5,000 μg/mL of streptomycin, Gibco/Invitrogen) stored in aliquots of 10 mL at –20°C.
5. Trypsin (0.25%, Gibco/Invitrogen).
6. Phosphate-buffered saline (PBS, Gibco/Invitrogen).
7. Thermanox plastic coverslips (diameter: 13 mm, Nalge Nunc International, Rochester, NY).
8. 75 cm² cell culture flask (Corning, Corning, NY).
9. 35 × 10 mm Petri dish (BD Biosciences, Bedford, MA).
10. CHO cells (American Type Culture Collection, Rockville, MD) expressing the HERG cardiac K+ channel.

2.2. Perfusion System

1. Teflon tubing (ID 1/32″, Cole-Parmer Instrument Company, Vernon Hills, IL).
2. Recording Chamber (see Note 1).
3. Stopcock (Harvard Apparatus, Holliston, MA).

2.3. Electrophysiology

1. Micropipette puller (Sutter Instruments Co., Novato, CA).
2. Glass capillary tubes (TW 150F-4, World Precision Instruments, Sarasota, FL).
3. Computer (IBM Personal Computer).
4. Inverted microscope (Nikon TE300, Tokyo, Japan).
5. Macromanipulator (Narishige MMN-1, Tokyo, Japan).
6. Micromanipulator (Narishige MW-3).
7. Axopatch 200B amplifier and corresponding headstage/hardware (Danahar Corporation, Union City, CA).
8. pCLAMP software (Clampex, Danahar Corporation).

2.4. Experiment Solutions

1. Internal (pipette) solution: 120 mM potassium aspartate, 20 mM KCl, 4 mM Na_2ATP, 5 mM HEPES, and 1 mM $MgCl_2$ (pH 7.2 adjusted with 8 N KOH). Solutions are prepared in deionized water. Generally 100 mL are made and stored in aliquots of 1–2 mL at $-20°C$.

2. External recording solution: A physiological saline solution (PSS) which contains 130 mM NaCl, 4 mM KCl, 2.8 mM sodium acetate, 1 mM $MgCl_2$, 10 mM HEPES, 10 mM glucose, and 1 mM $CaCl_2$ (pH 7.4 adjusted with 10 N NaOH). Usually, several liters of solutions are prepared in deionized water and stored refrigerated.

3. Methods

Electrophysiologists are sometimes reluctant to use a method developed in another laboratory. One reason for this is that patch clamp electrophysiology is a complex and delicate procedure that can be described as part science and part art form. Over time, each laboratory discovers their own set of "tricks" that seem to improve the accuracy, reliability, and success rate of their experiments. In the following methods section, we describe many basic electrophysiolgical techniques for the successful recording of the HERG channel currents as well as insights gained from our own particular experience. These methods have been employed by our laboratory, usually for screening drug effects, since we began measuring the HERG channel currents more than 10 years ago. After testing thousands of compounds, we have found the assay to be sensitive, reproducible and, as far as patch-clamping goes, relatively easy.

3.1. Cell Preparation

1. The CHO cell line is used to express the HERG channel since the cell line is easy to grow, lends itself quite well to patch clamp electrophysiology, and does not have significant endogenous potassium channel currents (8). CHO cells were transfected with cDNA encoding the HERG channel using Lipofectamine (Gibco/Invitrogen). The selection was carried out using 400 mg/mL Geneticin. Expression of HERG channels in the selected cell lines was confirmed by recording outward potassium currents that had biophysical and pharmacological properties characteristic of the HERG channel using patch clamp electrophysiology (8). One selected cell line was expanded and many vials of cells were frozen in a liquid nitrogen tank for long-term storage and future use using Recovery Cell Culture Freezing Medium (Gibco/Invitrogen).

2. Place one tube (50 mL) of FBS, one tube (10 mL) of penicillin/streptomycin, one bottle of Geneticin, and one bottle (500 mL) of F-12 (Ham) in a bath of warm water (approximately 37°C – exact temperature is not critical).

3. Use a biological safety cabinet, serological pipettes, and pipette-aid to add 5 mL of Geneticin, 10 mL of penicillin/streptomycin mixture, and 50 mL of FBS into 500 mL of F-12 nutrient mixture (Ham). Cells will be grown in this culture medium. This culture medium can also be kept in the refrigerator for later use.

4. Add about 30 mL of culture medium to a 50-mL tube. Remove a vial containing the CHO cells stably expressing the HERG channel from the liquid nitrogen storage tank and immediately place the vial into a bath of warm water (approximately 37°C – exact temperature is not critical). Gently shake the vial. As soon as the contents have thawed, remove the cap and place the contents of the vial into the 50 mL tube containing the culture medium.

5. At room temperature, centrifuge the cell suspension at approximately 3,000 RPM for 3 min. Remove and discard the supernatant by aspirating. Add 10 mL of culture medium to the tube and gently resuspend the cell pellet.

6. After the resuspension, plate the cells directly on coverslips in a 35×10 mm Petri dish for patch-clamp experiments the next day (see step 8–9 for more details) or seed cells into a 75 cm² cell culture flask for expansion for 1–3 days.

7. If expanding the cells, grow them to approximately 75% confluency in 75 cm² cell culture flasks. At this time, discard the media by aspirating, add 10 mL of PBS to washout the culture medium and discard the PBS. Add 2 mL of 0.25% Trypsin, and gently shake the flask for about 2 min, then discard the Trypsin by aspirating. Then, add 10 mL of culture medium to the flask and gently resuspend the cells. Seed the cells in suspension for further expansion (see Note 2) or plate them on coverslips for electrophysiological experiments.

8. Put 3–4 coverslips in each of 2–8, 35×10 mm Petri dishes. To the Petri dishes, add culture medium and the cell suspension, in a ratio to achieve the desired cell density (~4,000 cells/mL – a microscope is useful for assessing the cell density, which is not critical but should be sufficiently low so that single cells can be easily found after 1–2 days of growth). Use forceps to push down the coverslips to the bottom of the Petri dishes.

9. Put the culture dishes into an incubator gassed with 95% air/5% CO_2 and set at 37°C. Cells can be used for electrophysiological recordings after approximately 12 h of growth.

3.2. Electrophysiology

1. Conduct electrophysiology experiments at room temperature (see Note 3).

2. Using the micropipette puller, fabricate several electrodes from capillary tubes (TW150F-4). The resistance of the electrodes should be approximately 2–4 MΩ (see Note 4).

3. Set up a simple perfusion apparatus to deliver external recording solution to the cells (Fig. 1). Fill the solution reservoir with PSS and initiate the perfusion by suction (see Note 5). Set flow speed at approximately 2–3 mL/min (adjusted using the stopcock). Do not change flow speed during the course of the experiment since change in flow speed can result in a change in the HERG current amplitude.

4. Place a coverslip with CHO cells into the chamber using a pair of forceps. Gently tamp the coverslip down to prevent it from floating or drifting.

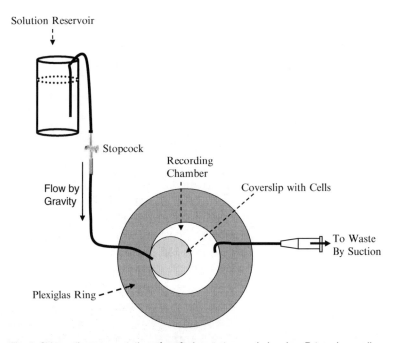

Fig. 1. Schematic representation of perfusion system and chamber. External recording solution bathes the cells that are grown on coverslips and placed in the chamber (Plexiglas ring). A shelf is affixed to the inside of the Faraday cage used for patch clamp recording. This shelf holds the solution reservoir. Solution flows via gravity to the chamber, where it is suctioned off by the use of small tubing connected to a vacuum source. This particular schematic shows a very basic perfusion system. The system can be modified to accommodate several reservoirs (that for example contain multiple drug concentrations) that can be connected thus enabling the conduct of concentration-response studies.

5. Identify a single cell suitable for patch clamp experiments (see Note 6).

6. Back-fill an electrode with internal solution using a fine needle (Microfil made by World Precision Instruments, Inc., Sarasota, FL) attached to a 1-mL syringe. Insert the electrode into the holder of the headstage, and place the tip of the electrode into the PSS flowing through the chamber.

7. Set the holding potential at 0 mV. At a rate of 5–10 Hz, apply a short (approximately 10 ms) 5 mV pulse. Examine the rectangular waveform that is generated. Make sure that the electrode resistance is approximately 2–4 MΩ. If not, inspect the electrode under the microscope to see if it is clogged or broken. If clogged or broken, prepare a new one.

8. Using the macro- and micromanipulators, move the electrode tip near the cell. Zero the current using the amplifier's offset knob. Move the electrode tip to touch the cell surface using the micromanipulator (Fig. 2). Apply gentle suction to the electrode by using the tubing connecting to the electrode holder, while watching the rectangle wave whose amplitude is inversely proportional to the seal resistance. When the amplitude begins to decrease, switch the holding potential from 0 to –80 mV and release the negative pressure from the electrode (switching the holding potential to –80 mV and releasing the negative pressure of electrode will help seal formation). If a gigaohm seal (seal resistance >1 GΩ) is not formed within 15–20 s, apply gentle suction 2–3 more times to aid seal formation. If still unsuccessful, try a new cell with a new electrode.

9. When a gigaohm seal is established, the rectangular wave will disappear and two small spikes emerge as capacity transients.

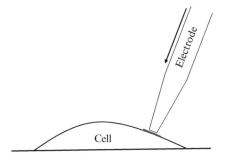

Fig. 2. Schematic representation of electrode/cell interaction during seal formation. The Figure assumes that the manipulators are mounted on the right-hand side of the microscope. The *arrow* indicates the direction in which the electrode is moving. The angle of the electrode relative to the bottom of the chamber should be as steep as possible, but at least greater than 45° (in practice, this angle is limited by the working distance of the microscope). In order to get high resistance seals, move the electrode in a perpendicular direction to that of the patching area to touch the membrane.

Cancel the spikes so that the waveform appears as a flat line by using the amplifier's Pipette Capacitance Compensation (fast and slow) knobs.

10. Break the cell membrane inside the pipette tip to obtain a whole-cell configuration by applying a stronger suction to the electrode, or by disrupting the membrane using the ZAP function on the amplifier. When the membrane is broken and the whole-cell configuration is established, two large capacity transient spikes will appear.

11. Adjust both whole cell capacitance and series resistance control knobs on the amplifier simultaneously to minimize the capacity transients. When the transients are minimized, record the cell capacitance and access resistance from the whole cell capacitance control and series resistance control, respectively.

12. To record currents at room temperature, a two-step protocol is used. From a holding potential of –80 mV, the cell is depolarized to +20 mV for 2 s. The cell is then immediately repolarized to –40 mV for 1.6 s to generate large outward tail currents, before again being returned to –80 mV. The protocol is repeated every 10 s. Currents should be recorded for 1–2 min to allow stabilization prior to any experiment. Figure 3 illustrates what acceptable HERG currents should look like using this recording protocol.

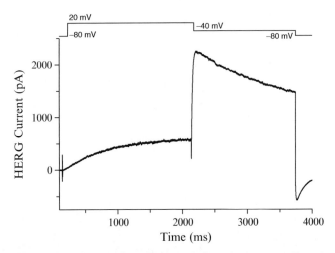

Fig. 3. HERG channel currents. Following the establishment of a gigaohm seal and rupture of the membrane to obtain the whole-cell configuration, HERG currents are generated from a holding potential of –80 mV. Upon depolarization to +20 mV, a slowly rising current appears. At this potential, both channel activation as well as fast, voltage-dependent inactivation processes are occurring. Upon repolarization to –40 mV, inactivation is relieved resulting in a large outward current characteristic of HERG. Peak amplitude of the current at –40 mV should be approximately three- to fourfold higher than the current amplitude obtained at the end of the +20 mV pulse. The –40 mV tail current decays slowly until the cell is finally repolarized back to –80 mV.

13. Three common problems we encounter when recording HERG channel currents are (a) excessive leak (*see* **Note 7** and Fig. 4), (b) series resistance errors (*see* **Note 8** and Fig. 5), and (c) spontaneous current run-down (*see* **Note 9** and Fig. 6). All of these variables should be carefully checked and monitored before starting an experiment and during its conduct.

4. Notes

1. Our chamber consists of a Plexiglas ring approximately 4 cm in diameter and 0.5 cm high. A small hole is drilled into the side to allow the insertion of the perfusion tubing and a piece of thin glass is glued to the bottom to form a water-tight seal (Fig. 1).

2. Cells can be passed several times and still retain suitable HERG current density. However, multiple passages can result in reduced HERG channel current density. When this occurs, it is necessary to thaw out a new vial of cells and begin the cell plating process anew.

3. A debate exists whether it is better to run HERG experiments at room temperature or at elevated (35–37°C) temperatures. The argument for elevated temperatures is that they are more physiological. Furthermore, it has been shown that erythro-

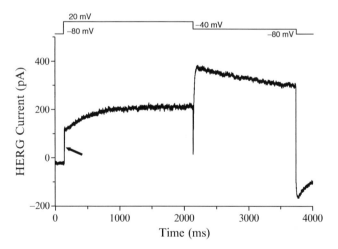

Fig. 4. Excessive leak during HERG channel recordings. This Figure illustrates a large leak current superimposed upon a HERG channel current. Note the large current observed instantaneously upon depolarization of the cell to +20 mV (*arrow*), and the fact that the tail current is not approximately three- to fourfold larger than the current at the end of the +20 mV pulse.

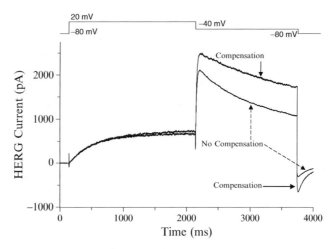

Fig. 5. Series resistance compensation during HERG channel recordings. HERG channel current traces from the same cell before and after series resistance compensation are shown. Note the large increase in current after compensation as well as the change in the shape of the current waveform.

mycin has several-fold higher affinity for blocking HERG currents at elevated temperature compared to room temperature (9). However, with the possible exception of erythromycin (which in our hands shows little temperature sensitivity if allowed extra equilibration time at room temperature), few if any drugs have been shown to display significant temperature-dependent affinity on HERG (10). On the other hand, we do find that currents recorded at room temperature have much less spontaneous run-down compared to currents recorded at elevated temperatures and that our seals remain stable and leak less for longer periods of time. Since both of these parameters can significantly impact the quality and accuracy of the recordings, we have chosen room temperature recording for the vast majority of our experiments.

4. The resistance (i.e., size) of the electrodes used will depend in part upon the amplitude of the current you are studying. For our cells, we typically have peak currents that measure between 0.5 and 2 nA. We find electrodes with resistances between 2 and 4 MΩ large enough to minimize series resistance errors, yet small enough to have a high success rate for forming gigaohm seals with the membrane.

5. Many different types of perfusion systems are available for patch clamp recordings. We use a simple system where a reservoir (for example a 50 mL glass test tube) flows into the cell chamber via gravity where the perfusate is removed by a tube connected to a vacuum source (Fig. 1). In practice, perfusion systems are usually more complex than that outlined in Fig. 1 utilizing multiple reservoirs. These multiple reservoirs allow

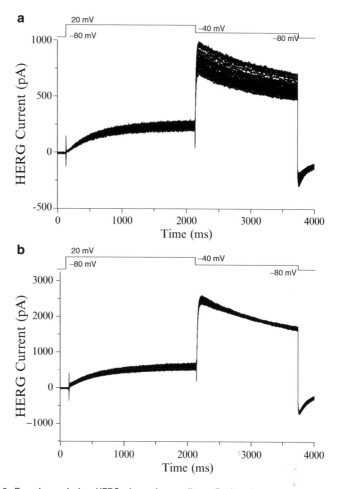

Fig. 6. Run-down during HERG channel recordings. During the course of whole-cell patch-clamping experiments, HERG channel current amplitude tends to spontaneously decline. (a) Shows HERG channel current traces every 30 s over a time period of 15 min. In this cell, current amplitude did not overlap from trace to trace, even at the beginning of the experiment. HERG current amplitude decayed by approximately 30% over the course of 15 min, an amount that may be unacceptable for some experiments. (b) Illustrates a cell with much less run-down. In this cell, HERG current amplitude decayed by approximately 7% during 15 min of recording, thereby minimizing any error related to spontaneous current run-down.

for different solutions (e.g., multiple drug concentrations for conducting concentration-response studies) to be delivered to the same cell. Those unfamiliar with patch clamp electrophysiology are encouraged to visit a laboratory in which it is run to see first-hand the details involved in setting up a perfusion system for patch-clamp recording.

6. Choose a single spherical cell located in the perfusion stream. If testing drugs, the response to test article is faster if the cell is located in the perfusion stream. This can reduce experimental time and minimize current rundown. For CHO cells, we pick

cells with relatively clear cytoplasm and dark edges. We like to patch small to middle size cells (capacitance 10–40 pF), but the choice of cell size may ultimately be decided by the current density in the clone that is being used (assuming that larger cells contain more current).

7. Typically, some amount of leak is introduced when the gig-ohm seal is ruptured to obtain the whole-cell configuration. In addition, leak current can increase with time during the course of an experiment as the integrity of the seal begins to decrease. The amount of leak that is acceptable depends upon the type of experiment being performed. However, leak currents should never be a significant component of the overall current amplitude (Fig. 4). Leak subtraction as provided on patch clamp amplifiers or software can overcome some amount of leak, but it is not a substitute for high quality recordings.

8. Series resistance errors during HERG recordings can be minimized. Always use electrodes that have a suitable resistance (size) for the amount of current you are recording and use the series resistance correction available on the amplifier (see Fig. 5 for example). Also be sure to check that the electrode is not clogged with debris.

9. During the course of whole-cell patch clamping experiments, the HERG channel current amplitude tends to decrease. This spontaneous "run-down" can vary from cell to cell (Fig. 6). As in the case for leak, there is no rule for determining how much run-down is too much. However, if current amplitude consistently drops from pulse to pulse with little or no overlapping of the traces, the cell should probably be discarded in favor of one with a more stable current.

Acknowledgments

The authors would like to thank Dr. Tony Lacerda (ChanTest, Inc.,) for his critical review of the manuscript.

References

1. Sanguinetti, M.C., Jiang, C., Curran, M.E., and Keating, M.T. (1995) A mechanistic link between and inherited and an acquired cardiac arrhythmia: HERG encodes the I_{Kr} potassium channel. *Cell* **81**, 299–307.

2. Sanguinetti, M.C., and Tristani-Firouzi, M. (2006) hERG potassium channels and cardiac arrhythmia. *Nature* **440**, 463–469.

3. Pearlstein, R., Vaz, R., and Rampe, D. (2003) Understanding the structure-activity relationship of the human *ether-a-go-go*-related gene cardiac K+ channel: A model for bad behavior. *J. Med. Chem.* **46**, 2019–2022.

4. Sanguinetti, M.C., Chen, J., Fernandez, D., Kamiya, K., Mitcheson, J., and Sanchez-Chapula, J.A. (2005) Physiochemical basis for

binding and voltage-dependent block of hERG channels by structurally diverse drugs. *Novartis Found. Symp.* **266,** 159–166.

5. Guo, L., and Guthrie, H. (2005) Automated electrophysiology in the preclinical evaluation of drugs for potential QT prolongation. *J. Pharmacol. Toxicol. Methods* **52,** 123–135.

6. Chaudhary, K.W., O'Neal, J.M., Mo, Z.L., Fermini, B., Gallavan, R.H., and Bahinski, A. (2006) Evaluation of the rubidium efflux assay for preclinical identification of HERG blockade. *Assay Drug Dev. Technol.* **4,** 73–82.

7. Hamill, O.P., Marty, A., Neher, E., Sakmann, B., and Sigworth, F.J. (1981) Improved patch clamp techniques for high resolution current recording from cells and cell free membrane patches. *Pfleug. Arch. Eur. J. Physiol.* **391,** 85–100.

8. Kang, J., Wang, L., Cai, F., and Rampe, D. (2000) High affinity block of the HERG cardiac K+ channel by the neuroleptic pimozide. *Eur. J. Pharmacol.* **392,** 137–140.

9. Kirsch, G.E., Trepakova, E.S., Brimecombe, J.C., Sidach, S.S., Erickson, H. D., Kochan, M.C., Shyjka, L.M., Lacerda, A.E., and Brown, A.M. (2004) Variability in the measurement of hERG potassium channel inhibition: effects of temperature and stimulus pattern. *J. Pharmacol. Toxicol. Methods* **50,** 93–101.

10. Yao, J.A., Du, X., Lu, D., Baker, R.L., Daharsh, E., and Atterson, P. (2005) Estimation of potency of HERG channel blockers: impact of voltage protocol and temperature. *J. Pharmacol. Toxicol. Methods* **52,** 146–153.

Part V

Investigative Toxicology

Chapter 10

Generation and Analysis of Transcriptomics Data

Philip D. Glaves and Jonathan D. Tugwood

Abstract

Transcript profiling ("Transcriptomics") is a widely used technique that obtains information on the abundance of multiple mRNA transcripts within a biological sample simultaneously. Therefore, when a number of such samples are analysed, as in a scientific experiment, large and complex data sets are generated. Here, we describe the use of one method commonly used to generate transcriptomics data, namely the use of Affymetrix GeneChip microarrays. Data generated in transcriptomics experiments can be analysed using a multitude of approaches, but a common goal is to identify those transcripts whose abundance is altered by the experimental conditions, or which differ between sets of samples. Here, we describe a simple approach, the calculation of the volcano score, which identifies transcripts with altered abundance, taking into account both the magnitude of the alteration and its statistical significance.

Key words: Transcriptomics, Transcript profiling, Genomics, Volcano plot, Microarray

1. Introduction

Transcript profiling, or "Transcriptomics", is defined as the simultaneous quantitation of multiple messenger RNAs in a biological sample. As many thousands of gene transcripts can be quantified, transcriptomics provides a means of gaining experimental information on the biology of a system relatively quickly. Typically, transcriptomics has been used to obtain comparative information on tissues or cells with different characteristics, for example, leukaemia subtypes (1), or to gain information on the effects of drugs or chemicals on cells or tissues, that is, "Toxicogenomics" (2).

The gene expression "microarray" is the most commonly used tool in transcriptomics experiments. In their simplest form, microarrays consist of gene sequences, either oligonucleotides or cDNA fragments, immobilised on a solid support. These sequences

Jean-Charles Gautier (ed.), *Drug Safety Evaluation: Methods and Protocols*, Methods in Molecular Biology, vol. 691,
DOI 10.1007/978-1-60761-849-2_10, © Springer Science+Business Media, LLC 2011

can be hybridised with labelled cDNA or cRNA from the sample
of interest, and the label detected by some form of scanner. The
extent of hybridisation to each gene fragment is proportional to
the abundance of the mRNA in the original sample. The Affymetrix
GeneChip® system (http://www.affymetrix.com) is a commonly
used example of a gene expression microarray, and use of this
system will be described in this chapter.

Microarray development has reached the point where experiments with material from many different species are possible.
Indeed, for human, rat and mouse, "whole-genome" arrays are
available which allow the analysis of the entire "transcriptome" of
the organism. Clearly, such analyses will generate large volumes
of data, and there are a number of ways of approaching the analysis of large data sets (3). The initial goal of transcriptomics data
analysis is the identification of "dysregulated" transcripts, that is,
those which have changed in abundance in the experiment or
study, either between samples with different characteristics, or in
response to a chemical or drug treatment. This chapter will
describe the generation of a transcriptomics data set, and outline
a simple method to obtain a list of dysregulated transcripts, which
then form the basis of further study.

The following sections describe the preparation of labelled
cRNA using a starting quantity of 100 ng total RNA per sample
extracted from human cells cultured in 100 mm dishes. Labelling
reactions are performed using the Genechip® 3′ IVT Express Kit
(Affymetrix) which contains sufficient reagent quantities for up to
30 labelling reactions. When alternative RNA sources or starting
quantities are used, certain steps may vary slightly and these variations are referred to in the Notes section.

2. Materials

2.1. Total RNA Extraction

1. RNeasy Plus Mini Kit (Qiagen) containing gDNA Eliminator
   Columns, RNeasy Mini Spin Columns, Buffer RLT Plus,
   Buffer RW1, Buffer RPE (concentrate), RNAase-free water,
   1.5 and 2 mL collection tubes (see Notes 1 and 2).

2. QIAshredder Kit (Qiagen) containing cell lysate homogeniser
   columns and 1.5 mL collection tubes.

3. Ethanol, 96–100% (v/v).

4. Ethanol, 70% (v/v).

5. 14.3 M β-mercaptoethanol.

6. Dilute the Buffer RPE (concentrate) with four volumes ethanol (96–100%) before use.

2.2. RNA Quantification and Quality Assessment

1. Nanodrop ND-1000 Spectrophotometer (Thermo Fisher).

2. 2100 Bioanalyzer System (Agilent Technologies).

3. RNA 6000 Nano Kit (Agilent Technologies) containing RNA Nano Chips, RNA Nano Gel Matrix, RNA Nano Dye Concentrate, RNA 6000 Nano Marker, RNA 6000 ladder, Spin column filters, 1.5 mL centrifuge tubes and a syringe (for the Chip Priming Station).

4. Bioanalyzer 2100 Chip Priming Station (Agilent Technologies).

5. Vortexer with mixer adapter (Agilent Technologies).

2.3. aRNA Target Preparation

2.3.1. First-Strand cDNA Synthesis

1. GeneChip® 3′ IVT Express Kit Box 2 (Affymetrix). The required components from this kit for this step are First-Strand Buffer Mix, First-Strand Enzyme Mix, Poly-A Control Stock and Poly-A Control Dilution Buffer. Poly-A RNA Control Stock must be diluted with Poly-A RNA Control Dilution Buffer before use. The required dilution is dependent on the starting quantity of total RNA. For a starting quantity of 100 ng perform a four-step serial dilution of 1:20, 1:50, 1:50 and 1:10. Use 2 µL of the fourth dilution in the reaction.

2. For First-Strand Reaction Mix: 4 µL First-Strand Buffer Mix, 1 µL First-Strand Enzyme Mix.

3. Thin-walled 500 µL PCR tubes (Anachem).

2.3.2. Second-Strand cDNA Synthesis

1. GeneChip® 3′ IVT Express Kit Box 2 (Affymetrix). The required components from this kit for this step are Second-Strand Buffer Mix, Second-Strand Enzyme Mix and Nuclease-free Water.

2. Thin-walled 500 µL PCR tubes.

2.3.3. In Vitro Transcription

1. GeneChip® 3′ IVT Express Kit Box 2 (Affymetrix). The required components from this kit for this step are IVT Biotin label, IVT labeling Buffer and IVT Enzyme Mix.

2. Thin-walled 500 µL PCR tubes.

2.3.4. Biotin-Labelled aRNA Purification

1. GeneChip® 3′ IVT Express Kit Box 2 (Affymetrix). The required components from this kit for this step are aRNA Binding Buffer Concentrate, RNA Binding Beads, aRNA Wash Solution Concentrate, aRNA Elution Solution, Nuclease-free Water, U-Bottom 96-well plate.

2. Ethanol, 96–100% (v/v).

3. Magnetic Stand-96 (Ambion)

2.3.5. aRNA Quantification

1. Nanodrop ND-1000 Spectrophotometer (Thermo Fisher).

2.3.6. Fragmentation of labelled aRNA

1. GeneChip® 3′ IVT Express Kit Box 1 (Affymetrix). The required components from this kit for this step are 5× Fragmentation Buffer and nuclease-free water.

2. Nanodrop ND-1000 Spectrophotometer (Thermo Fisher).

3. 2100 Bioanalyzer (Agilent Technologies).

4. RNA 6000 Nano Kit (Agilent Technologies) containing RNA Nano Chips, RNA Nano Gel Matrix, RNA Nano Dye Concentrate, RNA 6000 Nano Marker, RNA 6000 ladder, spin filters, 1.5 mL centrifuge tubes and a syringe (for the Chip Priming Station).

5. 2100 Bioanalyzer Chip Priming Station (Agilent Technologies).

6. Vortexer with Bioanalyzer Chip adapter (Agilent Technologies).

7. Thin-walled 500 μL PCR tubes.

2.4. GeneChip Hybridisation

1. GeneChip® 3′ IVT Express Kit: Box 2 (Affymetrix). The required components from this kit for this step are 20× Hybridization Controls and Control Oligonucleotide B2.

2. GeneChip® Hybridization, Wash and Stain Kit (Affymetrix): Hybridization Module (Box 1). The required components from this kit for this step are Pre-Hybridization Mix, 2× Hybridization Mix, DMSO and Nuclease-free water.

3. Affymetrix Human Genome HG_U_133A Plus2.0 GeneChip.

4. Affymetrix GeneChip Hybridisation Oven 320.

2.5. Washing and Staining

1. GeneChip® Hybridization, Wash and Stain Kit (Affymetrix): Stain Module (Box 1). Stain Cocktail 1, Stain Cocktail 2 and Array Holding Buffer.

2. GeneChip® Hybridization, Wash and Stain Kit (Affymetrix): Hybridization Module (Box 2). Wash Buffer A and Wash Buffer B.

3. Affymetrix Fluidics Station 450.

4. Affymetrix GeneChip Scanner 3000 with Autoloader and External Barcode Reader.

2.6. Scanning

1. Wash Buffer A.

2. Tough Spots (Anachem).

3. Affymetrix GeneChip Scanner 3000 with Autoloader and External Barcode Reader.

3. Methods

3.1. Total RNA Extraction from Cultured Cells

1. Remove all culture media from cells grown and treated in 100 mm culture dishes.

2. Add 600 μL of Buffer RLT Plus (containing 10 μL/mL β-mercaptoethanol) directly to each monolayer to lyse cells. Use a cell scraper to aid cell detachment if necessary.

3. Transfer the lysates to separate QIAshredder spin columns placed in a 2 mL collection tubes. Spin in a bench top centrifuge at maximum speed for 2 min.

4. Transfer the homogenised lysates to separate gDNA Eliminator columns placed in 2 mL collection tubes and spin (30 s at ≥8,000×g).

5. Discard the gDNA Eliminator column and add 600 μL 70% Ethanol to the flow-through. Mix by pipetting.

6. Transfer 700 μL of each sample to separate RNeasy Mini spin columns placed in a 2 mL collection tubes. Close the lids and spin (15 s at ≥8,000×g). Repeat with any remaining sample discarding the flow-through after each spin.

7. Add 700 μL Buffer RW1 to each RNeasy spin column. Close the lids and spin (15 s at ≥8,000×g). Discard the flow-through.

8. Add 500 μL Buffer RPE to each RNeasy spin column. Close the lid and spin (15 s at ≥8,000×g). Discard the flow-through.

9. Add a further 500 μL Buffer RPE to each RNeasy spin column. Close the lids and spin (2 min at ≥8,000×g).

10. Transfer each RNeasy spin column to a new 2 mL collection tube and spin at maximum speed for 1 min.

11. Transfer each RNeasy spin column to a 1.5 mL collection tube.

12. Add 50 μL RNAase-free water directly to each column membrane.

13. Spin the column for 1 min at ≥8,000×g.

14. Transfer each flow-through back onto appropriate column membrane and spin again for 1 min at ≥8,000×g.

3.2. RNA Quantitation and Quality Assessment

3.2.1. Nanodrop Spectrophotometer

1. Take a small aliquot of total RNA and prepare a 1:10 dilution with RNAase-free water.

2. Set the Nanodrop to measure RNA and set the blank using 1 μL RNAase-free water.

3. Use 1 μL diluted total RNA to determine the concentration and the 260:280 ratio (see Note 3).

3.2.2. Agilent 2100
Bioanalyzer

1. Thaw the RNA 6000 ladder on ice and denature by heating at 70°C for 2 min in a heat block. Store denatured ladder on ice until required (see Note 4).

2. Allow RNA 6000 Nano Dye Concentrate to equilibrate to room temperature.

3. Spin 550 µL RNA 6000 Nano gel matrix in a spin filter column (10 min at 1,500×*g*, room temperature) (see Note 5).

4. Combine 1 µL RNA 6000 Nano Dye Concentrate with 65 µL of filtered gel matrix in a microcentrifuge tube. Mix by vortexing.

5. Spin the gel-dye mix (10 min at 13,000×*g*, room temperature).

6. Place a RNA 6000 Nano Chip into the Chip Priming Station.

7. Pipette 9 µL of gel-dye mix into the well on the chip marked with a black G (immediately to the right of sample well 9).

8. Position the syringe plunger at 1 mL and close the Chip Priming Station.

9. Press the syringe plunger until it is held by the clip. Release the clip after 30 s and pull the plunger back to the 1 mL position after a further 5 s.

10. Open the Chip Priming Station and pipette 9 µL of gel-dye mix in the two wells marked with a white G (immediately to the right of sample wells 3 and 6).

11. Pipette 5 µL of RNA 6000 Nano marker into each sample well (marked 1–12) and into the ladder well (immediately to the right of sample well 12).

12. Pipette 1 µL of denatured ladder into the ladder well, 1 µL of each sample into separate sample wells and 1 µL of RNA 6000 Nano Marker into each unused sample well.

13. Place the chip into the Bioanalyzer vortex adapter and vortex (1 min at 2,400 rpm).

14. Place the chip into the 2100 Bioanalyzer and commence electrophoresis using the Eukaryote Total RNA Nano Series II Assay to determine the integrity of each RNA sample (see Notes 6 and 7). A typical electrophoresis trace of RNA is shown in Fig. 1.

3.3. aRNA Target
Preparation

3.3.1. First-Strand cDNA
Synthesis

1. For each sample combine 2 µL of poly-A control (fourth dilution) with 100 ng total RNA in a 0.5 mL PCR tube. Make up to 5 µL using RNase free water and keep on ice.

2. Prepare First Strand Master Mix: 4 µL First Strand Buffer Mix, 1 µL First strand Enzyme Mix per sample. Mix and spin down. (See Note 8).

3. Transfer 5 µL master mix to each RNA / Poly A sample tube. Mix gently spin down.

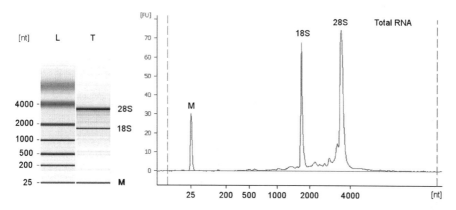

Fig. 1. A Bioanalyzer 2100 trace of a good-quality total RNA sample (RIN = 9.8). The *left-hand panel* is a gel image. Shown is a RNA size ladder (L) with fragment lengths given in nucleotides (nt), and the total RNA image (T) shows the two 28S and 18S ribosomal RNA bands, and the RNA 6000 Nano Marker (M). The *right-hand panel* is the electropherogram of the same total RNA sample. The bands corresponding to 28S and 18S rRNAs and the RNA 6000 Nano Marker are labelled. RNA fragment lengths in nucleotides are shown on the *x*-axis. "FU" on the *y*-axis refers to fluorescence units (arbitrary units of RNA concentration).

4. Incubate at 42 °C in a thermal cycler for 2 hours. (See Note 9).

5. Spin down and place on ice.

3.3.2. Second-Strand cDNA Synthesis

1. Prepare a second-strand synthesis master mix on ice: 13 μL RNase free water, 5 μL second-strand synthesis buffer mix and 2 μL second-strand synthesis enzyme mix per sample in a RNase free microcentrifuge tube.

2. Gently mix and spin down.

3. Transfer 20 μL of the master mix to each first strand cDNA sample.

4. Gently mix and spin down.

5. Set a thermal cycle to 16 °C for 1 hour and then at 65 °C for 10 min. Allow the thermal cycler to reach 16 °C.

6. Place the tubes in the thermal cycler and incubate as described in the previous step.

7. Spin the contents down and place on ice while preparing the reagents for the next step. Alternatively, the samples can be stored overnight at –20 °C.

3.3.3. Synthesis of biotin labelled aRNA by In Vitro Transcription

1. Prepare an IVT Master Mix: 4 μL IVT Biotin Label, 20 μL IVT Labelling Buffer, 6 μL IVT Enzyme Mix per sample in a 1.5 mL RNase free microcentrifuge tube.

2. Mix gently and spin down. Place on ice.

3. Add 30 μL of the IVT Master Mix to each double-stranded cDNA sample. Mix gently and spin down.

4. Place the tubes in a thermal cycler and incubate at 40 °C for 16 hours to synthesise biotin labelled aRNA (See Note 10). After the incubation is complete, place the aRNA samples on ice and proceed to the aRNA Purification step. Alternatively store overnight at –20°C.

3.3.4. Biotin Labelled aRNA Purification

1. Prepare the working aRNA wash solution by adding 100% ethanol to the aRNA Wash Solution Concentrate.

2. Transfer the total required volume of aRNA Elution Solution (55 µL per sample) to a RNase free microcentrifuge tube and heat at 55 °C for 15 min.

3. Meanwhile, prepare aRNA Binding Mix at room temperature by combining 10 µL aRNA Binding Beads (resuspended by vortexing) with 50 µL aRNA Binding Buffer Concentrate per sample in a RNase free microcentrifuge tube.

4. Dispense 60 µL aRNA Binding Mix to each aRNA sample.

5. Transfer each sample to a well of a U-bottom 96 well plate and mix by pipetting up and down several times.

6. Add 120 µL 100% ethanol to each sample.

7. Mix again by pipetting and shake the plate very gently for 2 min using a plate shaker.

8. Capture the beads by sitting the plate the magnetic stand for 5 min.

9. Once the beads have formed a pellet and the solution is transparent carfully aspirate the supernatant. Avoid disturbing the pellet.

10. Remove the place from the magnetic stand.

11. Add 100 µL aRNA Wash Solution to each sample well.

12. Shake the plate for 1 minute at a medium speed in a plate shaker.

13. Transfer the plate back to the magnetic stand and leave beads for 5 min to form another pellet.

14. Aspirate the supernatant. Avoid disrupting the pellet.

15. Repeat the washing steps.

16. Aspirate and discard the supernatant.

17. Place the plate back on the plate shaker and shake vigorously for 1 minute to allow any remaining ethanol to evaporate.

18. Add 50 µL of the preheated aRNA Elution Soltuion to each sample to elute the purified aRNA.

19. Shake the plate vigourous in the plate shaker for 3 min until the binding beads are fully dispersed.

20. Transfer the plate back to the magnetic stand until the beads form a pellet and the supernatant is transparent. The purified biotin labelled aRNA is now in the supernatant.

21. Transfer the supernatant to a RNase free PCR tube.

22. Place on ice if proceeding directly to aRNA Quantitation otherwise store at −20 °C

3.3.5. aRNA Quantification

1. Remove 1 µL of each sample, dilute 1/10 in RNAase-free water and determine the cRNA concentration using a Nanodrop ND-1000 Spectrophotometer.

2. Retain the 1/10 dilution for analysis on a Bioanalyzer 2100 (see Subheading 3.3.6).

3.3.6. Fragmentation of labelled aRNA

1. Transfer 15 mg of aRNA to a PCR tube in a maximum volume of 32 µL (see Note 11).

2. Add 8 µL 5× Array Fragmentation Buffer and adjust to 40 mL with RNAase-free water.

3. Incubate at 94 °C for 35 min in a thermal cycler and store the samples on ice.

4. Check for successful fragmentation by running 1 mL of each unfragmented sample (1/10 dilution) adjacent to 1 mL of the corresponding fragmented sample with the 2100 Bioanalyzer, using the mRNA Nano Series II Assay. A typical electrophoresis trace of aRNA fragmentation is shown in Fig. 2.

5. The size of fragmented samples should be in the range of 35–200 bases with a peak at approximately 100–120 nucleotides.

6. Store undiluted fragmented aRNA samples at −80 °C.

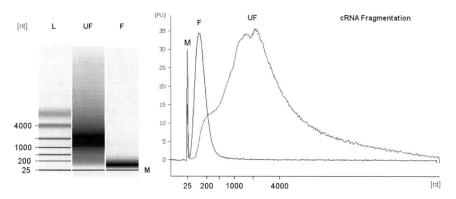

Fig. 2. A Bioanalyzer 2100 trace of unfragmented and fragmented cRNA. The *left-hand panel* is a gel image showing the RNA size ladder (L), and a comparison of the cRNA before fragmentation (UF) and after (F). The *right-hand panel* shows a corresponding electropherogram, with the traces for the unfragmented (UF) and fragmented (F) cRNA superimposed on the same figure for clarity.

3.4. GeneChip
Hybridisation

1. Allow microarrays to equilibrate to room temperature and label each with a unique sample ID.

2. Heat the 20× Hybridization Controls to 65°C for 5 min to ensure complete resuspension.

3. Ensure that the DMSO is completely thawed.

4. Prepare a Hybridisation Cocktail Master Mix: 4.2 µL Control Oligonucleotide B2, 12.5 µL 20× Hybridization Controls, 125 µL 2× Hybridization Mix, 25 µL DMSO and 50 µL RNase Free Water per sample in a RNase free tube. Mix well and centrifuge briefly.

5. Transfer 33.3 µL (12 µg) of each fragmented aRNA sample to a separate RNase free PCR tube and add 237.5 µL of the hybridization cocktail master mix to each tube giving a total volume of 250 µL.

6. Insert a 200 mL pipette tip into the top rubber septum on the back of the GeneChip and fill with 200 µL Pre-Hybridisation Mix from the bottom septum using another 200 mL pipette tip.

7. Remove the pipette tips from the rubber septa and pre-incubate the GeneChips at 45°C in hybridisation oven with rotation set at 60 rpm.

8. Meanwhile, heat the samples at 99°C for 5 min and then at 45°C for 5 min in a thermal cycler.

9. Spin the samples at maximum speed for 5 min to pellet any insoluble material.

10. Insert a 200 mL pipette tip into the top septum of the GeneChip. Remove the Pre-Hybridisation buffer through the bottom septum and replace with 200 mL of appropriate sample.

11. Ensure the bubble will move freely and cover each septum with a Tough Spot.

12. Place the GeneChips back in the hybridisation oven and incubate at 45°C with rotation at 60 rpm for 16–18 h (see Note 12).

13. Remove Tough Spots and remove the hybridisation cocktail from each GeneChip through the bottom septum. This can be stored at –20°C and used again up to five times. Fill the GeneChip completely with non-stringent buffer and store at 4°C while the fluidics stations are being primed.

3.5. Washing
and Staining

3.5.1. Fluidics Station
Priming

1. Turn on the Fluidics Station.

2. Place an empty 1 L bottle and three 500 mL bottles containing 500 mL Buffer A, Buffer B and water in the appropriate spaces to the right of each fluidics station.

3. Place the tubes into the appropriate bottles.

4. Pull the needle lever for each required module into the up position and place an empty 1.5 mL microcentrifuge tube into the three holders located beneath each module.

5. Ensure that the large blue levers on each require module is pulled out so that the Genechip holding compartments are closed.

6. Open the AGCC software and select AGCC Fluidics Control.

7. In the fluidics control window select the 'Master' tab and tick all the wash station modules that will be required.

8. With the 'List all protocols' option selected, select the Prime_450 protocol from the drop down menu. Leave the 'Probe Array Type' box empty.

9. Click the 'Copy to all modules' button.

10. Click the Run button.

11. When prompted to "load vials 1-2-3", push the needle lever down into the locked position to commence priming. Ensure that each needle is inserted into an empty microcentrifuge tube.

12. Once priming is complete lift the needle level into the up position.

3.5.2. Sample Registration

1. Open the AGCC Launcher and select the AGCC Portal.

2. Click Sample > Register.

3. To register chips individually fill in the fields for Sample File Name, Probe Array Type and Array Name.

4. Select the Barcode box and scan the GeneChip barcode using a barcode scanner.

5. Click Save.

6. Sample (.ARR) files for each sample are saved in the default location using the specified sample name as a prefix.

7. To register multiple chips click Sample > Batch Registration

8. An excel template can be downloaded from this window. Fill in the required fields (including sample name and chip type). Barcodes can also be scanned directly into this template.

9. Save the template.

10. Click upload, select the template file and click ok to save the resulting .ARR files to the default location.

3.5.3. Washing and Staining

1. For each sample, aliquot 600 µL of Stain Cocktail 1, 600 µL of Stain Cocktail 2 and 800 µL Array Holding Buffer into three separate 1.5 µL microcentrifuge tubes.

2. Insert a GeneChip into a module using the cartridge lever to open and close the GeneChip holder.

3. In the AGCC software, open the Fluidics Control Window.

4. Select the appropriate fluidics station from the available tabs and for the required module select the corresponding sample name for the inserted Genechip.

5. Select the EukGE-WS2v5_450 wash protocol (see Note 13) from the "Protocol" drop down menu.

6. Click Run.

7. Remove the empty microcentrifuge tubes in the three sample holders located below the needle lever and replace with tubes of Stain Cocktail 1, Stain Cocktail 2 and Arry Holding Buffer in positions 1, 2 and 3 respectively.

8. When prompted to 'load vials 1-2-3' push the needle lever down until it locks into position to start the washing and staining procedure. Check that each needle is inside the relevant tube.

9. Repeat this process in separate modules for all the samples.

10. Once washing and staining are complete, remove each GeneChip from the modules and check the glass window for the presence of air bubbles inside the GeneChip cartridge. If bubbles are present manually refill the GeneChip with Array Holding Buffer. Ensure the buffer is free from bubbles before scanning as they may give rise to inaccuracies.

11. Close the GeneChip holder. The module will "re-prime" itself and at this point is ready to receive another chip if required. Once the fluidics stations are no longer required they should be shutdown by placing all external tubing into an empty 1 L waste bottle and running the "Shutdown" wash protocol on all used modules.

12. Place a Tough Spot over each septum to prevent any leakage during the scanning process. Ensure the Spots are securely adhered to the back of the GeneChip.

3.6. Scanning GeneChips

1. Turn on the GeneChip scanner. The scanner laser will require a warm up period of approximately 20 min.

2. Ensure the surface of the GeneChip is free from dust or dirt. Wipe with a soft tissue if necessary.

3. Place each GeneChip into the scanner autoloader (starting at position 1).

4. Open the Scan Control window via the AGCC Launcher.

5. Start the scanner by clicking the Start button at the top of the screen.

6. The scanner will automatically detect the GeneChip and associate it with the appropriate .ARR file created earlier. A scanned image is saved as a .DAT file prefixed by its sample name. Once the scan is complete, the software will automatically generate a .CEL file for that sample.

3.7. GeneChip Data Generation

1. Open the Expression Console software.

2. Select File > New Study > Add Intensity Files.

3. Navigate to the folder containing the .CEL files to be analyzed, highlight the required .CEL files and click 'Open'. The .CEL file names will appear in the Study window.

4. Select the .CEL files to be analyzed and click the 'Run Analysis' Button.

5. Select the MAS5 algorithm (RMA and PLIER algorithms are also available to use.) A box appears in which an optional suffix can be added to the resulting .CHP files.

6. Click OK to start the analysis.

3.8. Quality Control

1. From AGCC launcher, open the AGCC Viewer.

2. Open a .DAT file.

3. On the image, check that the grid has aligned to the GeneChip title, to the centre cross and to each corner of the image (see Fig. 3). If it has not aligned correctly the grid can be realigned by clicking on "image processing" and then "realign all grids".

4. Select Report > View Full Report from the menu at the top of the screen.

5. In the table, check the 3′-5′ ratios for β-Actin and GAPDH. Ideally, these should be below 3. Values above 3 may indicate

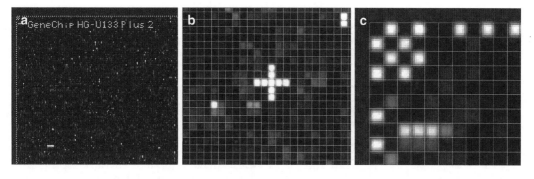

Fig. 3. GeneChip images. (**a**) GeneChip title (*top left-hand corner* of chip, low magnification), (**b**) cross (*centre* of chip, medium magnification) and (**c**) corner (high magnification). Panels (**b, c**) show the grid to which the images should be aligned.

suboptimal RNA quality, and such samples should be excluded from the subsequent analysis.

6. In the same way, once multiple samples have been scanned, check for atypical samples ("outliers") amongst the sample sets under Scaling Factor, % Present, and Noise. You may wish to exclude these outliers from the subsequent data analysis.

3.9. Data Export

1. Open the Expression Console Software.

2. Click File > Open Study.

3. Navigate to the Study file and click open.

4. Click 'Export' in the menu at the top of the screen.

5. Click "Export Probe Set Results (Pivot Table) as TXT" and save as a .txt file.

6. Open the .txt file in Excel.

3.10. "Volcano" Analysis

A typical transcriptomics experiment will consist of a number of samples, grouped according to treatment received, time of sampling, etc. The principal goal of the data analysis is to identify the transcripts that are differentially regulated between sample groups and/or individual samples. Using the simple example of a comparison of an experimental sample set that have been treated with an experimental compound versus an untreated sample set, this section will outline a method for identifying a list of transcripts that are differentially regulated between the two sample sets.

The "volcano score" takes into account of both the magnitude of the change in transcript abundance (fold change – FC) and the statistical significance of the change (p-value). To establish statistical significance, it is important to build in replicate samples into the experimental design. Typically, a transcript profiling experiment will have a minimum of five biological replicates per experimental condition – in this example, this would mean five independent samples that have received compound treatment, plus five untreated samples.

The volcano score is defined as $v = \log FC \times \log p$-value. Typically, transcripts are identified as dysregulated when $v \le -0.339$, a score derived when $FC = 2$ and $p = 0.05$. This approach allows the identification of transcripts that exhibit a large fold change but low statistical significance, and vice versa.

The following method involves the use of an MS Excel spreadsheet to calculate and plot the volcano scores for transcript profile data obtained from five untreated samples, and five compound treated samples:

1. From the Excel spreadsheet generated in Subheading 3.9, copy and paste the probeset identifiers from Column A into

column A on a new worksheet. For the Affymetrix HG_U133_Plus2.0 GeneChip, there are 54,613 probesets, excluding the quality control probesets. Row 1 should have a "column header", for example, "probeset ID".

2. In columns B–F, copy and paste the signal values from the five untreated samples. In columns G–K, copy and paste the signal values from the five compound treated samples. Assign column headers in row 1, for example, sample 1, etc. (see Note 14).

3. In column L, calculate the mean signal value for the five untreated samples in columns B–F, row 2. This is done by using the Excel "Average" function. Copy this formula for all cells L2–L54,614. In column M, perform the same procedure for the five compound treated samples in columns G–K.

4. In column N row 2, calculate the fold change for the first probeset by dividing the contents of cell M2 by that in L2: "=M2/L2". Copy this formula for all cells N2–N54,614.

5. In column O row 2, calculate the significance (p-value) of the difference between the untreated and treated samples. This is done using the students' t-test (TTEST in the Excel function menu). The correct formula is "TTEST(B2:F2,G2:K2,2,3)". The "2" figure defines a two-tailed t-test and the "3" figure defines the comparison of two sets of samples with unequal variance. Copy this formula for all cells O2–O54,614.

6. The FC values calculated in step 4 will be <1 if the probeset is down-regulated by the compound treatment. It is necessary to convert all FC values to ≥1 (i.e. absolute FC). In column P row 2, insert the formula "=IF(N2>1,N2,1/N2)". Copy this formula for all cells P2–P54,614.

7. The next step is to calculate the log FC values. In column Q row 2, insert the formula "=Log10(P2)". Copy this formula for all cells Q2–Q54,614.

8. Similarly, calculate the log p-values. In column R row 2, insert the formula "=Log10(O2)". Copy this formula for all cells R2–R54,614.

9. The volcano score, v, is obtained by multiplying log FC by log p. In column S row 2, insert the formula "=(Q2*R2)". Copy this formula for all cells S2–S54,614. Table 1 shows an example of the correct format with data from 10 probesets.

10. Open a new worksheet, and copy and paste the values from columns A (probeset IDs), N (fold changes), O (p-values) and S (volcano scores). Select the four columns and use the "data sort" function to arrange the data in ascending order of the volcano score (column S). This will allow identification of the probesets with a volcano score of ≤−0.339.

Table 1

Example data set for 10 probesets, showing spreadsheet layout for the v score calculation

Probeset ID	Control 1	Control 2	Control 3	Control 4	Control 5	Treated 1	Treated 2	Treated 3	Treated 4	Treated 5	Control Mean	Treated Mean	FC	p-value	|FC|	log|FC|	log$p$-value	v score
1007_s_at	71	139.4	80.3	99.5	131	114.3	98.1	105.1	77.6	109.5	104.24	100.92	0.96815	0.832066	1.032897	0.014057	−0.079842	−0.00112
1053_at	45.5	8.4	51.9	30	66.9	61.3	80.8	51.9	59.6	65.4	40.54	63.8	1.573754	0.082357	1.573754	0.196937	−1.084301	−0.21354
117_at	51.1	82.1	49.8	478.5	387	64.6	45.4	31.9	694.1	597.8	209.7	286.76	1.367477	0.671865	1.367477	0.13592	−0.172718	−0.02348
121_at	345.5	747.2	327.1	204.2	289.1	385.9	478.4	499.3	269.8	219.1	382.62	370.5	0.968324	0.915165	1.032713	0.013979	−0.038501	−0.00054
1255_g_at	2.9	3.4	1.3	9.4	32	1	15.1	11	107	2.4	9.8	8.04	0.820408	0.790704	1.218905	0.08597	−0.101986	−0.00877
1294_at	117.5	59.5	107.5	97.5	66.8	97.9	129.4	154.1	102.6	138.5	89.76	124.5	1.387032	0.056757	1.387032	0.142087	−1.24598	−0.17704
1316_at	55.6	64.8	34.4	34.2	84.7	34.1	56	56	40.9	51.4	54.74	47.68	0.871027	0.529246	1.14807	0.059969	−0.276342	−0.01657
1320_at	4.9	8.9	3.7	17.9	4.6	24.4	5.4	16.7	6.7	27.5	8	16.14	2.0175	0.164911	2.0175	0.304814	−0.782752	−0.23859
1405_i_at	23.3	26.3	35.5	33.6	106.7	29.2	14	17.5	110.9	137.7	45.08	61.86	1.372227	0.597796	1.372227	0.137426	−0.223447	−0.03071
1431_at	903.4	666.6	878.1	491.6	602.2	904.5	1,376.5	1,032.2	419.5	456.6	708.38	837.86	1.182783	0.538391	1.182783	0.072905	−0.268902	−0.0196

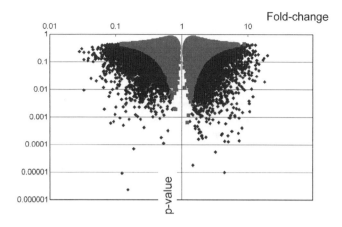

Fig. 4. Volcano plot. Individual *v* scores for each probeset are plotted against log fold change (*x*-axis) and log *p*-value (*y*-axis). Dysregulated probesets, that is, those with a *v* score of ≤−0.339, are coloured *black*. Non-regulated probesets (*v* ≥ −0.339) are coloured *grey*.

11. A "volcano plot" can be generated using the Excel chart function. This plots fold change (*x*-axis) versus *p*-value (*y*-axis), and if the *x*-axis is located centrally then the characteristic volcano shape is obtained (Fig. 4). From the Excel chart wizard, select the XY (scatter) plot.

12. In the "chart source data" field, choose the "add series" option. For series 1, select the values in columns N and O that correspond to *v* ≥ −0.339, that is, the probesets that are not dysregulated by treatment. For series 2, select the values in columns N and O that correspond to *v* ≤ −0.339. On the scatter plot, the two series will appear in different colours.

13. The probesets identified in step 10 in this example are those that are potentially dysregulated by compound treatment. Those that have the lowest (i.e. most negative) *v* scores will be the most significantly dysregulated, and a priority for further analysis.

14. Further analysis can include identification of biological pathways and functions that the dysregulated genes belong to – there are a number of publicly available analytical tools available to assist with this, for example, the KEGG Pathway database (http://www.genome.ad.jp/kegg/pathway.html).

15. It is advisable to verify the dysregulation of genes that have been prioritised for analysis by some independent means, for example, quantitative RT-PCR ("TaqMan").

4. Notes

1. When using mammalian tissue as a starting material, Affymetrix recommend using Trizol for the extraction of RNA followed by cleaning with the Qiagen RNeasy columns. However, we have extracted total RNA at a sufficient quantity and quality for gene expression analysis from most tissue types (up to 30 μg) using the Qiagen RNeasy Plus Mini Kits and a Polytron homogeniser (we increase the volume of RLT buffer for the homogenisation process to reduce frothing). For successful extractions, the sample must be well homogenised and the increased volume of homogenate can be passed through the RNeasy column in multiple steps to ensure all RNA is captured by the column membrane. It is also worth noting that Qiagen also supply specific RNeasy kits for the extraction of RNA from fibrous (e.g. muscle), or lipid-rich (e.g. brain) tissues.

2. Use RNAase-free pipette tips, microcentrifuge tubes and reagents throughout the entire procedure.

3. Starting RNA should be of high quality with a 260:280 ratio of 1.9–2.1.

4. Denatured ladder should be divided into aliquots and stored at −80°C.

5. Filtered gel matrix can be stored at 4°C for up to 1 month.

6. RNA Nano Chips should be used within 5 min of preparation.

7. High-quality total RNA should produce clear 18S and 28S rRNA peaks on the Bioanalyzer trace, ideally with a 28S:18S ratio of 1.9–2.1 and a RNA Integrity Number (RIN) of 7 or above. The presence of low molecular weight RNA often indicates sample degradation.

8. When labelling multiple samples always prepare a master mix and include enough reagents for at least $n + 1$ samples to account for minor pipetting errors.

9. Perform reactions in a thermal cycler. Temperatures and times for each step can be pre-set in advance and stored for future use.

10. Time the start of the IVT step so that it will end at a convenient time the following morning (e.g. 5 p.m. start, 9 a.m. finish). The thermal cycler can be set to stand at 4°C once the IVT step is complete but avoid leaving the samples at 4°C for long periods.

11. Alternative array formats may require different quantities of fragmented aRNA for hybridisation, and therefore reagent volumes should be scaled up or down accordingly.

12. Time the start of the 16–18 h hybridisation so that it ends at a convenient time the following morning.

13. The wash protocol described is appropriate for the human HG_U133_Plus2.0 GeneChip. The wash protocol may vary slightly for other GeneChip types.

14. Periodically, ensure that all columns have the same number of rows by navigating to the bottom of the worksheet.

References

1. Golub, T.R., Slonim, D.K., Tamayo, P., Huard, C., Gaasenbeek, M., Mesirov, J.P., Coller, H., Loh, M.L., Downing, J.R., Caligiuri, M.A., Bloomfield, C.D., and Lander, E.S. (1999) Molecular classification of cancer: class discovery and class prediction by gene expression monitoring. *Science* **286**, 531–537.

2. Huby, R. and Tugwood, J.D. (2005) Gene expression profiling for pharmaceutical safety assessment. *Expert Opin. Drug Metab. Toxicol.* **1**, 247–260.

3. Chen, J.J. (2007) Key aspects of analysing microarray gene-expression data. *Pharmacogenomics* **8**, 473–482.

Chapter 11

Protocols of Two-Dimensional Difference Gel Electrophoresis to Investigate Mechanisms of Toxicity

Emmanuelle Com, Albrecht Gruhler, Martine Courcol, and Jean-Charles Gautier

Abstract

In recent years, several global omics technologies have been increasingly used to better understand the molecular mechanisms of drug toxicity. Two-dimensional difference gel electrophoresis (2D-DIGE) is a large-scale proteomics high-resolution gel-based quantitative method widely used to detect protein expression alterations after drug treatment. The 2D-DIGE technology is based on the labeling of proteins with different fluorescent dyes, allowing the separation of different samples on the same gel with the use of an internal standard, thus reducing the complexity of spot pattern comparison and providing a reliable method applied to toxicology studies for the detection of modulated proteins in targeted organs.

Key words: Two-dimensional difference gel electrophoresis, Relative quantification, Toxicology, Drug development, Liver, Kidney

1. Introduction

In preclinical drug safety evaluation, the preliminary risks of a new compound to human safety are classically assessed by using *in vivo* studies on animals together with histopathology and biochemical parameters. The prediction of toxic effects of new drugs and the understanding of their molecular mechanisms of toxicity is one of the major challenges in drug development. Another challenge is the identification of new toxicity biomarkers which could be more sensitive and predictive than current ones. To answer these challenges, proteomics technology such as two-dimensional (2D) electrophoresis has been applied in the past few years to toxicological studies to detect global effect of compound

Jean-Charles Gautier (ed.), *Drug Safety Evaluation: Methods and Protocols*, Methods in Molecular Biology, vol. 691,
DOI 10.1007/978-1-60761-849-2_11, © Springer Science+Business Media, LLC 2011

on protein expression in target organs (1–3). The 2D technology is based on the separation of proteins according to their isoelectric points in the first dimension (isoelectric focusing) and their apparent size in the second dimension by sodium dodecyl sulfate–polyacrylamide gel electrophoresis (SDS–PAGE). Due to its high resolution, 2D-PAGE allows the resolution of complex protein mixtures and the visualization of thousands of proteins on a single gel. Thus, this technique is a powerful tool to study global changes in protein expression pattern following exposure of an organism to a toxicant. Another advantage of 2D gels is to provide information about protein modifications due to toxicants such as posttranslational modifications or proteolytic products. Two-dimensional difference gel electrophoresis (2D-DIGE) is a newly developed technology that greatly improves quantitative proteomics by 2D gel electrophoresis (4, 5). This technique is based on the use of three mass- and charge-matched, spectrally resolvable fluorescent dyes (Cy2, Cy3, and Cy5) which are covalently linked to lysine residues of intact proteins. This allows analyzing a mixture of three differently labeled protein samples in one gel, thus greatly improving the comparison of different samples. Typically, one of the samples is an internal standard which is a pool of all the samples of an experiment. Adding the internal standard to each gel has a twofold advantage: firstly, it enhances the matching of proteins between different gels because the spot pattern of the standard is the same for each gel and secondly, it is used to calculate protein abundances for the two other samples separated on the same gel. In addition, the internal standard allows the normalization of the abundances of each protein spots across several gels, leading to a more accurate and reliable quantification of altered protein expression with greater statistical power. 2D-DIGE minimizes gel-to-gel variations and variations due to sample preparation and processing and thereby improves the detection of biologically relevant changes in protein expression between differentially treated samples. It can be easily adapted to toxicological *in vivo* studies, comparing protein expression profiles of targeted organs such as liver or kidney from animals treated with toxicants. In this chapter, we describe the 2D-DIGE methodology used in preclinical studies with rats performed in the PredTox (predictive toxicology) consortium, which is a collaborative effort funded partly by the EU as part of the Framework 6 program, to understand mechanisms of toxicity.

2. Materials

2.1. Protein Extraction

1. Buffer 1B: 32 mM Tris–HCl pH 8.18 and 1.2% (w/v) Triton X-100. The solution is aliquoted and frozen at –20°C (see Notes 1 and 2).

2. RNAse solution: 2 mg/mL RNAse A (Sigma, R5500), 500 mM Tris pH 7.4, and 50 mM $MgCl_2$. The solution is prepared on ice by upside-down shaking, aliquoted and frozen at –20°C.

3. DNAse solution (Roche, 776 785).

4. CHAPS buffer: 21.4% (w/v) CHAPS in H_2O. The solution is aliquoted and frozen at –20°C.

5. EDTA (Sigma, E-1644) stock solution: 100 mM EDTA in H_2O. The solution is aliquoted and frozen at –20°C.

6. Pefabloc: 100 mM Pefabloc (Merck, 124839) in H_2O. The solution is aliquoted and frozen at –20°C.

7. DNAse/RNAse solution: Mix 5.32 μL DNAse and 32 μL RNAse solution. This solution must be prepared freshly.

8. Pefabloc/EDTA solution: Mix 50 μL Pefabloc and 100 μL EDTA. This solution must be prepared freshly.

9. Urea (Merck KgaA, 108484).

10. Thiourea (Merck KgaA, 107979).

11. Potter-elvehjem-type tissue grinder with teflon pestle (Thomas scientific).

12. Bradford protein assay.

13. Lyophilizer, for example, Freeze Dryer GAMMA 2-16 LSC (Martin Christ Gefriertrocknungsanlagen GmbH, Germany).

2.2. DIGE Labeling

1. N,N-Dimethylformamide (DMF) (see Note 3).

2. CyDye™ DIGE fluors (minimal dyes) 1 mM stock solution (GE Healthcare, RPK0272, RPK0273, RPK0275): reconstitute the 25 nmol dry CyDye™ in 25 μL DMF. This stock solution can be aliquoted in a sufficient volume for one experiment and frozen at –80°C.

3. 10 mM lysine quenching solution. The solution is aliquoted and frozen at –20°C.

4. 2× sample buffer (2× SB): 7 M urea, 2 M thiourea, 4% (w/v) CHAPS, 2% (w/v) DTT, 2% (v/v) Pharmalytes™ 3-10 (GE Healthcare, 17-0456-01), and 0.2% (v/v) Triton X-100. The solution is aliquoted and frozen at –20°C (see Note 4).

2.3. Two-Dimensional Electrophoresis

2.3.1. Isoelectric Focusing (First Dimension)

1. Immobiline™ DryStrip Reswelling tray (GE Healthcare, 80-6371-84).

2. Isoelectric Focusing (IEF) Multiphor™ II apparatus (GE Healthcare, 18-1018-06).

3. Immobilized pH gradient (IPG) strips (Immobiline™ DryStrip gels 18 cm, pH 5.5–6.7, GE Healthcare, 17-6001-87) (see Note 5).

4. Rehydration buffer: 6 M urea, 2 M thiourea, 1% (w/v) CHAPS, 0.4% (w/v) DTT, and 0.5% (v/v) Pharmalytes™ pH 3–10 (GE Healthcare, 17-0456-01). Aliquots may be stored for several weeks at –20°C.

5. Mineral oil (Aldrich, 16140-3).

6. 1.5 cm width electrode papers cut in 5 mm filter paper.

7. Equilibration buffer: 100 mM Tris–HCl pH 6.8, 8 M urea, 30% (v/v) glycerol, and 1% (w/v) SDS. This solution must be prepared freshly (see Note 6).

8. DTT (Prolabo, 33630-135).

9. Iodoacetamide (Sigma, I-6125).

2.3.2. SDS–PAGE (Second Dimension)

1. Gel caster IsoDalt system (Hoefer, 80-6330-61).

2. Low-fluorescence glass plates 25×20 cm (GE Healthcare, 80-6448-98).

3. Bind silane solution: 2 mL bind silane (GE Healthcare, 17-1330-01) in 500 mL water acidified with three drops of glacial acetic acid. Shake at least 15 min until complete dissolution (see Note 7).

4. Picking Reference markers (GE Healthcare, 18-1143-34).

5. Gel solution for 24 large format gels (25×20 cm): 844 mL PROTOGEL (30% (w/v) acrylamide/methylenebisacrylamide solution – 37.5:1 ratio, National Diagnostics, EC-890-1L), 500 mL 1.5 M Tris–HCl, 0.4% SDS pH 8.6, 100 g Glycerol, 564 mL water, and 800 μL *N*,*N*,*N'*,*N'*-Tetramethylethylene diamine (TEMED). Prepare fresh prior to use.

6. Ammonium persulfate: 10% (w/v) solution in water. Prepare fresh prior to use.

7. Displacement solution: 50% (w/v) glycerol in water with trace amount of bromophenol blue (GE Healthcare, 17-1329-01) (see Note 8). Approximately 100 mL/cast is needed.

8. 0.1% SDS solution prepared freshly.

9. Mark12™ unstained molecular weight standard (Invitrogen, LC5677).

10. IsoDalt SDS–PAGE tank (Hoefer, 80-6068-98).

11. SDS–PAGE running buffer: 24 mM Tris, 200 mM Glycine, and 0.1% SDS.

12. Low melting point (LMP) agarose sealing solution: 1% (w/v) dissolved in running buffer with trace amount of bromophenol blue (see Note 8).

13. Sypro Ruby protein gel stain (BioRad, 170-3125).

14. Fixing solution: 30% ethanol, 7.5% acetic acid, and 0.01% SDS.

15. Destain solution: 10% methanol and 6% acetic acid.

2.4. Image Acquisition and Analysis

1. ProXPRESS™ CCD camera (Perkin Elmer) or Diversity CCD camera (Syngene) equipped with lasers and filters that are compatible with the emission/excitation spectra of CyDyes™ or Typhoon™ scanner (GE Healthcare).
2. DeCyder™ 2D 6.5 software (GE Healthcare).

3. Methods

3.1. Sample Preparation from Targeted Organs (Kidney and Liver)

3.1.1. Protein Extraction from Kidney

1. Transfer frozen kidney in the precooled Potter-elvehjem-type tissue grinder with teflon pestle.
2. According to the weight of the tissue, add corresponding volume of precooled buffer 1B (40 µL for 35 mg of tissue), Pefabloc/EDTA solution (3.25 µL for 35 mg of tissue), and DNAse/RNAse solution (9.3 µL for 35 mg of tissue).
3. Homogenize at 2,000 rpm on ice.
4. Transfer in a microtube and incubate for 10 min on ice.
5. Add at room temperature corresponding amounts of urea (52.5 mg for 35 mg of tissue), thiourea (19.25 mg for 35 mg of tissue), and CHAPS buffer (23.5 µL per 35 mg of tissue).
6. Gently mix by upside-down shaking until dissolution of urea and thiourea. This can take several minutes. Do not vortex nor heat the solution (see Note 9).
7. Centrifuge for 45 min at $100,000 \times g$ at 20°C.
8. Discard the pellet and transfer the supernatant into a new tube.
9. Determine the protein concentration using a Bradford assay. The protein concentration is generally between 20 and 30 mg/mL.
10. Aliquot the supernatant and store at –80°C (see Note 10).

3.1.2. Protein Extraction from Liver

1. Frozen liver tissues are lyophilized using the conditions indicated in Table 1.
2. The lyophilized tissue is ground to a fine powder with a pestle in a mortar between sheets of weighing paper. The ground tissue is stored at –80°C.
3. Buffer 1B is heated to 100°C.
4. 160 µL of heated buffer 1B are added to 20 mg of lyophilized tissue powder, and samples are vortexed vigorously. It is important that all of the tissue powder comes in contact with the buffer. The resulting solution is very viscous (see Note 11).
5. The samples are incubated at 100°C for 5 min and are regularly mixed by a fast vortex during this incubation.

Table 1
Lyophilization protocol for liver

Process phase	Time (h)	Temperature (°C)	Vacuum (mbar)
Freezing	1	–50	
Sublimation	2	–50	0.009
Sublimation	2	–40	0.011
Sublimation	2	–30	0.03
Sublimation	30	–20	1.03
Sublimation	4	0	1.03
Second drying	8	20	0.001

6. The sample tubes are cooled on ice for 5 min. Then, 15 μL of the Pefabloc/EDTA solution is added and the sample is vortexed.

7. 37.2 μL of the DNAse/RNAse mix are added.

8. Degradation of nucleic acids is carried out for 30 min on ice.

9. 210 mg urea, 76 mg thiourea, and 94 μL CHAPS buffer are added directly to the solution at room temperature.

10. The sample is gently mixed (not vortexed) until dissolution of the urea/thiourea (see Note 9). This can take several minutes. Alternatively, the samples can also be rotated for 20–30 min at ambient temperature.

11. The protein extract is centrifuged for 45 min at $100,000 \times g$ at 20°C (see Note 12).

12. The supernatant is removed from the pellet, aliquoted and stored at –80°C (see Note 10).

13. Protein concentration is determined with a Bradford assay.

3.2. Experimental Design and Protein Preparation and Labeling

3.2.1. Experimental Design

1. Control and treated protein extracts were labeled with Cy2 and Cy5 in a reciprocal manner (i.e., dye swapping), so that both the control and the treated group contain samples that were labeled with either Cy2 or Cy5 (see Note 13).

2. A pooled internal standard which is a mix of all the control and treated protein extracts is labeled with Cy3 (see Note 14). It allows the calculation of the expression ratios within a gel and the normalization of these ratios between several gels.

3. A mix of a Cy2-labeled sample type 1, a Cy3-labeled standard, and a Cy5-labeled sample type 2 is run on each gel.

4. At least four different analytical gels corresponding to biological replicates are required for a good statistical confidence.

5. In each experiment, two preparative gels for spot picking and MS identification are run in parallel in order to facilitate the spot matching between analytical and preparative gels by minimizing experimental variations. On one gel, 500 μg of a mix of the control samples are loaded allowing the picking of the downregulated spots in the treated samples, and on the other one 500 μg of a mix of the treated samples are loaded allowing the picking of upregulated in the treated samples.

6. A quality control is performed for each experiment where samples from internal standard are labeled with Cy2, Cy3, and Cy5 and run on the same gel. Analysis of pair images is performed using the DIA module of DeCyder™ software, and quality criteria of the protein labeling are checked: frequency distribution of the log of spot volume ratios very close to normality and less than 5% of the spots detected as false up- or downregulated with a cutoff value of their modulation factors ≥1.3 in absolute value (Fig. 1).

7. Each experiment (analytical gels, preparative gels, and quality control gel) is performed in duplicate and the experiment showing the best images and quality control is kept for further analysis.

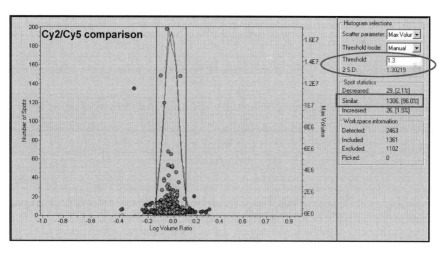

Fig. 1. Frequency distribution of the modulation factors of spots in a quality control gel. In this example, the Cy2 and Cy5 images are compared. The *black* and *white circles* correspond to the modulation factor of each protein calculated after a logarithmic transformation of the pixel volume ratios Cy5 versus Cy2. This transformation is achieved to get a Gaussian distribution and is helpful to select the modulation factor threshold. The two curves which correspond to the theoretical distribution and the observed distribution are merged in this case. In this example, the 2 SD (standard deviation) value of 1.302 means that 95% of the spots have a modulation factor (in absolute value) equal or below this threshold value. Here, the threshold, represented by the *solid black* lines, was adjusted to 1.3 and as a result, 96% of the spots are considered to be similar in terms of modulation (*white circles* inside the *solid black lines*) and about 2% of the spots were found upregulated (*black circles* in the right of the *solid black line*) or downregulated (*black circles* in the left of the *solid black line*).

3.2.2. Protein Preparation and Labeling

1. Prepare the pooled internal standard by mixing equal protein amounts from all samples from the two conditions (control and treated) to be compared.

2. Prepare control and treated samples for preparative gels by mixing equal protein amounts from all the control samples and from all the treated samples, respectively.

3. Prepare prior to use the 400 μM CyDye™ working solution by adding 1 volume of 1 mM CyDye™ stock solution to 1.5 volumes of DMF.

4. Add 1 μL CyDye™ working solution (400 pmol) to 50 μg of each protein sample (see Notes 15 and 16).

5. Gently mix and spin briefly in a microcentrifuge.

6. Incubate for 30 min at room temperature in darkness.

7. Add 1 μL of 10 mM lysine, mix gently, and spin briefly in a microcentrifuge. Incubate for an additional 10 min at room temperature in darkness to stop each reaction.

8. Add to each reaction tube an equal volume of 2× SB.

9. Gently mix and spin briefly in a microcentrifuge.

10. Incubate for 15 min at room temperature in darkness.

11. One aliquot each of Cy2-, Cy3-, and Cy5-labeled samples are mixed (i.e., 150 μg total protein) and used for IEF.

12. In parallel label 5 μL of molecular weight standard with 1 μL (40 pmol) of 40 μM CyDye™ in the same manner than the sample. After adding 1 μL of 10 mM lysine quenching solution, the Cy2-, Cy3-, and Cy5-labeled molecular weight standards are mixed and stored at 4°C in the dark until using for the SDS–PAGE.

3.3. Two-Dimensional Electrophoresis

3.3.1. Isoelectric Focusing (First Dimension)

IEF should be performed according to the manufacturer's instructions. Refer to the user's manual for general details. We describe here only specific steps of our protocol:

1. Rehydrate IPG strips in the Immobiline™ DryStrip Reswelling tray with 400 μL rehydration buffer. Overlay each strip with 2 mL mineral oil and incubate at 22°C for at least 8 h.

2. Transfer the IPG strips (gel side up) directly onto the Immobiline™ DryStrip tray which is positioned on the cooling plate of the Multiphor™ II. The temperature of the cooling plate is set to 22°C.

3. Soak 1.5 cm width electrode papers with water (see Note 17), place these moistened papers across the anodic and cathodic ends of the strips, and place the electrode over these papers.

4. Place the sample cups at the anodic side of the strip, pour mineral oil into the tray to completely cover the strips and the cups (see Note 18).

Table 2
Migration parameters for isoelectrofocalisation

Step	Voltage	Duration (h)	Voltage gradient type	Duration (kVh)
1	50	2	Step and hold	
2	100	2	Step and hold	
3	300	2	Step and hold	
4	2,000	16	Step and hold	
5	3,500	18	Step and hold	95.9

5. Load the CyDye™ labeled samples in the cups and run on Multiphor™ II with the parameters indicated in Table 2 (see Note 19).

6. Replace electrode papers soaked with water once after 10 h at 2,000 V and once at the beginning of the 3,500 V step (see Note 17).

7. After the run is complete, the voltage is ramped down to 100 V to maintain focusing until equilibration steps are performed.

8. Carefully remove the maximum of mineral oil by aspiration, remove the electrode papers, and replace by dried ones.

9. Add 100 mL of equilibration buffer containing 0.5% DTT in the Immobiline™ DryStrip tray and incubate for 10 min at room temperature with gentle agitation. In this step, the cysteine sulfhydryl groups of the focused proteins are reduced.

10. Replace the DTT equilibration solution by 100 mL of equilibration buffer containing 4.5% iodoacetamide and incubate for an additional 10 min with gentle agitation. This step corresponds to the alkylation of the reduced sulfhydryl groups of cysteine, leading to cysteine S-carbamidomethyl residue.

11. After equilibration, IPG strips can be stored at –80°C up to 2 weeks on a rigid support and under a sealed plastic film.

3.3.2. SDS–PAGE
(Second Dimension)

3.3.2.1. Preparation
of the Preparative Gels

Picking reference markers are used by the spot picking software to determine spot coordinates. Gels for spot picking (preparative gels) are cast with picking reference markers and have to be bound with bind silane to the back glass plate. The preparation of the bind silane plate and the assembly of plates must be performed under a fume hood to ensure that dusts or particles do not settle on the plate:

1. Wash the low-fluorescence glass plates with water and dried them with a nonfluffy paper.

2. Add at least 70 mL of bind silane solution on one plate for each gel and let it contact for at least 1 h. Be careful that the whole surface of the plate is recovered by the solution.

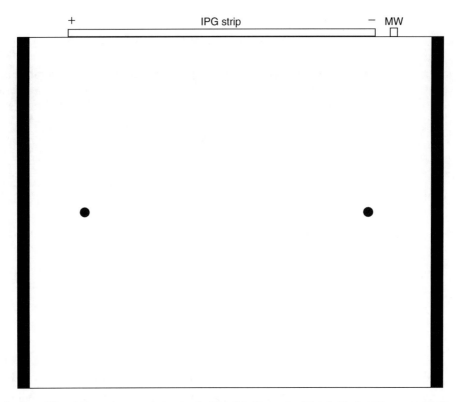

Fig. 2. Position of the picking reference markers and of the IPG strip on the 2D gel. *Black circles* represent the picking reference markers. The acid (+) and the basic (−) ends of the IPG strip are annotated. *MW* position of the molecular weight standards. The *black rectangles* represent the spacers.

3. Remove the excess of solution, wash plates with water, and dry the plates for at least 1 h.

4. Place the reference markers on the bind silane-treated plate. The reference markers must be positioned in the middle of the plate at the left and the right side of the plate close to the spacer, so that they cannot interfere with protein spots (see Note 20 and Fig. 2).

5. Assemble the front plate and the bind silane-treated plate with the 1 mm thick spacers and place them in the gel caster. The assemblage of the silane-treated plate must be performed just prior to cast the gels to avoid transfer of bind silane vapors on the nontreated plate which will make difficult the turning out of the gels.

3.3.2.2. Preparation of the Gel Solution and Cast of the SDS–PAGE Gels

1. Wash the low-fluorescence glass plates with water and dried them with a nonfluffy paper.

2. Assemble the glass plates with the 1 mm thick spacers, place them on the gel caster, and assemble it.

3. At the same time, prepare the gel solution and degas it under gentle agitation.

4. Add 10 mL of freshly prepared 10% APS.

5. Introduce the gel in the gel caster until 1–2 cm before the top of the plates.

6. Replace by the displacement solution which will balance with the gel solution to the desired height.

7. Immediately pipet 1 mL of 0.1% SDS solution onto each gel to create a level interface.

8. Allow the gel to polymerase for at least 1 h at room temperature before disassembling the caster. Rinse thoroughly the gels with water and check that the top of the gels are linear, allowing a good contact between the strip and the polyacrylamide gel. The gels can be stored horizontally in an airtight container covered with tissue paper soaked with water at 4°C for several days.

3.3.2.3. SDS–PAGE Procedure

1. If polyacrylamide gels are stored at 4°C, let them warm at room temperature.

2. Heat 1% LMP agarose in a microwave until liquefaction and keep it in heated water (max. 60°C) to avoid solidification.

3. Just after equilibration, rinse the IPG strip with SDS–PAGE running buffer.

4. Cut about 8 and 5 mm at the anodic and cathodic side of the strip, respectively, in order to discard the precipitation area of the proteins at the acidic and basic end of the strip that could interfere with image acquisition and analysis. The size of the piece of strip to cut could vary in function of the localization of the electrode papers during the IEF. The areas of precipitation are slightly visible with white strokes and therefore must be cut accordingly.

5. Fill the top of the polyacrylamide gel with LMP agarose without bubbles and immediately place the IPG strip onto the polyacrylamide gel, center it in regards to the reference markers, so that all the strips are aligned in the same manner on the 2D gels (Fig. 2).

6. Ensure that the strip is in direct contact with the polyacrylamide gel by carefully pushing the plastic side of the strip with the end of a thin spatula. If enough LMP agarose is used, there are no bubbles formed between strip and gel or glass plates.

7. Wait several minutes that agarose is solidified.

8. Load 2 μL of labeled molecular weight standards on a small filter paper pad (5 × 5 mm) and place it near the basic end of the IPG strip (Fig. 2).

9. Fill the SDS–PAGE tank with running buffer which is prepared the day before and kept at 4°C. The buffer should be stirred constantly at 10°C (see Note 21).

10. Place the gels in the electrophoresis tank and run electrophoresis with the following parameters: 50 mA for 1.5 h, 100 mA for 1.5 h, and 25 mA/gel for an overnight migration, until the migration front reaches the bottom of the gels (see Note 22).

3.3.2.4. Poststaining of the Preparative Gels

1. Carefully remove the front glasses (untreated with bind silane) of the preparative gels, as the IEF strip and the agarose sealing gel.

2. Fix the preparative gels in the fixing solution for 2 h at room temperature under gentle agitation.

3. Stain with the Sypro Ruby solution overnight at room temperature under gentle agitation.

4. Destain 1 h at room temperature under gentle agitation with the destain solution.

3.4. Image Acquisition and Analysis

3.4.1. Image Acquisition of Analytical Gels

Immediately after SDS–PAGE, analytical gels are scanned at a resolution of 100 μm using a ProXPRESS™ CCD camera with the Cy2, Cy3, and Cy5 filters indicated in Table 3 (see Note 23):

1. Perform a prescan during 1,000 ms and note for each channel the intensity of the maximum pixel value. Ensure that this value corresponds to a protein spot and not to a dust particle.

2. Calculate the exposure time needed for reaching a maximum pixel value of 55,000 and scan the gels accordingly.

3. Repeat the operation for each gel (see Note 24).

Table 3
Filter parameters used for image acquisition using ProXPRESS™ CCD camera

	Excitation		Emission	
	Peak (nm)	Bandwidth (nm)	Peak (nm)	Bandwidth (nm)
Cy2	480	35	530	30
Cy3	540	25	590	35
Cy5	625	35	680	30
Sypro Ruby	480	35	633	40

3.4.2. Image Acquisition of Preparative Gels

Immediately after destaining, preparative gels are scanned at a resolution of 100 µm using a ProXPRESS™ CCD camera with the filters indicated in Table 3 for Sypro Ruby.

1. Reassemble the gels.

2. Scan each preparative gel so that the maximum pixel value is close to the value obtained for the analytical gels.

3. Store the preparative gels in the destain solution at 4°C until spot picking.

3.4.3. Image Analysis Using DeCyder™ 6.5 Software

Image analysis is performed according to the software user manual.

3.4.3.1. Quality Control of the CyDye™ Labeling

1. Perform the image analysis with the Differential In-gel Analysis (DIA) module of the software which allowed the intragel analysis.

2. Create a workspace with the Cy2, Cy3, and Cy5 images of the quality control gel.

3. Perform spot detection with an estimated number of spots of 2,500 (see Note 25).

4. Carefully remove the nonprotein spots from the analysis by performing spot exclusion according to the software user manual. The following parameters could be set for a first filtering: slope > 1.2, area < 100, height < 200, and volume < 10,000 that should be completed by manual inspection.

5. Check that the frequency distribution of the log volume ratio for the Cy2/Cy3 and Cy5/Cy3 image analyses is close to the normality in the histogram view.

6. Check also in the histogram view that for a threshold of 1.3, at least 95% of the detected spots are considered as similar (the 2 SD (standard deviation) value should be under the 1.3 value) (Fig. 1).

7. If all these criteria are fulfilled, the quality of the labeling is good enough to perform the analysis with the analytical gels.

3.4.3.2. Analysis of the Analytical Gels

1. The DIA module of the software should be used first for the intragel analysis (see Note 26).

2. Create a workspace for all the analyzed gels.

3. Perform spot detection with an estimated number of spots of 2,500 (see Note 25).

4. Create a workspace in the Biological Variation Analysis (BVA) module for the intergel analysis with each DIA of the analytical gels.

5. Perform the intergel matching and check that the master gel corresponds to the Cy3 (standard) image of the gel with the most important number of spots.

6. Manually check the matching between each gel, merge or divide spots if necessary.

7. In the experimental design view of the spot map table, define each group (control, standard, and treated) and assign each image of each gel to one of these groups.

8. In the protein statistics dialog box, choose the options of the statistical analysis:

   (a) Independent tests

   (b) Average ratio

   (c) Student's t-test

   (d) Population 1: control

   (e) Population 2: treated

   And perform the statistical t-test analysis.

9. Define protein of interest in the protein filter toolbox: spots with a p-value (t-test)≤ 0.01 and a volume ratio ≥ 1.3 or ≤ -1.3.

10. Among the protein of interest, manually check the spots and if they are correct select the "Pick" check box.

3.4.3.3. Processing the Preparative Gels and Generating a Picking List

The preparative gels have to be matched to the analytical gels in the BVA module in order to pick in the preparative gels the spots corresponding to those showing differential expression in the analytical gels:

1. Create a DIA workspace for each preparative gels (one with the pooled control samples for the downregulated proteins and one with the pooled treated samples for the upregulated proteins).

2. Perform spot detection with an estimated number of spots of 2,500 and the "autodetected picking references" check box selected (see Note 25).

3. Include these DIA analyses in the previous BVA analysis.

4. For each spot map corresponding to each preparative gel, deselect the default "Analysis" check box and select the "Pick" one.

5. Match the preparative gels with the analytical ones.

6. Manually check that spots assigned with a Pick status are present with sufficient intensity and are matched in the preparative gels. If it is not the case, deselect the "Pick" check box of the corresponding spot.

7. Export the picking list in an appropriate file extension for further spot picking.

8. Transfer the picking list and the corresponding preparative gel to an appropriate picking system for the excision of spots which could then be processed for identification by mass spectrometry.

4. Notes

1. All the solutions should be prepared with 18.2 MΩ water, stored at 4°C if not frozen, and filtered with a 0.45 μm filtration device.

2. Wear powder-free gloves (preferably latex-free) and mobcap at each steps of the protocol to avoid keratin contamination which prevents further optimal protein identification by mass spectrometry.

3. Should not be used for more than 3 months once opened.

4. IPG buffer pH 5.5-6.7 can be used in the 2× SB buffer.

5. Different pH ranges for IPG strips from wide range (i.e., pH 3–10) to narrow range (i.e., pH 5.5–6.7) are commercially available. We recommend using high-resolution narrow-range IPG strips in order to detect more faint proteins and to limit the comigration phenomenon (6). Indeed when several proteins comigrate in the same spot, after MS identification it is almost impossible to know which protein is really modulated. Moreover, comigration of several proteins could prevent high confidence MS identification.

6. Alternative protocol: keep the equilibration solution for up to 6 months on the shelf and add DTT/iodoacetamide fresh.

7. Alternative protocol for bind silane solution: 8 mL 70% ethanol, 200 μL acetic acid, and 10 μL Bind Silane. Use 4 mL per glass plate, spread the solution evenly with a lint-free cloth, and let it dry for at least 2 h.

8. Use products compatible with fluorescence staining (e.g., bromophenol blue) and do not use products which could interfere with fluorescence staining (such as color markers).

9. Never heat urea solutions above room temperature as this leads to the carbamylation of proteins and to charge trains in 2D gels.

10. It is important to store the extracted proteins at –80°C to avoid the viscosity observed at a –20°C storage.

11. Alternatively, the protein extraction can be done using the Sample Grinding Kit (GE Healthcare) with lysis buffer (7 M urea, 2 M thiourea; 30 mM Tris–HCl pH 8.5; 4% (w/v) CHAPS).

12. Alternative protocol: If necessary, the ultracentrifugation step could be replaced by two centrifugations at $20,000 \times g$ at 20°C.

13. The labeling of one sample type (i.e., control or treated) with only one CyDye™ could lead to the detection of false-positive modulated spots which has been estimated to 15% in our experiment.

14. Alternative protocol: in most DIGE studies, Cy2 is used for the labeling of internal standard because it is structurally a little different from Cy3 and Cy5, leading to very subtle migration differences for some proteins in SDS–PAGE (particularly when high current is applied for a quick run). We had never observed any differences in labeling efficiency nor dye bias between the three dyes and we decided to use Cy3 for internal standard labeling.

15. Manufacturer (GE Healthcare) states that the labeling efficiency is also dependent on protein concentration which should be between 5 and 10 mg/mL. However in our conditions, an efficient labeling is achieved above 10 mg/mL and the protocol described here has been used successfully to label proteins up to 30 mg/mL.

16. For an efficient labeling, it is essential that the pH of the protein solution is between pH 8.0 and 9.0. Usually with the protocol described here, the pH of the protein solution has not to be changed.

17. During IEF, the change of electrode paper damped with distilled water is performed to avoid electroendosmosis. Electrode papers must be damp, not wet. Blot with tissue paper to remove excess of water which may cause streaking.

18. If the oil leaks into the sample cups, suck the oil up, adjust the leakage, and check for leakage again.

19. The IEF parameters described here are optimized for 18 cm pH 5.5–6.7 IPG strips run on a Multiphor™ II apparatus. Changes in IEF apparatus, pH ranges, strips lengths, or samples need other optimization for the IEF parameters.

20. It could be useful to use a schema of the plate with a cross to locate the position of the reference markers, so that these positions are always the same for all the gels.

21. It is often recommended to perform migration at higher temperature to increase the resolution of the spots. It could be applied when gels are run at constant power, so that the heat input is constant during the migration. When gels are run at constant current, the heat input increases during migration and the running buffer needs to be cooled.

22. A slight difference in the migration of Cy2- and Cy5-labeled samples has been observed when high current is applied for a quick run. The consequence is that the same spot could be detected as two different ones by the image analysis software, leading to the detection of false-positive differential spots.

23. The scanning procedure is rather long. So during this procedure, the gels must be kept in the migration buffer cooled at 10°C to prevent them from drying.

24. The maximum pixel intensity of each image in a gel and between each gel of an experiment should not differ by more than 5,000–10,000 and the most intense spots should not be saturated. This is crucial to obtain meaningful quantitative comparison between all the gel images.

25. For spot detection, it is recommended to slightly overestimate the number of spots detected on the gel in order to compensate the detection of nonprotein spots (such as dust particles). For a kidney or a liver lysate run on an 18 cm pH 5.5–6.7 Immobiline™ DryStrip and a large format gel, around 1,700 protein spots are detected and a value of 2,500 for the estimated number of spots is satisfactory.

26. The batch processing function of the DeCyder™ software can be used to create automatically both the individual DIA and the BVA workspaces. Removal of a lot of the noise can easily be done by filtering for the spot volume, for example, only spots with volume >30,000 are used. In this case, it is not necessary to estimate the number of spots because the maximum number of 10,000 can be used for the spot detection.

Acknowledgments

The authors would like to acknowledge Jean-François Léonard for insightful discussions and critical reading of the manuscript and Claire Mariet for advice and technical assistance. This work was supported by the EU FP6 Integrated Project InnoMed PredTox.

References

1. Charlwood, J., Skehel, J. M., King, N., Camilleri, P., Lord, P., Bugelski, P., and Atif, U. (2002) Proteomic analysis of rat kidney cortex following treatment with gentamicin. *J Proteome Res.* **1**, 73–82.

2. Léonard, J. F., Courcol, M., Mariet, C., Charbonnier, A., Boitier, E., Duchesne, M., Parker, F., Genet, B., Supatto, F., Roberts, R., and Gautier, J.-C. (2006) Proteomic characterization of the effects of clofibrate on protein expression in rat liver. *Proteomics* **6**, 1915–1933.

3. Friry-Santini, C., Rouquie, D., Kennel, P., Tinwell, H., Benahmed, M., and Bars, R. (2007) Correlation between protein accumulation profiles and conventional toxicological findings using a model antiandrogenic compound, flutamide. *Toxicol. Sci.* **97**, 81–93.

4. Unlu, M., Morgan, M. E., and Minden, J. S. (1997) Difference gel electrophoresis: a single gel method for detecting changes in protein extracts. *Electrophoresis* **18**, 2071–2077.

5. Alban, A., David, S. O., Bjorkesten, L., Andersson, C., Sloge, E., Lewis, S., and Currie, I. (2003) A novel experimental design for comparative two-dimensional gel analysis: two-dimensional difference gel electrophoresis incorporating a pooled internal standard. *Proteomics* **3**, 36–44.

6. Com, E., Evrard, B., Roepstorff, P., Aubry, F., and Pineau, C. (2003) New insights into the rat spermatogonial proteome: identification of 156 additional proteins. *Mol. Cell. Proteomics* **2**, 248–261.

Chapter 12

Protocols and Applications of Cellular Metabolomics in Safety Studies Using Precision-Cut Tissue Slices and Carbon 13 NMR

Gabriel Baverel, Sophie Renault, Hassan Faiz, Maha El Hage, Catherine Gauthier, Agnès Duplany, Bernard Ferrier, and Guy Martin

Abstract

Numerous xenobiotics are toxic to human and animal cells by interacting with their metabolism, but the precise metabolic step affected and the biochemical mechanism behind such a toxicity often remain unknown. In an attempt to reduce the ignorance in this field, we have developed a new approach called cellular metabolomics. This approach, developed *in vitro*, provides a panoramic view not only of the pathways involved in the metabolism of physiologic substrates of any normal or pathologic human or animal cell but also of the beneficial and adverse effects of xenobiotics on these metabolic pathways. Unlike many cell lines, precision-cut tissue slices, for which there is a renewed interest, remain metabolically differentiated for at least 24–48 h and allow to study the effect of xenobiotics during short-term and long-term incubations. Cellular metabolomics (or cellular metabonomics), which combines enzymatic and carbon 13 NMR measurements with mathematical modeling of metabolic pathways, is illustrated in this brief chapter for studying the effect of insulin on glucose metabolism in rat liver precision-cut slices, and of valproate on glutamine metabolism in human renal cortical precision-cut slices. The use of very small amounts of test compounds allows to predict their toxic effect and eventually their beneficial effects very early in the research and development processes. Cellular metabolomics is complementary to other omics approaches, but, unlike them, provides functional and dynamic pieces of information by measuring enzymatic fluxes.

Key words: Toxicology, Liver, Kidney, Cellular metabolomics, Carbon 13 NMR

1. Introduction

Tissue slices, used since the 1920s (1), have proved to be a very useful *in vitro* tool to identify most of the cellular metabolic pathways. With the availability of collagenase in the seventies (2),

Jean-Charles Gautier (ed.), *Drug Safety Evaluation: Methods and Protocols*, Methods in Molecular Biology, vol. 691,
DOI 10.1007/978-1-60761-849-2_12, © Springer Science+Business Media, LLC 2011

they have been progressively replaced by cells isolated from a great variety of tissues. Thanks to technical improvements that made the preparation of automatically thinner slices possible (3), there has been a renewed interest in the use of precision-cut tissue slices starting about 30 years ago, particularly for pharmaco-toxicology studies (4–6). The latter model presents a number of advantages over other cellular models used *in vitro*: maintenance of the *in vivo* tissue architecture, of the heterogeneity of cell populations, and of cell–cell and cell–matrix interactions; use of the same cellular model for short-term (for up to some hours) and long-term (for at least up to 48 h) incubations; possibility of histological studies and preservation of differentiated metabolic functions.

Numerous xenobiotics are toxic to various tissues and cells because they interact negatively with cellular energy metabolism but, in most cases, the precise adverse mechanism involved remains unknown. This is why it is desirable to understand the precise biochemical step(s) altered and responsible for these toxic effects. For this, the development of methods that provide a panoramic view of cellular metabolic pathways is needed.

Because this has been comprehensively covered by other authors (7–12), the objectives of this chapter are not to explain in detail how to prepare and incubate precision-cut tissue slices and how this experimental model can be used for toxicology and drug metabolism studies. Rather, we wish to illustrate our experience with the use of precision-cut liver and kidney slices in combination with what we call "cellular metabolomics" to understand how hepatotoxic and nephrotoxic drugs may interfere with cellular metabolic pathways. Indeed, traditional metabolomics, which uses either the mass spectrometry (MS) or the nuclear magnetic resonance spectrometry (MRS) techniques, is a large-scale method that allows to identify and quantify metabolites present in body fluids (mainly urine and plasma) (13); metabolomics is of great diagnostic and prognostic value, but rarely allows to identify the mechanisms behind the biomarkers identified. This is why we have developed a cellular metabolomic approach that combines the use of enzymatic and carbon 13 MRS measurements with mathematical modeling of metabolic pathways. This new approach provides a panoramic view not only of all the pathways involved in the metabolism of any given substrate in any human or animal cell type *in vitro*, but also of the beneficial and adverse effects of xenobiotics on these metabolic pathways. For this, only small amounts of test compounds are needed, which explains why it is possible to predict both the beneficial and toxic effects of these compounds at a very early stage of the research and development processes.

2. Materials

2.1. Reagents and Incubation Media

1. Enzymes, coenzymes, and L-lactate were supplied by Roche Molecular Biochemicals (Meylan, France). L-glutamine, D-glucose, and valproate were obtained from Sigma Chemicals (St. Louis, MO, USA). L-[3-^{13}C]glutamine, [2-^{13}C]glycine, deuterated water, and D-[2-^{13}C]glucose were obtained from Euriso-Top (St. Aubain, France). These ^{13}C-labeled compounds had a 99% isotopic abundance.

2. Krebs–Henseleit buffer (see Note 1 for the composition of this buffer).

3. William's Medium E was obtained from Invitrogen (Cergy-Pontoise, France; see Note 2 for the composition of this medium).

2.2. Liver and Kidney-Cortex Samples

1. Fresh human normal kidney cortex was obtained from the uninvolved pole of kidneys removed for neoplasm from 18-h-fasted patients.

2. Fed or 48-h-fasted male Wistar rats (250–300 g) were obtained from Charles River (Saint Germain sur l'Arbresle, France) and anesthetized with sodium pentobarbital (35 mg/kg body weight, i.p.). The portal vein was catheterized and the inferior vena cava was severed; then, ice-cold well-oxygenated Krebs–Henseleit buffer was infused for 3 min before removal of the liver and kidneys. The kidneys were sagitally opened and the medulla discarded.

2.3. Preparation of Precision-Cut Liver and Renal Cortical Slices and Incubations

1. Tissue coring tool (Alabama R&D, Alabama, USA).
2. Krumdieck tissue slicer (Alabama R&D, Alabama, USA).
3. Teflon rollers (Vitron Inc., Tucson, Arizona, USA).
4. HClO$_4$.

2.4. ^{13}C-NMR

1. Bruker AM-500 WB spectrometer.

3. Methods

This section describes the preparation of precision-cut liver and renal cortical slices, incubation procedures, metabolic characterization of precision-cut liver and kidney slices, and applications of cellular metabolomics to safety problems.

3.1. Preparation of Precision-Cut Liver and Renal Cortical Slices

1. Cylindrical cores of 5 or 8-mm diameter were prepared from renal cortical or liver sections with a tissue coring tool from the kidneys and the liver, respectively.

2. The cores were maintained in oxygenated (5% CO_2 and 95% O_2) ice-cold Krebs–Henseleit buffer and transferred to a Krumdieck tissue slicer filled with oxygenated ice-cold Krebs–Henseleit buffer and set to produce slices of 200–250-μm thickness.

3.2. Incubation Procedures

1. Short-term incubations were performed for up to 4 h at 37°C in 2 or 4 mL of Krebs–Henseleit medium in a shaking water bath in 25-mL stoppered Erlenmeyer flasks with an atmosphere of 5% CO_2 and 95% O_2. Slices were incubated with either unlabeled or ^{13}C-labeled substrate (glutamine, glucose, lactate, alanine, etc.) in the absence and the presence of the effector (agonist or antagonist) of interest (see Notes 1 and 3).

2. When "long-term" incubations were performed, the slices were floated on to Teflon rollers which were carefully loaded into scintillation vials containing 2 mL of William's medium E supplemented with the unlabeled or ^{13}C-labeled substrate of interest in the absence and the presence of the effector. The vials were closed with a cap having a central hole, placed horizontally on a vial rotator in a humidified incubator and set at 37°C and gassed with 40% O_2, 5% CO_2 and 55% N_2 (see Notes 2–4). Then, the slices were incubated either between 0 and 24 h or between 24 and 48 h after a prior 24-h incubation period.

3. Incubations were terminated by removing the slices and adding $HClO_4$ [2% (v/v) final concentration] to the incubation medium. In the flasks in which lactate dehydrogenase (LDH) activity was measured, slices were used for intracellular LDH activity measurement and the medium was collected for extracellular LDH measurement before $HClO_4$ addition. In all experiments, zero-time flasks were prepared with slices by adding $HClO_4$ before the slices. In all experiments, each experimental condition was performed at least in duplicate.

3.3. ATP and Protein Content

1. After the incubation, two slices were homogenized in 0.2 mL of cold 7% (v/v) $HClO_4$ using an Ultraturrax homogenizer at 9,500 rpm, and after centrifugation of the homogenate for 5 min at $3,000 \times g$, the supernatant was neutralized with 20% KOH before ATP measurement. The slice ATP content was quantified using the method of Lamprecht and Trautschold (14).

2. Pellets were solubilized in 0.5 M NaOH for protein determination. Total protein was determined according to the method of Lowry et al. (15) using bovine serum albumin as internal standard.

3.4. LDH Release

At the end of the incubation period, the slices were removed, frozen in liquid nitrogen, and thawed three times to release intracellular LDH. Enzyme leakage, a marker of the integrity of the cellular plasma membrane, was determined in the incubation medium and compared with total LDH activity (extracellular and intracellular LDH). LDH activity was determined using the method described by Bergmeyer and Bernt (16).

3.5. Metabolite Assays

After removing the denatured protein by centrifugation (3,000×g for 5 min), the supernatant was neutralized with 20% KOH and used for metabolite determinations. Glutamine, glutamate, ammonia, urea, alanine, glucose, aspartate, pyruvate, lactate, glycogen, triglycerides, acetoacetate, and β-hydroxybutyrate were measured by the enzymatic methods described previously elsewhere (17, 18).

3.6. ¹³C-NMR Techniques

1. Data were recorded at 125.75 MHz on a Bruker AM-500 WB spectrometer using a 5-mm broadband probe thermostated at 8°C. Magnet homogeneity was adjusted using the deuterium lock signal. Supernatants containing the ¹³C-labeled substrates were lyophilized. The lyophilized material was redissolved in deuterated water containing [2-¹³C]glycine as internal standard and centrifuged (5,000×g at 4°C for 5 min).

2. To obtain quantitative results, special care was taken for data acquisition. Acquisition parameters were as follows: spectral width, 25,000 Hz; tilt angle, 90°C; data size, 32 k; repetition time, 50 s; number of scans, 420. We used a standard (WALTZ 16) pulse sequence for inverse-gated proton decoupling (19). We did not use the NOESY during proton decoupling to avoid the use of the corresponding correction factors. A 1-Hz line broadening was applied prior to Fourier transformation. Peak areas were determined by Lorentzian fitting. Chemical shifts were expressed as ppm with respect to tetramethylsilane. Assignments were made by comparing the chemical shifts obtained with those given in the literature (20, 21).

3.7. Calculations and Statistical Analysis

1. Net substrate utilization and product formation were calculated as the difference between the total flask contents at the start (zero-time flasks or rollers) and after the period of incubation.

2. When [¹³C]glutamine or [¹³C]glucose was the substrate, the transfer of the ¹³C of glutamine or glucose to a given position in a given metabolite was calculated using the formula: (Lm – lm)/(Es – es); Lm is the amount of ¹³C measured in the corresponding NMR resonance, lm is the natural ¹³C abundance (1.1%) multiplied by the amount of metabolite assayed enzymatically, Es is the ¹³C abundance of the ¹³C of glutamine or glucose, and es is the ¹³C natural abundance. Note that (Es–es) is the specific enrichment of the corresponding species.

3. When absolute fluxes through metabolic pathways were calculated, they were obtained by replacing the parameters of the equations developed in the mathematical models of substrate metabolism by the enzymatic and ^{13}C NMR values measured. The models were developed in-house as described in several publications from this laboratory (22–25).

4. Values presented as means $\pm$ SEM are expressed in μmol of substrate removed or metabolite produced: (per gram of protein/ incubation time). Comparison of two groups were made by the paired Student's t-test. $P < 0.05$ was considered to be statistically significant.

3.8. Metabolic Characterization of Precision-Cut Liver and Kidney Slices

Figure 1 is a general scheme of the renal metabolism of lactate and glutamine carbons. Lactate is converted into pyruvate by lactate dehydrogenase. Then, pyruvate (a) can be converted into alanine by cytosolic or mitochondrial alanine aminotransferase except in the rat kidney in which this enzyme is present at a very low activity; (b) can enter the gluconeogenic pathway, thanks to the action of the key gluconeogenic enzymes (pyruvate carboxylase, phosphoenolpyruvate carboxykinase, fructose 1,6-bisphosphatase, and glucose 6-phosphatase); or (c) can be converted into acetyl-CoA which binds to oxaloacetate to form citrate, which is further metabolized in the tricarboxylic acid cycle. Note that in the presence of ammonia, α-ketoglutarate can be partly converted into glutamate and glutamine, thanks to the glutamate dehydrogenase and glutamine synthetase reactions. Note also that in slices from

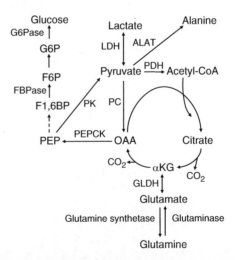

Fig. 1. Scheme of hepatic and renal metabolism of lactate and glutamine in the rat. *αKG* α-ketoglutarate, *LDH* lactate dehydrogenase, *PDH* pyruvate dehydrogenase, *PC* pyruvate carboxylase, *PEPCK* phosphoenolpyruvate carboxykinase, *F1,6BP* fructose 1,6-bisphosphatase, *G6Pase* glucose 6-phosphatase, *GLDH* glutamate dehydrogenase, *ALAT* alanine aminotransferase.

the liver of fed animals, glycogen is degraded and is partly converted into glucose, pyruvate, and lactate; this does not occur in slices from the kidney of fed rats because the kidney does not accumulate glycogen.

Both in the liver and the kidney, the metabolism of glutamine (Fig. 1) is initiated by glutaminase which forms glutamate and ammonia. In the rat kidney, glutamate is converted into α-ketoglutarate by glutamate dehydrogenase, which also gives ammonia. By contrast, in the rat liver, glutamate is converted into α-ketoglutarate by aspartate aminotransferase which also forms aspartate; then, the latter aspartate and the ammonia released by glutaminase provide the two nitrogens needed to synthesize urea via the urea cycle. The α-ketoglutarate formed both in the liver and the kidney can be converted either into glucose by the gluconeogenic pathway or can be completely oxidized to CO_2 as a result of the conversion of phosphoenolpyruvate into pyruvate by pyruvate kinase and the subsequent operation of pyruvate dehydrogenase and the tricarboxylic acid cycle.

Tables 1–3 show the results of enzymatic measurements of the removal of physiological substrates (lactate, glutamine, and glucose) and of the production of metabolites by precision-cut liver and kidney slices from fed or fasted rats. Such preliminary measurements are required before performing experiments with ^{13}C-labeled substrates to make sure that substrate removal and, therefore, product formation are sufficiently high to obtain reliably quantifiable resonances in ^{13}C NMR spectra and, therefore, to allow the application of our cellular metabolomic approach.

Table 1 shows that precision-cut kidney and liver slices from fed and fasted rats removed lactate and synthesized glucose at high rates, although these rates substantially decreased during 24 h of incubation. Carbon balance calculations indicate that irrespective of the experimental condition, a large fraction of the lactate removed by kidney slices was completely oxidized to CO_2. By contrast, in liver slices from fasted rats, the lactate removed was almost completely converted into glucose, leaving little room for lactate complete oxidation. It is important to emphasize that, in liver slices from fed rats, a large fraction of the glucose produced arose from the degradation of glycogen which also gave lactate. A cellular metabolomic approach using ^{13}C-lactate allows to differentiate the glucose arising from lactate from that synthesized from glycogen; this approach also allows to determine the ^{13}C-lactate removal and therefore the lactic acid synthesized from glycogen. Concomitantly, it is possible to evaluate the lactate oxidized in mitochondria. Thus, any xenobiotic interaction with all the pathways of lactate and glycogen metabolism in the liver (glycogen synthesis and glycogenolysis, glycolysis, lactic acid formation, lactate removal, lactate gluconeogenesis, and glycogen and lactate oxidation in mitochondria) can be assessed concomitantly.

Table 1
Metabolism of 5 mM L-lactate in precision-cut slices from the renal cortex and liver of fed or 48 h-fasted Wistar rats

Tissue	Nutritional state	Number of experiments (n)	Incubation (h)	Metabolite removal (−) or production		
				Lactate	Pyruvate	Glucose
Kidney	Fed	3	4	−1,751 ± 348	147 ± 56	168 ± 31
Kidney	Fasted	3	4	−1,698 ± 223	90 ± 15	308 ± 34
Kidney	Fasted	4	24	−7,091 ± 1,100	−	563 ± 87
Liver	Fed	4	4	−764 ± 231	311 ± 48	1,451 ± 194
Liver	Fasted	4	4	−1,379 ± 82	54 ± 7	592 ± 106
Liver	Fasted	4	24	−3,299 ± 139	−26 ± 6	1,470 ± 83

Values, expressed in $\mu mol/(g\,protein)/(incubation\ time)$, are means ± SEM for n (3 or 4) experiments. In the experiments with liver slices from fed rats incubated for 4 h, lactate removal was a net removal because lactic acid (like pyruvic acid) was concomitantly produced from glycogen. In experiments with liver slices from fasted rats incubated for 24 h, alanine removal (−424 ± 47) also occurred. Incubations for 4 h were performed in Krebs–Henseleit buffer and those for 24 h in William's medium E without glucose

Table 2
Metabolism of 5 mM L-glutamine in precision-cut slices from the renal cortex and liver of fed or 48 h-fasted Wistar rats

Tissue	Nutritional state	Number of experiments (n)	Incubation (h)	Metabolite removal (−) or production		
				Glutamine	Glutamate	Glucose
Kidney	Fed	3	4	−2,299 ± 258	671 ± 99	140 ± 21
Kidney	Fasted	3	4	−1,453 ± 92	626 ± 44	178 ± 103
Kidney	Fasted	4	24	−4,259 ± 309	681 ± 70	298 ± 48
Liver	Fasted	4	4	−827 ± 66	65 ± 10	426 ± 33
Liver	Fasted	4	24	−2,634 ± 334	28 ± 14	1,318 ± 141

Values, expressed in $\mu mol/(g\ protein)/(incubation\ time)$, are means ± SEM for n (3 or 4) experiments. In the experiments with slices from fasted rats incubated for 24 h, alanine removal (−370 ± 44) and pyruvate removal (−48 ± 5) also occurred. Incubations for 4 h were performed in Krebs–Henseleit buffer and those for 24 h in William's medium E without glucose

Table 2 shows that precision-cut kidney and liver slices from fasted rats also removed glutamine and synthesized glucose at high rates, but again these rates greatly declined during 24 h of incubation. As observed with lactate as substrate, carbon balance calculations reveal that in kidney slices, most of the glutamine carbon removed was completely oxidized to CO_2 with a small

Table 3
Metabolism of D-glucose in precision-cut slices from the renal cortex and liver of fed Wistar rats

Tissue	Nutritional state	Number of experiments (n)	Glucose (mM)	Incubation (h)	Metabolite removal (−) or production			
					Glucose	Pyruvate	Lactate	Glycogen
Kidney	Fed	4	5	4	−411±121	24±6	94±34	–
Kidney	Fed	4	5	24	−2,996±270	−82±24	242±53	–
Kidney	Fed	4	10	24	−3,413±534	−80±6	236±50	–
Liver	Fed	5	5.5	24	1,761±106	−36±9	396±62	−3,791±366
Liver	Fed	5	11	24	562±142	3±14	710±90	−3,780±367

Values, expressed in $\mu mol/(g\ protein)/(incubation\ time)$, are means±SEM for n (4 or 5) experiments. In the experiments with liver slices in the presence of 5.5 and 11 mM glucose as substrate, alanine removal (−253±23 and −148±34, respectively) also occurred. Glycogen removal is expressed in glucosyl units

fraction converted into glucose. By contrast, in liver slices from fasted rats, glucose explained virtually all the glutamine removed both after 4 and 24 h of incubation. It is important to note that in our hands, the rate of removal of 5 mM glutamine and of glutamine gluconeogenesis in precision-cut liver slices from fasted rats that were incubated for 4 h were approximately the same as those measured in isolated hepatocytes from fasted rats incubated for 1 h (see (26)) and Table 2. Similar rates of glutamine removal were also observed in precision-cut kidney slices incubated for 4 h and isolated proximal tubules from fed rats incubated for 1 h, but the rate of glutamine gluconeogenesis was lower in slices than in isolated tubules (for comparison, see (27) and Table 2).

Figure 2 is a general scheme of the metabolism of glucose. In the liver and the kidney, glucose can be both removed and metabolized, or synthesized and released. During a short fast, the glucose released by the liver arises both from glycogenolysis and gluconeogenesis (from lactate, alanine, glutamine, and glycerol), whereas the glucose released by the kidney arises only from gluconeogenesis. After a prolonged fast (longer than 24 h), the glucose released by the liver and the kidney is formed only by the gluconeogenic pathway. The liver, but not the kidney, has the capacity to synthesize, store, and degrade substantial amounts of glycogen. When glycogen is degraded, it is converted into glucose, lactic acid, and CO_2 in the mitochondria. The pentose phosphate pathway provides NADPH for fatty acid synthesis in the liver and

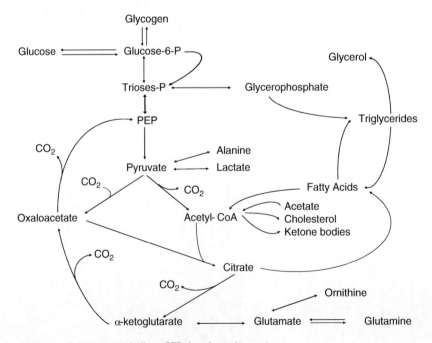

Fig. 2. General scheme of glucose metabolism. *PEP* phosphoenolpyruvate.

the reduced form of glutathione in the kidney which, unlike the liver, is not able to synthesize fatty acids. Both the liver and the kidney can synthesize and degrade triglycerides, the fatty acids needed to synthesize renal triglycerides being taken up from the circulating blood by the kidney. Numerous mitochondria, present in both the renal cortex and the liver, can oxidize glucose to CO_2; glycogen can also be oxidized to CO_2 in liver mitochondria. Fatty acids taken up from the circulating blood can be oxidized to CO_2 both in the liver and the renal cortex, or can be converted into ketone bodies only in liver mitochondria.

Table 3 shows the characteristics of glucose metabolism in kidney and liver slices from fed rats. Kidney slices removed glucose at high rates both during 4 and 24 h and this rate did not diminish during 24 h of incubation. The elevation of glucose concentration from 5 to 10 mM did not increase the rate of glucose removal during 24 h of incubation. Under all experimental conditions, the glucose removed was almost completely oxidized to CO_2 in the mitochondria, as revealed by carbon balance calculations. In the presence of 5.5 and 11 mM glucose, liver slices from fed rats did not remove, but rather produced, glucose in net amounts because the large amounts of glucose formed as a result of the degradation of glycogen masked the glucose removal. Under these conditions, the use of ^{13}C-glucose allowed not only to determine (data not shown) the removal of glucose but also to differentiate the lactic acid formed from glucose on the one hand and, on the other hand, the lactic acid formed from glycogen; it also allowed to determine the CO_2 produced from glucose in mitochondria, and the glycogen and triglycerides synthesized from glucose.

3.9. Effect of Insulin on ^{13}C-Glucose Metabolism in Precision-Cut Rat Liver Slices

Hyperglycemia, the hallmark of type 1 and type 2 diabetes, results from the deficit of insulin secretion and/or action. This leads to a deficit of hepatic glucose removal and an excess of hepatic glucose production. The following example illustrates how cellular metabolomics can be applied not only to safety but also to efficacy problems related to the effect of insulin on the hepatic metabolism of glucose. Table 4 shows the results of enzymatic measurements when 11 mM [2-^{13}C]glucose was used as substrate in the absence and the presence of 100 nM insulin.

Table 4 shows that, in liver slices incubated between 24 and 48 h, insulin converted a net glucose production into a net glucose removal. Insulin inhibited the net degradation of glycogen and the small accumulation of ammonia, and stimulated alanine removal. Insulin also converted the net degradation of triglycerides into a net production. The other parameters measured (glutamate and glutamine accumulation, ureagenesis, and ketogenesis) remained unaltered by insulin.

Figure 3 shows a typical carbon 13 NMR spectrum of a perchloric extract of the incubation medium after incubation with

Table 4

Effect of insulin on the metabolism of [2-¹³C]glucose in Wistar rat liver slices incubated between 24 and 48 h (enzymatic data)

| Experimental condition | Metabolite removal (−) or production | | | | | | | | β-OH-butyrate | Triglycerides | Urea | Ammonia |
	Glucose	Glycogen	Lactate	Pyruvate	Alanine	Glutamate	Glutamine	Acetoacetate				
11 mM [2-¹³C] glucose	245±344	−193±49	968±69	52±22	−388±29	123±7	229±38	213±30	156±25	−35±10	653±34	40±3
11 mM [2-¹³C] glucose + 100 nM insulin	−725±472*	52±79*	941±74	47±22	−450±36*	125±9	203±34	170±24	121±17	17±10*	572±46	19±3*

The slices were incubated in William's medium E for 24 h prior to these experiments. Values, expressed in μmol/(g protein)/24 h, are means ±SEM for five experiments. *$P<0.05$

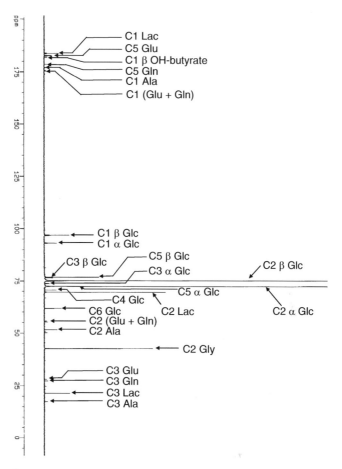

Fig. 3. Carbon 13 NMR spectrum of the medium incubated with liver slices between 24 and 48 h. [2-13C]glycine was used as internal standard.

11 mM [2-^{13}C]glucose. In this spectrum, it can be seen that, after incubation, glucose carbons other than the C-2 became labeled, which means that glucose resynthesis occurred, thanks to the glucose 6-phosphatase reaction.

Figures 4 and 5 show typical carbon 13 NMR spectra of the glycogen and triglycerides extracted from the slices incubated under the same condition. It can be seen that all significant peaks could be assigned and corresponded to carbons of the products determined enzymatically. From these spectra, it was possible to calculate the amounts of labeled products after correction for the 1.1% ^{13}C natural abundance.

As shown in Table 5, the results of these calculations indicate that, under the experimental conditions used, 100 nM insulin stimulated glucose removal without altering the resynthesis of ^{13}C-glucose or stimulating the production of lactic acid and triglycerides; insulin also stimulated the synthesis of ^{13}C-glycogen. In agreement with the absence of change in the production of CO_2 by

218   Baverel et al.

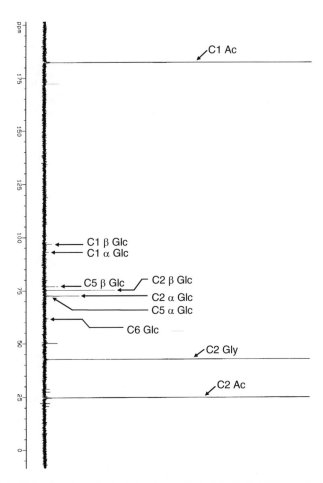

Fig. 4. Carbon 13 NMR spectrum of the glucose derived from glycogen accumulated in liver slices. [2-13C]glycine was used as internal standard.

liver mitochondria, there was no alteration of the β-hydroxybutyrate/ acetoacetate or of the lactate/pyruvate ratios, indicating that insulin did not modify the mitochondrial and cytosolic redox potentials, respectively.

It is easy to anticipate that this approach is applicable to assess early not only the efficacy and safety of any antidiabetic drug or drug candidate, but also the hepatic safety of any xenobiotic (drug, chemical, and environmental contaminant) that might stimulate lactic acid production (risk of lactic acidosis) or triglyceride accumulation (risk of steatosis), or inhibit mitochondrial functions (tricarboxylic acid cycle, respiratory chain, and β-oxidation), risk of energy restriction, ATP fall, and necrosis.

3.10. Effect of Valproate on ^{13}C-Glutamine Metabolism in Human Renal Cortical Precision-Cut Slices

Sodium valproate (n-dipropylacetic acid, sodium salt), a branched chain fatty acid, is a widely used and very effective antiepileptic drug in adult and children (28). Drug administration often induces a moderate hyperammonemia, especially when other anticonvulsants are taken in addition to valproate (29). Since this hyperammonemia

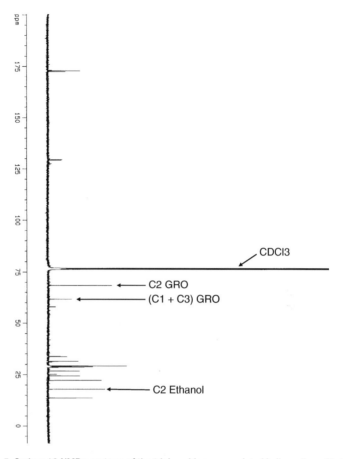

Fig. 5. Carbon 13 NMR spectrum of the triglycerides accumulated in liver slices. [2-13C] ethanol was used as internal standard. The resonances surrounding that of ethanol correspond to the fatty acid carbons of triglycerides.

is in some rare cases accompanied by clinical manifestations of liver dysfunction or of encephalopathy (30), it was of clinical importance to identify the origin of the valproate-induced elevation of blood ammonia levels.

Measurements on human and rat kidney *in vivo* have shown that valproate increases glutamine uptake and ammonia release (31–33).

In order to examine the possible mechanisms by which valproate stimulates the renal production of ammonia in the human kidney, we have employed our cellular metabolomic approach in which we have incubated human renal cortical precision-cut slices for 4 h in Krebs–Henseleit buffer containing 2 mM [1-^{13}C]- and [3-^{13}C]glutamine in the absence and presence of 1 mM valproate. The methods employed are described in detail in a recent publication from this laboratory which shows the typical carbon 13 NMR spectra obtained (34). Valproate did not increase the release of LDH from the human renal cortical slices used.

Figure 6 shows a panoramic view of the metabolism of glutamine obtained, thanks to the application of our cellular metabolomic

Table 5
Effect of insulin on the metabolism of [2-^{13}C]glucose in Wistar rat liver slices incubated between 24 and 48 h (^{13}C NMR data)

Experimental condition	Metabolite removal (−) or production									
	2-^{13}C-glucose	^{13}C-glucose	2-^{13}C-glycogen	^{13}C-lactate	^{13}C-alanine	^{13}C-glutamate	^{13}C-glutamine	^{13}C-β-OH-butyrate	^{13}C-triglycerides	^{13}CO$_2$
11 mM [2-^{13}C] glucose	−2,096±305	270±47	15±4	179±14	37±6	37±4	29±6	3±1	113±48	1,373±195
11 mM [2-^{13}C] glucose + 100 nM insulin	−2,279±189*	320±41	37±6*	197±19	39±6	55±7	33±6	4±1	140±59	1,399±90

Values, expressed in μmol of carbon 13/(g protein)/24 h, are means±SEM for five experiments. * $P<0.05$. The corresponding enzymatic results are presented in Table 4. The ^{13}C-pyruvate and ^{13}C-acetoacetate, which are destroyed during the lyophilization procedure, were calculated from the ^{13}C-lactate and ^{13}C-β-OH-butyrate, respectively. They were taken into account to calculate the production of ^{13}CO$_2$

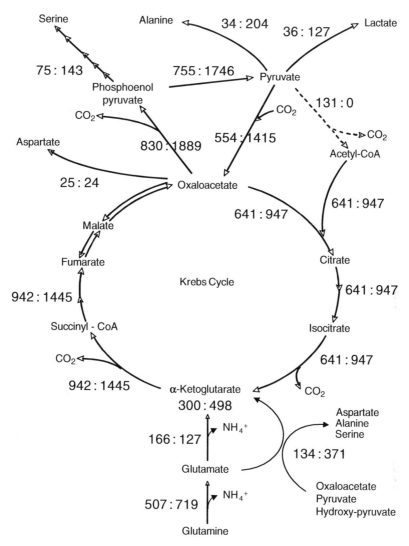

Fig. 6. Fluxes through the pathways of glutamine metabolism in human precision-cut renal cortical slices in the absence (*left*) and presence (*right*) of 1 mM valproate. Values are expressed in μmoles per gram tissue dry weight per 4 h.

approach in a representative experiment in which it was possible to measure flux through pyruvate dehydrogenase. Values are fluxes through the metabolic steps of glutamine metabolism in the absence (left) and presence (right) of 1 mM valproate. It can be seen that out of two ammoniagenic steps catalyzed by glutaminase and glutamate dehydrogenase, flux through the first but not through the second step was stimulated by valproate. Thus, it appears that glutaminase but not glutamate dehydrogenase is the target of valproate. In this experiment, the glutamate synthesized in greater amount by glutaminase was converted into α-ketoglutarate at increased rates not by a stimulation of flux through glutamate dehydrogenase but rather by a stimulation of fluxes through alanine aminotransferase and phosphoserine aminotransferase. Flux through the tricarboxylic acid cycle (Kreb's cycle) could also be measured, revealing that flux from α-ketoglutarate to oxaloacetate was greatly stimulated. It should also be underlined that the cellular metabolomic approach revealed that glutamine metabolism is much more complex than previously thought. Indeed, it involves the futile cycle "oxaloacetate-phosphoenolpyruvate-pyruvate-oxaloacetate" catalyzed by phosphoenolpyruvate carboxykinase, pyruvate kinase, and pyruvate carboxylase; it is of interest that this cycle was greatly stimulated by valproate. It should also be emphasized that valproate completely inhibited flux through pyruvate dehydrogenase; this explains why valproate increased the production of lactate and alanine as a result of an increased availability of pyruvate. The latter inhibition is in line with our demonstration that valproate is metabolized by renal cells and accumulates as valproyl-coenzyme A that leads to a depletion of cellular levels of coenzyme A, a substrate of the pyruvate dehydrogenase reaction (35, 36).

This example clearly shows that cellular metabolomics allowed to better understand the mechanism of the hyperammonemic effect of valproate and represents a screening method for other valproate-related antiepileptics. Again, it is easy to understand that this approach can be used for detecting, understanding, and, if possible, preventing the nephrotoxicity of any xenobiotic (drug, drug candidate, chemical, or metal).

4. Notes

1. The composition of Krebs–Henseleit buffer, which was gassed with 5% CO_2 and 95% O_2 for 20 min prior to utilization, was 118 mM NaCl, 4.7 mM KCl, 1.2 mM $MgSO_4$, 1.2 mM KH_2PO4, 25 mM $NaHCO_3$, and 2.5 mM $CaCl_2$.

2. The composition of this medium was l-alanine 90 mg/L, L-arginine 50 mg/L, L-asparagine H_2O 20 mg/L, L-aspartic acid 20 mg/L, L-cysteine 30 mg/L, L-cystine 40 mg/L, L-glutamic acid 50 mg/L, glycine 50 mg/L, l-histidine 15 mg/L, L-isoleucine 15 mg/L, L-leucine 75 mg/L, L-lysine HCl 87.5 mg/L, L-methionine 15 mg/L, L-phenylalanine 25 mg/L, L-proline 30 mg/L, L-serine 10 mg/L, L-threonine 40 mg/L, L-tryptophan 10 mg/L, L-tyrosine 35 mg/L, L-valine 50 mg/L, D-glucose 2,000 mg/L, ascorbic acid 2 mg/L, vitamin B12 (cobalamin) 0.2 mg/L, biotin 0.5 mg/L, choline chloride 1.5 mg/L, ergocalciferol 0.1 mg/L, folic acid 1 mg/L, L-inositol 2 mg/L, menadione sulfate 0.01 mg/L, pyridoxal hydrochloride (vitamin B6) 1 mg/L, riboflavin 0.1 mg/L, glutathione 0.05 mg/L, methyl linoleate 0.03 mg/L, phenol red 10 mg/L, sodium pyruvate 25 mg/L, $CaCl_2$ 2 H_2O 264 mg/L, $CuSO_4$ 5 H_2O

0.0001 mg/L, $Fe(NO_3)_3$ 9 H_2O 0.001 mg/L, KCl 400 mg/L, $MgSO_4$ 7H_2O 200 mg/L, $MnCl_2$ 4 H_2O 0.0001 mg/L, NaCl 6,800 mg/L, $NaHCO_3$ 2,200 mg/L, NaH_2PO_4 2 H_2O 158 mg/L, $ZnSO_4$ 7 H_2O 0.0002 mg/L.

3. Composition of the incubation media. We found it useless to add fetal or newborn bovine serum to the Krebs–Henseleit medium or to the William's Medium E; this did not change the metabolism of the substrates used. Similarly, the addition of Glutamax (the dipeptide alanylglutamine) did not improve the viability of the slices. In addition, both in liver and kidney slices, this dipeptide was rapidly hydrolyzed leading to the release and subsequent utilization of alanine and glutamine by the liver slices and of glutamine by the kidney slices. Therefore, the utilization of both alanine and glutamine was hardly evaluated with precision.

4. Oxygenation conditions. We found that 40% oxygen in the gas phase was sufficient to provide adequate amounts of oxygen to the slices during the 24–48-h incubation periods. When compared with the presence of 20% oxygen, this greatly decreased the lactic acid production from glucose but did not change the other characteristics of glucose metabolism. This allowed a good preservation of the slices whose metabolic functions were not improved with higher (up to 70%) oxygen percentages in the gas phase.

Acknowledgments

The authors would like to thank Claudie Pinteur, Rémi Nazaret, and Lara Koneckny for their technical assistance as well as Claire Morel for secretarial assistance. This work was supported by grants from the European Commission [project numbers: BIO4-CT97-2145(Euroslice) and STREP032731(CellNanoTox)] and from INSERM.

References

1. Warburg, O. (1923) Versuche an uberieben-dem Carcirnomgewebe. *Biochem. Z.* **142**, 317–333.

2. Berry, M. N., and Friend, D. S. (1969) High-yield preparation of isolated rat liver paren-chymal cells: a biochemical and fine structural study. *J. Cell. Biol.* **43**, 506–520.

3. Krumdieck, C. L., dos Santos, J. E., and Ho, K. J. (1980) A new instrument for the rapid preparation of tissue slices. *Anal. Biochem.* **104**, 118–123.

4. Hirsch, G. H. (1976) Differential effects of nephrotoxic agents on renal transport and metabolism by use of *in vitro* techniques. *Environ. Health Perspect.* **15**, 89–99.

5. Bach, P., and Lock, E. (1985) The use of renal tissue slices, perfusion and infusion techniques to assess nephrotoxicity related changes. In: (Bach, P. H., and Lock, E. A., eds.) Nephrotoxicity Assessment and Pathogenesis. Monographs of Applied Toxicology. Vol. 1. New-York: Wiley, pp. 505–518.

6. Berndt, W. O. (1987) Renal slices and perfusion. In: (Bach, P. H., and Lock, E. A., eds.) Nephrotoxicity: The Experimental and Clinical Situation. Martin Nijhoff Publishers, Boston, MA, USA pp. 301–316.

7. Bach, P. H., Vickers, A. E. M., Fisher, R., et al. (1996) The use of tissue slices for pharmacotoxicology studies. *Altern. Lab. Anim.* **24**, 893–923.

8. Parrish, A. R., Gandolfi, A. J., and Brendel, K. (1995) Precision-cut tissue slices: applications in pharmacology and toxicology. *Life Sci.* **57**, 1887–1901.

9. Lerche-Langrand, C., and Toutain, H. J. (2000) Precision-cut liver slices: characteristics and use for *in vitro* pharmaco-toxicology. *Toxicology* **153**, 221–253.

10. Vickers, A. E., and Fisher, R. L. (2004) Organ slices for the evaluation of human drug toxicity. *Chem. Biol. Interact.* **150**, 87–96.

11. Vickers, A. E., and Fisher, R. L. (2005) Precision-cut organ slices to investigate target organ injury. *Expert Opin. Drug Metab. Toxicol.* **1**, 687–699.

12. De Graaf, I. A. M., Groothuis, G. M. M., and Olinga, P. (2007) Precision-cut tissue slices as a tool to predict metabolism of novel drugs. *Expert Opin. Drug Metab. Toxicol.* **3**, 879–898.

13. Nicholson, J. K., Lindon, J. C., and Holmes, E. (1999) "Metabonomics": understanding the metabolic responses of living systems to pathophysiological stimuli via multivariate statistical analysis of biological NMR spectroscopic data. *Xenobiotica* **29**, 1181–1189.

14. Lamprecht, W., and Trautchold, I. (1974) Adenosine-5-triphosphate. Determination with hexokinase and glucose-6-phosphate dehydrogenase. In: (Bergmeyer, H., ed.) Methods of Enzymatic Analysis. Vol. 4. New York: Academic Press, pp. 2101–2110.

15. Lowry, O. H., Rosebrough, N. J., Farr, A. L., and Randall, R. J. (1951) Protein measurement with the Folin phenol reagent. *J. Biol. Chem.* **193**, 265–275.

16. Bergmeyer, H. U., and Bernt, E. (1974) Lactate dehydrogenase: UV assay with pyruvate and NADH. In: (Bergmeyer, H., ed.) Methods of Enzymatic Analysis. Vol. 2. New-York: Academic Press, pp. 574–579.

17. Baverel, G., Bonnard, M., D'Armagnac de Castanet, E., and Pellet, M. (1978) Lactate and pyruvate metabolism in isolated renal tubules of normal dogs. *Kidney Int.* **14**, 567–575.

18. Baverel, G., and Lund, P. (1979) A role for bicarbonate in the regulation of mammalian glutamine metabolism. *Biochem. J.* **184**, 599–606.

19. Shaka, A. J., Keeler, J., Frenkiel, T., and Freeman, R. (1983) An improved sequence for broadband decoupling: Waltz 16. *J. Magn. Reson.* **52**, 335–338.

20. Howarth, O. W., and Lilley, D. M. J. (1978) Carbon-13-NMR of peptides and proteins. *Prog. NMR Spectrosc.* **12**, 1–40.

21. Canioni, P., Alger, J. R., and Shulman, R. G. (1983) Natural abundance Carbon-13 nuclear magnetic resonance spectroscopy of liver and adipose tissue of the living rat. *Biochemistry* **22**, 4974–4980.

22. Martin, G., Chauvin M.F., Dugelay S., and Baverel G. (1994) Non-steady state model applicable to NMR studies for calculating flux rates in glycolysis, gluconeogenesis, and citric acid cycle. *J. Biol. Chem.* **269**, 26034–26039.

23. Martin G., Chauvin, M. F., and Baverel, G. (1997) Model applicable to NMR studies for calculating flux rates in five cycles involved in glutamate metabolism. *J. Biol. Chem.* **272**, 4717–4728.

24. Dugelay, S., Chauvin, M. F., and Megnin-Chanet, F., et al. (1999) Acetate stimulates flux through the tricarboxylic acid cycle in rabbit renal proximal tubules synthesizing glutamine from alanine: a ^{13}C NMR study. *Biochem. J.* **342**, 555–566.

25. Conjard, A., Dugelay, S., Chauvin, M. F., Durozard, D., Baverel, G., and Martin, G. (2002) The anaplerotic substrate alanine stimulates acetate incorporation into glutamate and glutamine in rabbit kidney tubules. A ^{13}C NMR study. *J. Biol. Chem.* **277**, 29444–29454.

26. Vincent, N., Martin, G., and Baverel, G. (1992) Glycine, a new regulator of glutamine metabolism in isolated rat-liver cells. *Biochim. Biophys. Acta.* **1175**, 13–20.

27. Vercoutere, B., Durozard, D., Baverel, G., and Martin, G. (2004) Complexity of glutamine metabolism in kidney tubules from fed and fasted rats. *Biochem. J.* **378**, 485–495.

28. Simon, D., and Penry, J. K. (1975) Sodium di-N-propylacetate (DPA) in the treatment of epilepsy. A review. *Epilepsia* **16**, 549–573.

29. Coulter, D. L., and Allen, R. J. (1980) Secondary hyperammonaemia: a possible mechanism for valproate encephalopathy. *Lancet* **1**, 1310–1311.

30. Powell-Jackson, P. R., Tredger, J. M., and Williams, R. (1984) Hepatotoxicity to sodium valproate: a review. *Gut* **25**, 673–681.

31. Warter, J. M., Marescaux, C., Chabrier, G., Rumbach, L., Micheletti, B., and Imler, M. (1984) Renal glutamine metabolism in man

during treatment with sodium valproate. *Rev. Neurol. (Paris)* **140**, 370–371.

32. Ferrier, B., Martin, M., and Baverel, G. (1988) Valproate-induced stimulation of renal ammonia production and excretion in the rat. *J. Clin. Chem. Clin. Biochem.* **26**, 65–67.

33. Elhamri, M., Ferrier, B., Martin, M., and Baverel, G. (1993) Effect of valproate, sodium 2-propyl-4-pentenoate and sodium 2-propyl-2-pentenoate on renal substrate uptake and ammoniagenesis in the rat. *J. Pharmacol. Exp. Ther.* **266**, 89–96.

34. Vittorelli, A., Gauthier, C., Michoudet, C., Martin, G., and Baverel, G. (2005) Characteristics of glutamine metabolism in human precision-cut kidney slices: a ^{13}C-NMR study. *Biochem. J.* **387**, 825–834.

35. Durozard, D, and Baverel, G. (1987) Gas chromatographic method for the measurement of sodium valproate utilization by kidney tubules. *J. Chromatogr.* **414**, 460–464.

36. Durozard, D., Martin, G., and Baverel, G. (1991) Valproate-induced alterations of coenzyme A and coenzyme A ester concentrations in human kidney tubules metabolizing glutamine. *Contrib. Nephrol.* **92**, 103–108.

Chapter 13

Statistical Analysis of Quantitative RT-PCR Results

Richard Khan-Malek and Ying Wang

Abstract

Real-time reverse transcription polymerase chain reaction (RT-PCR) represents a benchmark technology in the detection and quantification of mRNA. Yet, accurate results cannot be realized without proper statistical analysis of RT-PCR data. Here, we examine some of the issues concerning RT-PCR experiments that would benefit from rigorous statistical treatment, including normalization, quantification, efficiency estimation, and sample size calculations. Examples are used to illustrate the methods.

Keywords: RT-PCR, Relative quantification, Statistical analysis

1. Introduction

Real-time reverse transcription polymerase chain reaction (RT-PCR) has become one of the most widely used approaches in the detection and quantification of mRNA (1). Due to its high sensitivity, reproducibility, and wide dynamic range, RT-PCR is considered by many to be the "gold standard" for gene expression studies, and it is commonly used for the validation of results from microarray experiments (2).

Both absolute quantification and relative quantification can be achieved in RT-PCR (3). Absolute quantification determines precise copy numbers based on the construction of a standard curve with known copy numbers or concentrations. In relative quantification, gene expression is measured against a calibrator sample and expressed as an n-fold difference relative to the calibrator. In this chapter, we focus on relative quantification.

While there is an abundance of papers that discuss statistical analysis techniques for microarray data, there are notably less that present statistical methods for RT-PCR experiments. In this

Jean-Charles Gautier (ed.), *Drug Safety Evaluation: Methods and Protocols*, Methods in Molecular Biology, vol. 691,
DOI 10.1007/978-1-60761-849-2_13, © Springer Science+Business Media, LLC 2011

entry, we examine key elements of RT-PCR data analysis that would benefit from rigorous statistical treatment, including the selection of endogenous control genes, analysis of relative gene expression, efficiency estimation, and sample size calculations. In each section, an example is presented along with computational details. SAS (4) program code is provided for all of the examples.

2. Normalization

In a relative quantification RT-PCR experiment, a popular normalization method is to normalize the expression of a target gene against an endogenous control, or so-called housekeeping gene (5). A fundamental assumption in the use of housekeeping genes is that the expression level of the gene remains constant across different experimental conditions. Selecting a candidate housekeeping gene from the literature might not satisfy this assumption, resulting in biased relative expression of the target genes and erroneous conclusions (6). Therefore, we recommend that the selection of a housekeeping gene be included as part of the experimental protocol.

Various methods for selecting a suitable housekeeping gene have been described in the literature. Vandesompele et al. (7) defined a gene-stability parameter M as the average pairwise variation of a particular gene with all other control genes. Genes with small values of M are considered to be the most stable. Pfaffl et al. (8) proposed calculating the pairwise correlation of all pairs of candidate genes. The highly correlated genes are combined into an index. Subsequently, the pairwise correlation between each gene and the index is calculated. Genes that correlate well with the index are considered suitable housekeeping genes. In accordance with methods described by Abruzzo et al. (9), Andersen et al. (10), and Szabo et al. (11), we illustrate the use of statistical modeling, along with *analysis of variance* (ANOVA), to select a housekeeping gene. ANOVA is a technique of partitioning the variability in a set of data into component parts.

Let Y_{ij} represent the threshold cycle (Ct) observed on the jth animal of the ith dose group. The observed response can be modeled as

$$Y_{ij} = \mu_i + e_{ij} \qquad (1)$$

where μ_i denotes the mean of the ith treatment (dose group) and e_{ij} is residual error.

Table 1
ANOVA table for fixed-effects one-way model

Source	Sum of squares	df	Mean square	F
Treatment (Between)	$SS_{TREATMENT}$	$a-1$	MST	MST/MSE
Error (Within)	SS_{ERROR}	$N-a$	MSE	
Total	SS_{TOTAL}	$N-1$		

a no. of treatments; N no. of animals

An ANOVA table for the fixed-effects one-way model given in Eq. 1 is presented in Table 1 (12).

The ANOVA table for a one-way model partitions the total variance into two parts, between groups, due to *treatment* differences and within groups, due to *error*, i.e.,

$$SS_{TOTAL} = SS_{TREATMENT} + SS_{ERROR}$$

where $SS_{TREATMENT}$ is called the sum of squares due to treatments, and SS_{ERROR} is called the sum of squares due to error. To make the sources of variability comparable, we divide each by their respective degrees of freedom (df) to obtain mean squares. The ratio of the mean squares yields an F-statistic, i.e., $F = MST/MSE$. Values of the F-statistic close to 1 indicate that the two sources of variability, between treatment and within treatment, are approximately equal.

A housekeeping gene that remains constant across different experimental conditions, or treatments, will have a small F-statistic compared to other genes. Thus, we define an optimum housekeeping gene based on a non-significant ($p > 0.05$), minimum F-statistic. If none of the genes yield a nonsignificant F-statistic, we advise that none is suitable for use as a housekeeping gene.

Example. The ANOVA table for the HK001 data from Table 2 is given in Table 3, using the model given in Eq. 1.

Note that the F-statistic is 3.74. The F-statistics for both HK001 and HK002 are given in Table 4.

The minimum F-statistic is given by HK002, so this would be our choice for an optimum housekeeping gene. Alternatively, one can use the geometric mean of several optimum genes as suggested by Vandesompele et al. (7).

A SAS program to select an optimum housekeeping gene based on a minimum F-statistic is provided in Appendix 1.

Table 2
Ct values for two potential reference genes, HK001 and HK002

Animal	Dose group	HK001	HK002
1	A	20.30	19.68
2	A	20.57	19.69
3	A	20.54	19.80
4	A	20.20	19.95
5	A	20.20	19.93
6	B	20.57	19.97
7	B	20.95	19.93
8	B	20.78	20.02
9	B	20.88	20.27
10	B	20.87	19.93
11	C	20.80	19.88
12	C	20.83	19.90
13	C	19.97	19.91
14	C	19.92	19.98
15	C	20.33	20.57
16	D	19.70	19.68
17	D	19.72	19.95
18	D	19.47	19.85
19	D	20.58	20.27
20	D	20.57	20.08
21	E	20.41	20.07
22	E	20.58	20.10
23	E	20.85	20.07
24	E	20.48	20.10
25	E	20.30	20.25

3. Statistical Analysis of Relative Quantification Data

Relative quantification of RT-PCR data is based on the expression ratio of a target gene versus a reference (housekeeping) gene. In this section, we present two mathematical models used for the

Table 3
ANOVA table for HK001 data

Source	Sum of squares	df	Mean square	F
Dose group (between)	1.6919	4	0.4230	3.74
Error (within)	2.2633	20	0.1132	
Total	3.9552	24		

Table 4
F-statistics for HK001 and HK002 data

Gene	F-statistic
HK001	3.74
HK002	1.88

relative quantification of RT-PCR data, the $\Delta\Delta Ct$ model and the efficiency corrected model. We then discuss the use of statistical modeling techniques to analyze the relative quantification data.

The $\Delta\Delta Ct$ model (5) assumes the amplification efficiency for both the target and reference genes is 2 (indicating double the amount of PCR product in each cycle), and is given by the formula

$$\text{Ratio} = 2^{-\Delta\Delta Ct} \tag{2}$$

where $\Delta\Delta Ct = \Delta Ct_{\text{TREATED}} - \Delta Ct_{\text{CONTROL}}$, $\Delta Ct_{\text{TREATED}}$ is the Ct difference of a reference and target gene for a treated sample (i.e., $\Delta Ct_{\text{TREATED}} = Ct_{\text{TARGET}} - Ct_{\text{REF}}$) and $\Delta Ct_{\text{CONTROL}}$ is the Ct difference of a reference and target gene for a control sample (i.e., $\Delta Ct_{\text{CONTROL}} = Ct_{\text{TARGET}} - Ct_{\text{REF}}$).

The efficiency corrected model (13), which is a more general form of the $\Delta\Delta Ct$ model, is given by

$$\text{Ratio} = \frac{\left(E_{\text{TARGET}}\right)^{\Delta Ct_{\text{TARGET}}}}{\left(E_{\text{REF}}\right)^{\Delta Ct_{\text{REF}}}} \tag{3}$$

where E_{TARGET} is the target amplification efficiency, E_{REF} is the reference amplification efficiency, $\Delta Ct_{\text{TARGET}}$ is the Ct difference of a treated and control sample for the target gene (i.e., $\Delta Ct_{\text{TARGET}} = Ct_{\text{CONTROL}} - Ct_{\text{TREATED}}$), and ΔCt_{REF} is the Ct difference of a treated and control sample for the reference gene (i.e., $\Delta Ct_{\text{REF}} = Ct_{\text{CONTROL}} - Ct_{\text{TREATED}}$). The assessment of PCR efficiency is discussed in the next section.

One of the "early" references on the statistical analysis of relative expression data was Pfaffl et al. (14). They introduced a software tool (REST©) which used the efficiency corrected model to compute relative expression results; the expression results were then tested for significance using a randomization test. Fu et al. (15) proposed calculating the relative expression, $\Delta\Delta Ct$, using a generalized estimation equations (GEE) model. Following Yuan et al. (16), we discuss the use of ANOVA to calculate the relative expression.

Consider a simple experiment, the objective of which is to determine the gene expression across a single factor: treatment. Let Y_{ijk} represent the Ct value observed on the kth animal, jth gene (target or reference), and ith treatment (control or treated). The observed response can be modeled as

$$Y_{ijk} = \mu_{ij} + e_{ijk} \tag{4}$$

where μ_{ij} denotes the mean of the combination of treatment i and gene j, and e_{ijk} is residual error. $\Delta\Delta Ct$ can be estimated by a linear combination of cell means. The model given in Eq. 4 can easily be modified to accommodate a particular experimental design.

Example. Table 5 provides estimates of the $\Delta\Delta Ct$ and its standard error for the data given in Table 6, using the model given in Eq. 4. Technical replicates within animal (biological replicates) were averaged to increase precision. Target genes were normalized to the reference gene HK002. A significant treatment effect is indicated by $p \leq 0.05$.

A SAS program to perform $\Delta\Delta Ct$ analysis using ANOVA methodology is provided in Appendix 2.

For an amplification efficiency of less than two, the efficiency corrected model can be used, but to facilitate the statistical analysis, we must first rewrite Eq. 3. Given that for all positive values of x, if $x = a^y$, then $y = \log_a(x)$, we proceed as follows:

$$\text{Ratio} = \frac{\left(E_{\text{TARGET}}\right)^{\Delta Ct_{\text{TARGET}}}}{\left(E_{\text{REF}}\right)^{\Delta Ct_{\text{REF}}}} = \frac{2^{EA_{\text{TARGET}}(\Delta Ct_{\text{TARGET}})}}{2^{EA_{\text{REF}}(\Delta Ct_{\text{REF}})}} \tag{5}$$

$$= 2^{EA_{\text{TARGET}}(\Delta Ct_{\text{TARGET}}) - EA_{\text{REF}}(\Delta Ct_{\text{REF}})}$$

Table 5
Estimates of $\Delta\Delta Ct$ and fold change

Gene	$\Delta\Delta Ct$	SE	Ratio
TG001	−0.573	0.451	1.49
TG002	−2.508[a]	0.825	5.69

[a]Statistically significant with $p \leq 0.05$

Table 6
Ct values for two target genes (TG001 and TG002)
and reference gene (HK002)

Animal	Treatment	TG001	TG002	HK002
1	Control	23.22	29.08	19.68
1	Control	23.34	29.04	19.69
1	Control	23.12	29.39	19.80
2	Control	24.06	28.23	19.95
2	Control	24.15	28.01	19.93
2	Control	24.15	28.12	19.97
3	Control	23.18	28.79	19.93
3	Control	23.13	28.43	20.02
3	Control	23.10	28.49	20.27
4	Control	24.78	31.37	19.93
4	Control	24.45	30.74	19.88
4	Control	24.67	31.09	19.90
5	Treated	23.11	27.11	20.61
5	Treated	22.99	27.24	19.98
5	Treated	23.10	27.37	20.57
6	Treated	22.77	25.52	19.68
6	Treated	22.99	25.72	19.95
6	Treated	23.06	25.52	19.85
7	Treated	23.73	27.43	20.27
7	Treated	24.01	26.73	20.08
7	Treated	23.80	26.65	20.07
8	Treated	23.73	27.96	20.10
8	Treated	23.83	27.84	20.07
8	Treated	23.73	27.98	20.10

where we define EA as the "efficiency adjustment" given by $EA = \log_2(\text{efficiency})$.

Example. Let us revisit the data given in Table 6 using Eq. 5 assuming that the efficiency of the reference gene (HK002) was only 1.85. For an efficiency of 1.85, the $EA = \log_2(1.85) = 0.8875$ (note: for efficiencies of 2, the $EA = 1$). Using TG001 as the target gene, the fold change is

$$\text{Ratio} = \frac{2^{1(0.375)}}{2^{0.8875(-0.1983)}} = \frac{2^{(0.375)}}{2^{(-0.176)}} = 2^{(0.551)} = 1.465.$$

SAS code for the efficiency corrected model is also provided in Appendix 2.

4. Amplification Efficiency

If the assumptions behind the $\Delta\Delta$Ct method are not valid, the efficiency corrected model can be employed instead, in which case estimates of the amplification efficiencies are needed for the reference gene and any gene of interest (GOI). Common approaches used to assess PCR efficiency are the relative standard curve method as well as methods based on amplification kinetics.

The relative standard curve method requires running serial dilutions of cDNA for the reference gene and each GOI. Ct is then plotted against base 10 logarithm of cDNA and the PCR efficiency is calculated according to the relationship $E = 10^{(-1/\text{slope})}$ (13, 17).

There are a variety of methods based on amplification kinetics. A number of authors have suggested fitting a linear model to the log-linear portion of an amplification curve as a means of estimating efficiency (18, 19). Others have suggested fitting multiple models to the exponential portion of the amplification curve (20, 21) or modeling the amplification curve using sigmoidal or other models (22–25). Here, we present the linear model method and the method of Khan-Malek.

The linear model method fits a linear regression line to the points in the log-linear (base 10 logarithm) phase of the PCR amplification curve. The PCR efficiency is calculated according to the relationship $E = 10^{(\text{slope})}$. Figure 1 illustrates the linear model method using three points around the midpoint of the log-linear phase.

For these data, the fitted linear model yielded a $R^2 > 0.99$ and slope of 0.285 giving an efficiency estimate of $E = 10^{(0.285)} = 1.93$.

Instead of modeling the raw amplification curve, Khan-Malek fits a four-parameter logistic model of the form

$$f(x) = a + \frac{b}{1 + \exp{(c - x)}/d} \tag{6}$$

to the log10 transformed amplification curve. Here, $f(x)$ is the observed log10 fluorescence at cycle x, a is the lower asymptote, b is the difference between the lower and upper asymptote, c is a location parameter halfway between a and b, and d is a parameter relating to the slope; c, as a rule, falls in the middle of the log-linear phase (see Fig. 2).

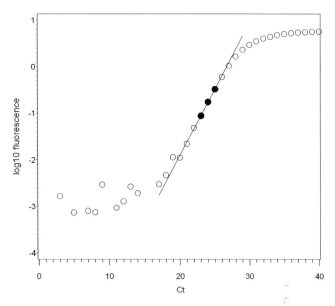

Fig. 1. Illustration of fitting a linear model to the log-linear portion of an amplification curve.

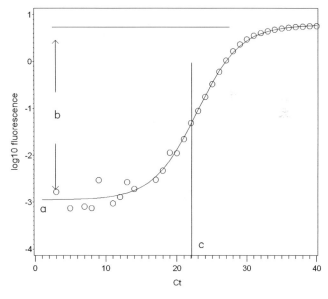

Fig. 2. Illustration of fitting a four-parameter logistic model to the log10 transformed fluorescence curve.

The parameters of the model given in Eq. 6 are solved using nonlinear regression. Substituting the parameter estimates into the first derivative of Eq. 6 at $x = c$ gives the slope of the tangent line of the function at c. The benefits of this approach are two-fold: first, the resulting efficiencies can be directly compared with

Table 7
Parameter estimates of
four-parameter logistic model

Parameter	Estimate
a	−2.9516
b	3.7290
c	22.8162
d	3.0980

"true PCR efficiency" although efficiencies can sometimes exceed the theoretical maximum of two, depending on model fit; second, this approach is easily programmable and can be used for high throughput screening with minimum user input. If the log10 transformed amplification curve lacks sufficient points in the lower and/or upper plateaus to permit modeling, the linear model method is recommended.

Example. Table 7 gives the parameter estimates of the four-parameter logistic model, fit to the data in Fig. 2.

If we substitute these estimates into the first derivative of Eq. 6, given by

$$f'(x) = (b / d) \frac{\exp(c - x) / d}{1 + 2\exp(c - x) / d + \exp2(c - x) / d} \qquad (7)$$

and solve for $x = 22.8162$, it yields a slope of 0.3009 giving an efficiency estimate of $E = 10^{(0.3009)} = 1.99$.

A SAS program to perform the four-parameter logistic model fit is provided in Appendix 3.

5. Power and Sample Size

Statistically speaking, *power* is the probability of rejecting the null hypothesis (H_0) when the alternative hypothesis (H_1) is valid. In other words, it is the probability of detecting a difference or treatment effect if one truly exists. Power is dependent on the sample size, significance criterion (α-level), effect size, and the sample standard deviation. Accordingly, prospective sample size calculations are important in the planning of an experiment as insufficient power may render any conclusions from an experiment as useless.

For simple comparative experiments comparing two treatment groups, power can be estimated using a two sample t-test assuming normal populations and equal variances. In Fig. 3, the

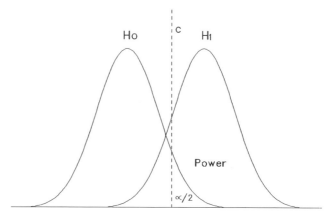

Fig. 3. Illustration of the two sample *t*-test (two-tailed) with equal variances under the null and alternative hypotheses.

Table 8
Sample size analysis

δ	SD	*n* (per group)
1.0	0.40	4
1.0	0.45	5
1.0	0.50	6

normal curve on the left represents a sampling distribution of no treatment effect (H_0: $\mu_1 - \mu_2 = 0$), whereas the normal curve on the right represents an alternate sampling distribution of an effect (H_1: $\mu_1 - \mu_2 = \delta$). The critical value c determines the point where H_0 is rejected. The power of the test is the area under the alternative curve beyond c. Notice that moving the alternative curve to the right increases the distance between the null and alternative hypothesis and thus increases the power.

Example. Suppose the objective is to determine the number of animals needed to achieve a power of at least 0.80 to detect a group mean difference of say $\delta = 1.0$ between treated and control Ct values. Based on historical data, you hypothesize that the common group standard deviation is between 0.40 and 0.50. The results for these parameters are given in Table 8 for an α-level of 0.05 (two-tailed).

A SAS program to perform the sample size calculations is provided in Appendix 4.

6. Appendix 1. SAS Code to Select an Optimum Housekeeping Gene Based on a Minimum F-statistic

```
data table2;
input ain dose$ gene$ Ct;
cards;
1 A HK001 20.30
2 A HK001 20.57
3 A HK001 20.54
4 A HK001 20.20
5 A HK001 20.20
.
Some data omitted for brevity
.
23 E HK002 20.07
24 E HK002 20.10
25 E HK002 20.25
;
proc sort;
    by gene;
    run;
ods listing close;
ods output OverallANOVA=ANOVA;
proc glm;
    by gene;
    class dose;
    model Ct=dose;
    run;
ods listing;
data ANOVA; set ANOVA;
if Source='Model';
proc print;
    var gene FValue;
    run;
```

7. Appendix 2. SAS Code to Perform the Relative Quantification Analysis Using ANOVA Methodology

```
data table6;
input ain treatment$ gene$ Ct;
cards;
1 Control TG001 23.22
1 Control TG001 23.34
1 Control TG001 23.12
2 Control TG001 24.06
2 Control TG001 24.15
2 Control TG001 24.15
.
```

Some data omitted for brevity
.
8 Treated HK002 20.10
8 Treated HK002 20.07
8 Treated HK002 20.10
;
```
proc summary nway;
    class ain treatment gene;
    var Ct;
    output out=out mean=;
    run;
proc sort data=out;
    by gene;
    run;
proc print data=out;
    run;
*~~~ The macro 'loop' allows Ct calculations
    for all the genes in the data set ~~~*;
%macro loop(gene);
proc mixed data=out;
    where gene in ("HK002","&gene");
    class treatment gene;
    model Ct=treatment*gene;
    lsmeans treatment*gene;
*~~~ The 'e' option for the 'estimate' statement allows a check of
the linear combination, which is dependent on the treatment
names ~~~*;
    estimate "delta delta Ct for &gene" treatment*gene 1 -1 -1
1 / cl e;
    *~~~ For an efficiency corrected estimate of the ratio, use the
estimate statement below instead ~~~*;
    * estimate "efficiency corrected for &gene" treatment*gene
-.8875 1 .8875 -1 / e;
    ods output estimates=estimates;
    title "&gene";
    run;
    %mend loop;
    *~~~ For additional target genes, simply add lines below
~~~*;
    %loop(TG001);
    %loop(TG002);
```

---

8. Appendix 3. SAS Code to Perform the Four-Parameter Logistic Model Fit

```
data raw_curve;
input x FL;
cards;
```

```
1 -0.00576
2 -0.00568
3 0.00166
Some data omitted for brevity

.
48 5.91043
49 5.95599
50 5.90091
;
data log_curve; set raw_curve;
    logFL=log10(FL); * <==== notice log10 ;
    ods listing close;
proc nlin method=newton;
    parms a=-10 to 0 by 1
        b=0 to 5 by 1
        c=25 to 30 by 1
            d=1 to 3 by 1;
    model logFL = a + b /(1+exp((c-x)/d));
    ods output parameterestimates=pe(keep=parameter estimate);
    output out=out p=p;
    run;
    ods listing;
    proc transpose data=pe out=est(rename=(col1=a  col2=b
col3=c col4=d));
    var estimate;
    run;
    data est; set est;
    x=c;
    slope=(b/d)*(exp((c-x)/d))/((1+2*exp((c-x)/d))
+exp(2*(c-x)/d));
    E=10**slope;
    run;
proc print data=est;
    run;
```

9. Appendix 4. SAS Code to Perform the Sample Size Calculations

```
*~~~ To calculate sample size ~~~*;
proc power;
    twosamplemeans
    meandiff = 1
    stddev = 0.40 0.45 0.50
    power = 0.8
    npergroup =.;
run;
```

References

1. Walker, N.J. (2002) Tech.Sight. A technique whose time has come. *Science* **296**, 557–579.

2. Wang, Y., Barbacioru, C., Hyland, F., Xiao, W., Hunkapiller, K.L., Blake, J., Chan, F., Gonzalez, C., Zhang, L., and Samaha, R. (2006) Large scale real-time PCR validation on gene expression measurements from two commercial long-oligonucleotide microarrays. *BMC Genomics* **7**, 59.

3. Wong, M.L. and Medrano, J.F. (2005) Real-time PCR for mRNA quantitation. *Biotechniques* **39**, 75–85.

4. SAS Institute Inc. (2004) *SAS/STAT 9.1 User's Guide*. Cary, NC: SAS Institute Inc.

5. Livak, K.J. and Schmittgen, T.D. (2001) Analysis of relative gene expression data using real-time quantitative PCR and the 2^{-CT} method. *Methods* **25**, 402–408.

6. Huggett, J., Dheda, K., Bustin, S., and Zumla, A. (2005) Real-time RT-PCR normalisation; strategies and considerations. *Genes Immun.* **6(4)**, 279–284.

7. Vandesompele, J., De Preter, K., Pattyn, F., Poppe, B., Van Roy, N., De Paepe, A., and Speleman, F. (2002) Accurate normalization of real-time quantitative RT-PCR data by geometric averaging of multiple internal control genes. *Genome Biol.* **3(7)**, RESEARCH0034.

8. Pfaffl, M.W., Tichopad, A., Prgomet, C., and Neuvians, T.P. (2004) Determination of stable housekeeping genes, differentially regulated target genes and sample integrity: bestKeeper – Excel-based tool using pairwise correlations. *Biotechnol. Lett.* **26**, 509–515.

9. Abruzzo, L.V., Lee, K.Y., Fuller, A., Silverman, A., Keating, M.J., Medeiros, L.J., and Coombes, K.R. (2005) Validation of oligonucleotide microarray data using microfluidic low-density arrays: a new statistical method to normalize real-time RT-PCR data. *BioTechniques* **38**, 785–792.

10. Andersen, C.L., Jensen, J.L., and Orntoft, T.F. (2004) Normalization of real-time quantitative reverse transcription-PCR data: a model-based variance estimation approach to identify genes suited for normalization, applied to bladder and colon cancer data sets. *Cancer Res.* **64**, 5245–5250.

11. Szabo, A., Perou, C.M., Karaca, M., Perreard, L., Quackenbush, J.F., and Bernard, P.S. (2004) Statistical modeling for selecting housekeeper genes. *Genome Biol.* **5**, R59.

12. Dean, A. and Voss, D. (1999) Design and Analysis of Experiments, Springer: New York.

13. Pfaffl, M.W. (2001) A new mathematical model for relative quantification in real-time RT-PCR. *Nucleic Acids Res.* **29(9)**, e45.

14. Pfaffl, M.W., Horgan, G.W., and Dempfle, L. (2002) Relative expression software tool (REST©) for group-wise comparison and statistical analysis of relative expression results in real-time PCR. *Nucleic Acids Res.* **30**, e36.

15. Fu, W.J., Hu, J., Spencer, T., Carroll, R., and Wu, G. (2006) Statistical models in assessing fold change of gene expression in real-time RT-PCR experiments. *Comput. Biol. Chem.* **30**, 21–26.

16. Yuan, J.S., Reed, A., Chen, F., and Stewart, C.N. (2006) Statistical analysis of real-time PCR data. *BMC Bioinform.* **7**, 85.

17. Applied Biosystems (2006) Amplification Efficiency of TaqMan® Gene Expression Assays: Application Note.

18. Peirson, S.N., Butler, J.N., and Foster, R.G. (2003) Experimental validation of novel and conventional approaches to quantitative real-time PCR data analysis. *Nucleic Acids Res.* **31**, e73.

19. Ramakers, C., Ruijter, J.M., Deprez, R.H., and Moorman, A.F. (2003) Assumption-free analysis of quantitative real-time polymerase chain reaction (PCR) data. *Neurosci. Lett.* **339(1)**, 62–66.

20. Tichopad, A., Dilger, M., Schwarz, G., and Pfaffl, M.W. (2003) Standardized determination of real-time PCR efficiency from a single reaction set-up. *Nucleic Acids Res.* **31**, e122.

21. Zhao, S. and Fernald, D. (2005) Comprehensive algorithm for quantitative real-time polymerase chain reaction. *J. Comput. Biol.* **12(8)**, 1047–1064.

22. Liu, W. and Saint, D. (2002) Validation of a quantitative method for real time PCR kinetics. *Biochem. Biophys. Res. Commun.* **294(2)**, 347–353.

23. Tichopad, A., Dzidic A., and Pfaffl, M.W. (2002) Improving quantitative real-time RT-PCR reproducibility by boosting primer-linked amplification efficiency. *Biotechnol. Lett.* **24(24)**, 2053–2056.

24. Rutledge, R.G. (2004) Sigmoidal curve-fitting redefines quantitative real-time PCR with the prospective of developing automated high-throughput applications. *Nucleic Acids Res.* **32(22)**, e178.

25. Khan-Malek, R. (2007) Application of logistic modeling to estimate RT-PCR efficiency. Preclinical and Research Biostatistics Report GV07053-EN-E01. Sanofi-aventis.

Chapter 14

Evaluation of Mitochondrial Respiration in Cultured Rat Hepatocytes

Jean-Pierre Marchandeau and Gilles Labbe

Abstract

Mitochondrial dysfunction is a major mechanism whereby drugs can induce liver injury and other serious side effects, such as lactic acidosis and rhabdomyolysis, in some patients. Several *in vitro* and *in vivo* investigations can be performed in order to determine if drugs can disturb mitochondrial fatty acid oxidation (FAO) and the oxidative phosphorylation (OXPHOS) process, deplete hepatic mitochondrial DNA (mtDNA), or trigger the opening of the mitochondrial permeability transition pore (MPT). Among these investigations, mitochondrial respiration is a relatively easy test to measure the potential toxicity of a drug. The use of cells instead of isolated mitochondria allows one to test the toxic effect of a parent compound and its metabolites. The use of rat hepatocytes can detect drugs involved in drug-induced liver injuries (DILI). The method consists in measuring oxygen consumption by using a Clark electrode in a chamber containing a suspension of hepatocytes pre-incubated with drug.

Key words: Mitochondrial respiration, Oxygen consumption, Clark electrode, Respirometer, Primary rat hepatocytes

1. Introduction

Drug-induced liver injury (DILI) is a major issue for pharmaceutical companies, as it is considered one of the frequent causes for the failure of a drug during the pre-marketing phase and for the withdrawal of a marketed medicine.

Although drugs can cause hepatotoxicity through different mechanisms (1), mitochondrial dysfunction is one such major mechanism of DILI (2). By hampering mitochondrial energy production and/or releasing mitochondrial pro-apoptotic proteins into the cytoplasm, drugs can trigger necrosis or apoptosis of hepatocytes, thus causing "cytolytic" hepatitis, which can evolve toward liver failure. Drug-induced mitochondrial dysfunction

Jean-Charles Gautier (ed.), *Drug Safety Evaluation: Methods and Protocols*, Methods in Molecular Biology, vol. 691,
DOI 10.1007/978-1-60761-849-2_14, © Springer Science+Business Media, LLC 2011

can also lead to steatosis and steatohepatitis, which can sometimes progress to cirrhosis (2–4). In addition, drug-induced mitochondrial dysfunction can also trigger diverse extrahepatic or general manifestations, such as hyperlactatemia, lactic acidosis, myopathy, rhabdomyolysis, pancreatitis, peripheral neuropathy, or lipoatrophy (5–7). Thus, because of its potential severity for patients, drug-induced mitochondrial dysfunction should be detected during the preclinical safety studies.

Mitochondria are able to oxidize many metabolites including fatty acids, pyruvate (generated from glycolysis), and several amino acids such as valine, leucine, and methionine (3, 8, 9). During the fasting state, fatty acid oxidation (FAO) in the liver is incomplete; the acetyl-CoA that is generated is not oxidized in the liver, but condenses into ketone bodies (mainly acetoacetate and β-hydroxybutyrate), which are released into the plasma for subsequent oxidation in extrahepatic tissues. In the kidney, heart, and brain, the ketone bodies are then cleaved into acetyl-CoA, which is oxidized through the tricarboxylic acid cycle (3, 8).

The intra-mitochondrial oxidation of fatty acids, pyruvate, and amino acids generates reducing "equivalents" ($FADH_2$ and NADH), which must be reoxidized by the mitochondrial respiratory chain (MRC) in order to regenerate the FAD and NAD^+ that are needed for the oxidative processes such as FAO, pyruvate dehydrogenation, and the activity of the tricarboxylic acid cycle. In addition to regenerating FAD and NAD^+, the MRC also creates a large electrochemical gradient across the inner mitochondrial membrane, the so-called mitochondrial transmembrane potential, or $\Delta\psi_m$. Indeed, the transfer of electrons along the different components of the MRC (for instance, complexes I, III, and IV when electrons come from NADH) is associated with the ejection of protons from the mitochondrial matrix to the intermembrane space, thus raising the $\Delta\psi_m$. The $\Delta\psi_m$ serves as a reservoir of potential energy. When cells need energy, the rise in ADP levels within the mitochondria induces the re-entry of protons into the mitochondrial matrix through the membrane-spanning F_0 portion of the ATP synthase complex (also referred to as the complex V of the MRC). This re-entry of protons partially dissipates the $\Delta\psi_m$, thus liberating energy, which is used by the F_1 portion of ATP synthase to phosphorylate ADP into ATP. Concomitantly, the transient decrease in $\Delta\psi_m$ unleashes the flow of electrons in the respiratory chain and increases mitochondrial respiration to restore the $\Delta\psi_m$. Hence, there is a tight coupling within the mitochondria between ATP consumption, mitochondrial respiration, and ATP synthesis (5, 9). A major dysfunction of this oxidative phosphorylation (OXPHOS) process can hinder cell metabolism and cellular function in the liver and elsewhere (2, 10).

Several *in vitro* assays can be used in order to detect drug-induced mitochondrial dysfunction either on hepatic cells or on isolated liver mitochondria. The mitochondrial respiration method will be described using primary rat hepatocyte cultures.

2. Materials

2.1. Anesthetic Used

Ketamine/xylazine mixture: Imalgene 1000/Rompun 2%™, 1.25/0.25 mL/kg, respectively, intraperitoneally.

2.2. Cell Preparation and Cell Culture

1. Culture medium (William's E with Glutamax, Invitrogen life Science).
2. Fetal calf serum (Invitrogen life Science).
3. Perfusion medium (Invitrogen life Science).
4. Digestion medium (Invitrogen life Science).
5. Wash medium (Invitrogen life Science).
6. Insulin/transferrin/selenium (ITS) (Invitrogen life Science) is stored at +4°C.
7. Penicillin/streptomycin mixture (10,000 units/mL of penicillin and 10,000 μg/mL of streptomycin, Sigma) is stored in aliquot fractions of 10 mL at –20°C.
8. Dexamethazone (Sigma) aliquots of 5 mL (1 μg/mL) are stored at –20°C.
9. Phosphate-buffered saline (PBS) (Invitrogen life Science).
10. Six-well plates coated with collagen I cellware (Biocoat cell environments, Becton Dickinson).

2.3. Respiration System

1. Oxytherm respirometer (Hansatek).
2. Clark electrodes.
3. Computer (HP Personal Computer).
4. Oxygraph Plus software (Hansatek).

2.4. Hepatocytes Viability, Cell Count

1. Inverted microscope (Axiovert 40C, Karl Zeiss).
2. Trypan blue (VWR).
3. Malassez hematimeter.

2.5. Cytotoxicity Study

1. 3-(4,5-dimethylthiazol-2-yl)-2,5-diphenyltetrazolium bromide (MTT) (Invitrogen life Science).
2. Neutral Red (Merck).
3. Spectramax M5 spectrophotometer (Molecular Devices).

2.6. Trypsinization

1. Trypsin 25% EDTA 1X (Gibco).
2. Deionized water.

2.7. Experiment Solutions

1. Attachment medium: to William's E Glutamax, add fetal calf serum (final concentration 5%), penicillin/streptomycin (final concentration 100 UI/mL and 100 μg/mL, respectively), dexamethazone (final concentration 1% in PBS), and ITS (5 mL of the commercial solution 100×).

2. Culture medium: to William's E Glutamax, add penicillin/streptomycin (final concentration 100 UI/mL and 100 μg/mL, respectively), dexamethazone (final concentration 1% in PBS), and ITS (5 mL of the commercial solution 100×).

3. Neutral Red solution: dissolve neutral red in water (concentration 4 mg/mL). After overnight dissolution, filter the solution and dilute into culture media without FCS (final concentration 50 μg/mL).

4. Destain the solution for neutral red assay: freshly prepared with 49 parts of water + 50 parts of ethanol + 1 part of acetic acid.

5. Respiration medium:

   Mix 85.58 g of sucrose, 0.27 g of KH_2PO_4, 2.38 g of HEPES, and 0.19 g of EGTA in 800 mL of deionized water. Adjust to pH 7.4 with 1N NaOH. Complete to 1,000 mL with deionized water. Slowly add 0.7 g of BSA while stirring gently to avoid foam (11). Store at +4°C.

3. Methods

3.1. Cell Preparation (Protocol is Approved by Local Ethical Committee)

1. An adult male Sprague–Dawley rat (200–300 g) is anesthetized with a mixture of ketamine/xylazine.

2. Abdomen is washed with 70% ethanol.

3. When the animal is anesthetized, a ventral midline incision is made from xiphisternum to pupic bone, and hepatic portal vein and vena cava inferior are exposed.

4. A loose ligature is placed around the portal vein. Vena cava inferior is clamped. Portal vein is catheterized and ligature is tightened.

5. The catheter is then attached to the perfusion tubing containing perfusion medium. Vena cava superior is cut.

6. Liver is perfused with 100 mL of perfusion medium at a flow rate of 20 mL/min.

7. The liver is then perfused with 200–500 mL of perfusion medium containing collagenase until it is considered to be sufficiently digested.

8. After dissection, the liver is transferred into a sterile dish containing 30 mL of digestion medium prewarmed at 37°C.

The digested liver is gently teased with a sterile fork to dissociate cells from connective tissue.

9. The cell suspension is filled up to 50 mL with wash medium at +4°C and is filtered through a 60-µm nylon sterilized filter.

10. The cell suspension is then centrifuged for 5 min at 50 g.

11. The supernatant is aspirated, 25 mL of wash medium at +4°C is added, and the cell suspension is centrifuged for 5 min at 50 g. This procedure is repeated twice.

12. After the last washing step, the wash medium is replaced by attachment medium at 37°C (from 10 to 20 mL, depending on the pellet size).

13. Viability is determined with trypan blue exclusion using Malassez hematimeter.

3.2. Cell Culture

1. Rat hepatocytes are seeded and incubated for 24 h for attachment in collagen-coated, 6-well plates in a humidified atmosphere containing 5% CO_2 and 95% air at 37°C. Cell density at the time of seeding is 1.5 million cells per well containing 1.5 mL of culture medium.

2. After the attachment period, the culture medium is removed and replaced by the treatment medium containing control articles or different concentrations of test articles.

3. The hepatocytes are then incubated for 24 h in a humidified atmosphere containing 5% CO_2 and 95% air at 37°C.

3.3. Cytotoxicity Study

1. MTT test
Cell viability is evaluated using a colorimetric assay based on the reduction of the 3-(4, 5-dimethylthiazol-2-yl)-2,5-diphenyltetrazolium bromide (MTT) by mitochondrial dehydrogenases to form insoluble blue formazan particles; this MTT test is an indicator of the activity of mitochondrial dehydrogenases (12).

   (a) At tfhe end of the incubation period with the test articles, the medium is removed and the cells are washed with 1 mL PBS.

   (b) The cells are incubated for 2 h in 1 mL per well of William's E containing 50 µg of MTT in a humidified atmosphere containing 5% CO_2 and 95% air at 37°C.

   (c) The blue formazan precipitates are dissolved in DMSO (1 mL/well in 6-well plates).

   (d) The plates are gently shaken for 10 min to ensure complete dissolution of the blue formazan.

   (e) Absorbance is then measured, using a SpectraMax M5 spectrophotometer from Molecular Devices at 570-nm wavelength.

(f) The impact on cell viability induced by test articles is assessed by comparing the absorbance obtained in cell cultures exposed to test articles with the one measured in cell culture exposed to solvent only. Results are expressed as percentage of viable cells compared to solvent controls (see Note 1).

2. Neutral red uptake test

Cell viability is also evaluated using a colorimetric assay based on the lysosomal uptake of neutral red (NR) by viable cells. This assay is an indicator of cell integrity (13).

(a) At the end of the incubation period with the test articles, medium is removed and the cells are washed with 1 mL of PBS.

(b) The cells are incubated for 3 h in 1 mL per well of a solution of William's E containing NR at a concentration of 50 µg/mL at 37°C.

(c) At the end of the incubation period, the medium is removed and the cells are washed with 1 mL of PBS.

(d) A destain solution (freshly prepared with 49 parts of water + 50 parts of ethanol + 1 part of acetic acid) is added (1 mL/well) to remove the NR from viable cells into solution.

(e) The plates are gently shaken for 10 min to ensure complete dissolution of NR.

(f) Absorbance is then measured, using a SpectraMax M5 spectrophotometer from Molecular Devices at 540-nm wavelength.

(g) Effect on cell viability induced by test substances is assessed by comparing the absorbance obtained in cell cultures exposed to test substances with the one measured in cell culture exposed to solvent only. Results are expressed as percentage of viable cells compared to solvent controls (see Note 1).

3.4. Trypsinization

1. At the end of the incubation period with the test articles, the treatment medium is removed and replaced with 1 mL of PBS prewarmed at 37°C.

2. The plate is slightly shaken.

3. PBS is removed and replaced with 0.5 mL of trypsin solution prewarmed at 37°C diluted to 1:2 (v/v) in PBS.

4. The plate is incubated for 8 min in a humidified atmosphere containing 5% CO_2 and 95% air at 37°C (see Note 2).

5. The trypsinization is stopped by rapid addition of 1 ml/well of treatment medium completed with 20% of FCS.

6. The plate is slightly shaken.

7. After several "backward and forward" motions into a pipette (from 5 to 10 times), the cell suspension is delivered into a conical vial.

8. An aliquot of 20 μL is mixed with 20 μL of trypan blue solution diluted 1:4 (v/v) in culture medium.

9. Viable cells are counted into Malassez hematimeter for at least 3 lines out of 10 (see Note 3).

10. N (number of alive cells/mL) = X (number of alive cells/number of counted lines) ×10 (total number of lines) ×2 (dilution factor) ×1,000 (hematimeter volume).

11. N' (total number of alive cells) = $N \times V$ (tube volume).

12. During the cell count step, the cells are centrifuged for 5 min at 50 g at room temperature.

3.5. Respiration

3.5.1. Clark Electrode

The oxygen electrode is a specialized form of electrochemical cell that consists of two electrodes immersed in an electrolyte solution. Typically, a 50% saturated solution of KCl is used in oxygen electrode systems. Application of a polarizing voltage of 700 mV ionized the electrolyte and initiated current flow via a series of electrochemical reactions. Oxygen is "consumed" during the electrochemistry; thus, the magnitude of the current flow is related to the oxygen concentration of the surrounding media. This type of electrode sensor was first developed by Clark (1956) to measure oxygen in blood samples. As a result, it is often referred to as the Clark Electrode.

3.5.2. Electrode Preparation

Before use, the electrode disc needs to be prepared in such a way that an electrolyte bridge is formed between the anode and cathode in order for current to flow in the presence of oxygen. The disc also requires a protective membrane that prevents any deposits from the reaction mixture from settling on the cathode, yet allowing oxygen to diffuse freely so as not to jeopardize the response time of the disc.

There are four preparation stages:

1. Place a small drop of electrolyte on top of the dome of the electrode disc.

2. Place a 1.5-cm^2 paper spacer over the electrolyte, ensuring that at least one corner of the spacer is in the electrode well to act as a wick. Cover this with a similar sized piece of polytetrafluoroethylene (PTFE) membrane.

3. Place the small electrode disc O-ring over the end of the applicator tool. Hold the applicator vertically over the dome and slide the applicator shaft down to push the O-ring over the dome.

4. Check that the membrane preparation is smooth and that there are no trapped air bubbles. Top the reservoir well up with several drops of electrolyte.

3.5.3. System Calibration

Before any measurements could take place, the electrode disc must be calibrated so that the electrical signal received from the disc is presented as actual calibrated units (nmol/mL). Calibrating the disc for liquid-phase measurements involves a two-step procedure in which the signal from the oxygen electrode is referenced to two known oxygen concentrations. The two calibration steps are

1. air line.
2. zero oxygen line.

3.5.4. Performing a Liquid–Phase Calibration

1. Connect the electrode disc to the rear of the control unit.

2. Place approximately 2 mL of air-saturated, deionized water into the reaction vessel. Air-saturated water is obtained by vigorously shaking a small quantity of deionized water (approximately 50 mL) in a large conical flask (approximately 1 L).

3. Connect the Peltier electrode chamber to the rear of the Oxytherm control unit and ensure that the sample and electrode disc equilibrate to the temperature required by the assay before starting calibration.

4. After setting temperature, atmosphere pressure, and stirring speed, the system starts recording the "air line" level corresponding to 100% of dissolved oxygen. After the signal plateau is reached, the system proceeds to the "zero oxygen phase." The "zero oxygen phase" can be achieved into three different ways:

   a. Addition of sodium dithionite, a strong oxygen reducing agent, in the reaction chamber. However, care must be taken to remove all traces of dithionite from the chamber before continuing the experiment.

   b. Carefully bubbling nitrogen into the reaction chamber in order to displace oxygen.

   c. Carefully bubbling argon into the reaction chamber in order to displace oxygen. Argon is more efficient than nitrogen for establishing the "zero oxygen line."

   Calibration must be done every day of experimentation and for every electrode preparation (the calibration is valid for 24 h).

5. Remove the medium from the reaction chamber and replace it with deionized water. The water should be stirred under air at 37°C in the reaction chamber for 10–15 min (see Note 4).

6. Close the reaction chamber and record the level of oxygen in the water. The normal value of oxygen is in the range of 200–250 nmol/mL.

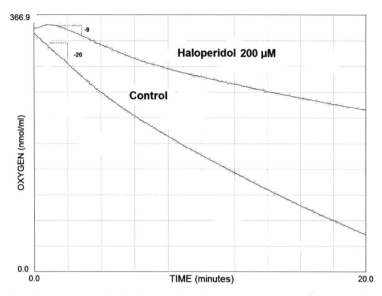

Fig. 1. Oxygen consumption in primary rat hepatocyte culture from control and haloperidol-treated cells. Hepatocytes are incubated for 24 h in the presence of haloperidol at a concentration of 200 μM or DMSO. The representation is a screenshot from the recording software. The slope calculation represents the rate of oxygen consumption expressed as nmol/mL/min. The rate of oxygen consumption is 20 nmol/mL/min for the control and 9 nmol/mL/min for the treated hepatocytes.

3.5.5. Hepatocytes Respiration Measurement

1. Remove the medium used to stop the trypsinization process and replace it by the respiration medium (see Note 5).

2. Adjust the volume so that it always has the same number of alive cells (e.g., 3 million cells in 1.9 mL, working volume in the reaction chamber).

3. Remove water from the respirometer reaction chamber and replace it by the previous hepatocyte suspension.

4. Close the chamber.

5. Start recording.

In these conditions, the oxygen concentration is decreasing as a function of time. After 10–15 min, the recording is stopped (see Note 6). The speed of oxygen consumption is calculated by determining the slope of the recording curve (Fig. 1). The speed is expressed in nmol oxygen/min/mL. This speed should be expressed in nmol oxygen/min/mL/million of viable cells to avoid variations depending on the number of cells in the chamber.

4. Notes

1. The MTT test (cytotoxicity study) may be replaced by another test of mitochondrial function such as Alamar blue or ATP

measurement. NR may be replaced by another test of cell integrity such as LDH. It is important to have at least two different tests, one testing the mitochondrial function and one testing the cell integrity.

2. The trypsinization step is a critical step as it leads to a great deal of cell destruction. The time of incubation with trypsin needs to be precisely respected. This time leads to a maximum cell death of 50%.

3. The viable cell count is a mandatory critical step. A minimum range of viable cells is necessary to have a good signal in the respirometer; it should at least be in the range of 1.5–3 million cells per measurement in the reaction chamber. A constant number of viable cells in the reaction chamber are important in order to compare the rates of oxygen consumption between samples.

4. An easiest way to saturate water with air is to shake deionized water at 37°C in a bottle (50 mL in a bottle of 1 L) and to pipette an aliquot into the reaction chamber.

5. The same interval of time must be respected between the counting after trypsinization and the beginning of oxygen consumption recording for every sample of a same experiment.

6. It is important to keep in mind that this protocol of respiration in hepatocytes measures spontaneous respiration as the consequence of the presence of the endogenous substrates and stimulated by the basic ATP consumption (11).

Acknowledgments

The authors would like to thank Delphine Hoët for her expertise and her support in hepatocyte culture.

References

1. Lee, W.M. (2003) Drug-induced hepatotoxicity. *N. Engl. J. Med.* **349**, 474–485.

2. Pessayre, D., Fromenty, B., Mansouri, A., and Berson, A. Hepatotoxicity Due to Mitochondrial Injury, in: Kaplowitz N. & DeLeve L.D. (Eds), *Drug-Induced Liver Disease* (second edition), Informa Healthcare, New York. 2007, pp.49–84.

3. Fromenty, B. and Pessayre, D. (1995) Inhibition of mitochondrial beta-oxidation as a mechanism of hepatotoxicity. *Pharmacol. Ther.* **67**, 101–154.

4. Pessayre, D., Mansouri, A., Haouzi, D., and Fromenty, B. (1999) Hepatotoxicity due to

mitochondrial dysfunction. *Cell Biol. Toxicol.* **15**, 367–373.

5. Igoudjil, A., Begriche, K., Pessayre, D., and Fromenty, B. (2006) Mitochondrial, metabolic and genotoxic effects of antiretroviral nucleoside reverse-transcriptase inhibitors. *Curr. Med. Chem. Anti-Infective Agents* **5**, 273–292.

6. Dykens, J.A. and Will, Y. (2007) The significance of mitochondrial toxicity testing in drug development. *Drug Discov. Today* **12**, 777–785.

7. Scatena, R., Bottoni, P., Botta, G., Martorana, G.E., and Giardina, B. (2007) The role of

mitochondria in pharmacotoxicology: a reevaluation of an old, newly emerging topic. *Am. J. Physiol. Cell Physiol.* **293**, C12–C21.

8. Salway, J.G. *Metabolism at a Glance* (first edition), Blackwell Scientific, London. 1994.

9. Pessayre, D. and Fromenty, B. (2005) NASH: a mitochondrial disease. J. *Hepatol.* **42**, 928–940.

10. Navarro, A. and Boveris A. (2007) The mitochondrial energy transduction system and the aging process. *Am. J. Physiol. Cell Physiol.* **292**, C670–C686.

11. Berson, A., Renault, S., Letteron, P., Robin, M.A., Fromenty, B., Fau, D., Le Bot, M.A., Riche, C., Durand-Schneider, A.M., Feldmann, G., and Pessayre, D. (1996) Uncoupling of rat and human mitochondria: A possible explanation for tacrine-induced liver dysfunction. *Gastroenterol.* **110**, 1878–1890.

12. Mosman, T. (1983) Rapid colorimetric assay for celullar growth and survival: application to proliferation and cytotoxicity assays. *J. Immunol. Methods* **65**, 55–63.

13. Borenfreund, E. and Puerner, J.A. (1985) Toxicity determined *in vitro* by morphological alterations and Neutral Red absorption. *Toxicology Lett.* **24**, 119–124.

Part VI

Screening Assays for Developmental Toxicity

Chapter 15

FETAX Assay for Evaluation of Developmental Toxicity

Isabelle Mouche, Laure Malesic, and Olivier Gillardeaux

Abstract

The Frog Embryo Teratogenesis Assay Xenopus (FETAX) test is a development toxicity screening test. Due to the small amount of compound needed and the capability to study organogenesis in a short period of time (96 h), FETAX test constitutes an efficient development toxicity alert test when performed early in drug safety development. The test is conducted on fertilized *Xenopus laevis* mid-blastula stage eggs over the organogenesis period. Compound teratogenic potential is determined after analysis of the mortality and malformation observations on larva. In parallel, FETAX test provides also information concerning embryotoxic effect based on larva length.

Key words: Embryo, FETAX, *Xenopus laevis*, Development, Toxicity, Teratogenesis, Teratogen

1. Introduction

Developmental toxicity represents an important issue for drug development in pharmaceutical companies. A teratogenic potential found prior to preclinical trials is a major benefit to initiate earlier appropriate *in vivo* studies to confirm or not the alert. However, in early development stage, the number of compounds to be tested is large and their available quantities are generally low. Regarding these requirements, Frog Embryo Teratogenesis Assay Xenopus (FETAX) is adapted to evaluate developmental toxicity potential using small drug quantities compared to *in vivo* studies. Furthermore, the main organogenesis nearly completed in a short time (96 h) constitutes a second advantage of FETAX test to obtain rapid development toxicity assessment compared to *in vivo* studies more time-consuming, even taking into account that FETAX assay should often be performed twice to conclude it positive or negative. An interlaboratory validation study based on

Jean-Charles Gautier (ed.), *Drug Safety Evaluation: Methods and Protocols*, Methods in Molecular Biology, vol. 691,
DOI 10.1007/978-1-60761-849-2_15, © Springer Science+Business Media, LLC 2011

a standard guide (1, 2) from the American Society for Testing and Materials (ASTM) showed advantages and difficulties to perform FETAX test. Herein, the method described is the FETAX method used as a routine test, in the lab, for several years, after an in-house validation period.

FETAX test is introduced as a developmental toxicity screening assay in this chapter, but it may be used as a mechanistic model to investigate developmental gene expression (3) which is not discussed herein. Indeed recent transcriptomic articles showed a great conservation of genes expressed in oocytes between *Xenopus laevis* and mouse (4). In that way, FETAX could be a tool for both developmental toxicity screening and development mechanistic model.

2. Materials

2.1. Xenopus laevis and Facilities

1. Twenty-four months to 3-years-old male and female *X. laevis* frogs are purchased from the Centre de Ressources Biologiques (CRB, Rennes, France) (see Note 1). The main problem one can face with *X. laevis* is the pathology called Red Leg Disease (see Note 2).

2. *X. laevis* are housed in *Xenopus* aquatic housing self-contained system (AQUANEERING, San Diego, USA) with 16-L tanks or 50-L tanks (see Note 3) maintained in a semi-darkness? environment at $20 \pm 2°C$.

3. Tanks have to be filled with chloride ion-free water obtained by filtration on 5 μm activated carbon cartridge (Millipore) (see Note 4).

4. Frozen stored mud worms are delivered to *Xenopus* twice a week.

2.2. Fertilization of Eggs

1. The Human chorionic gonadotrophin (hCG) lyophilisat of 5,000 IU (Sigma ref CG5) is dissolved with 5 mL sterile water to get a 1 IU/μL hCG solution.
The solution is stable 2 months at 2–8°C.

2. Leibovitz's L15 liquid media (1×) with L-glutamine and phenol red (Invitrogen).

2.3. Anesthesia

1. Ethyl 3-aminobenzoate methanesulfonate salt (MS-222, Sigma) is dissolved at 2% into chloride-free water and stored at around 4°C up to 3 months.

2. Ethyl 3-aminobenzoate methanesulfonate salt (MS-222, Sigma) is dissolved at 0.06% into FETAX medium and stored at around 4°C up to 3 months.

2.4. FETAX Culture and Treatment

1. FETAX medium: 10.7 mM NaCl, 1.14 mM NaHCO$_3$, 0.4 mM KCl, 0.1 mM CaCl$_2$, 0.35 mM CaSO$_4$, 2 H$_2$O, and 0.3 mM MgSO$_4$ in deionized water. Adjust pH to 7.6–7.9. FETAX medium can be purchased as a custom preparation (Xenopus medium, Invitrogen ref 041-94772M).

2. Dimethyl sulfoxyde Hybri-Max™ (DMSO, Sigma)

3. Thin forceps straight MORIA MC40 (11 cm) or MORIA 9980 (13 cm) (Fine Science Tools ref 11370-40 and 11399-80) and thin forceps curved MORIA MC40/B (11 cm) or MORIA 9987 (13 cm) (Fine Science Tools ref 11370-42 and 11399-87).

4. Binocular stereomicroscope WILD MZ8 (Leica), optical fibers with Intralux 5000-1 generator (volpi, Switzerland).

3. Methods

The test method is described in four main stages, starting with *in vitro* egg fertilization, following by egg selection, test article treatment, and then larva observation with the different developmental endpoints to assess. Finally, a section is dedicated to analysis and interpretation of the results. Timelines of FETAX test are shown in Fig. 1. *In vitro* egg fertilization leads to sacrifice *Xenopus* male to collect the sperm but provides a large amount of synchronized mid-blastula stage eggs to develop at the same time (see Note 5). Fertilization and egg selection are crucial steps to succeed in the test. Furthermore, the capability to identify accurately larva malformations needs much of experience acquired after many examinations of a very large number of larvae. This methodology is performed in-house under the approval from local ethical committee.

3.1. In Vitro Egg Fertilization

1. On the previous evening (T0 – 15/18 h) maintain the *Xenopus* frog with one hand on a benchkote paper or similar to perform a subcutaneous injection of 700 IU hCG to female and 300 IU hCG to the male from a 1 IU/μL hCG solution into the dorso-lymphatic sac (see Note 6).

2. At T0, about 15–18 h after hCG injection, anesthetize the *Xenopus* male putting it into the MS-222 2% solution

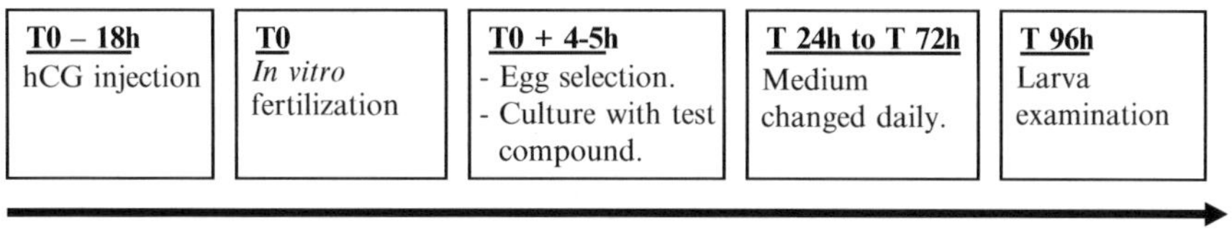

T0 – 18h	T0	T0 + 4-5h	T 24h to T 72h	T 96h
hCG injection	*In vitro* fertilization	- Egg selection. - Culture with test compound.	Medium changed daily.	Larva examination

Fig. 1. Timelines of the test.

260

odytarting now.

before lobotomize it. Make an abdominal incision to remove testes from the abdominal cavity and place them in leibovitz's L15 medium. Testes can be kept up to 4 days at 4°C in this medium.

3. *Xenopus* female generally does not release all the eggs. Therefore, it is necessary to make them get out from the cloaca. Therefore, maintain the *Xenopus* female firmly in one hand with its head placed toward the wrist, keeping its posterior legs folded up next to its body. With the thumb give an abdominal massage in the rostro-caudal direction carefully not to push too strongly on the *Xenopus* abdomen. Finally, put down the oocytes that are released from the cloaca on a 90-mm dry plastic Petri dish.

4. To fertilize oocytes, first, make multiple thin incisions with scissors and forceps in a piece of testis that is applied on the oocytes. Next, spread well oocytes on the Petri dish to obtain a monolayer, using the testis as a tool to make it. A few minutes later cover the oocytes with FETAX medium.

5. Incubate eggs at 25°C about 5 h to develop up to the mid-blastula stage. Check them regularly to ensure development that occurs correctly and not to miss the mid-blastula stage (see Note 7).

3.2. Egg Culture and Compound Treatment

3.2.1. Concentration Range Selection and Preparation

1. Determine the tested concentration range of the compound. According to the limit of solubility (see Note 8), compound is tested up to the limit of solubility or through a standard range of five concentrations 1 – 4 – 16 – 32 – 62.5 mg/L with a DMSO maximum concentration of 0.5% when this vehicle is used to dissolve the compound. When no effects are observed on *Xenopus* embryos with the standard dose range a second assay is performed up to a maximum of 400 mg/L even if the solubility is higher than 400 mg/L in FETAX medium. Upper concentration is generally toxic whatever the compound from experience.

2. At T0, dissolve compound in DMSO or in FETAX medium according to the solubility, under a laminar flow microbiological safety cabinet. The volume of this stock solution has to be sufficient for the entire assay.

3. Distribute the stock solution in identified dark flasks, such as the minimum volume of each final concentration is 32 mL FETAX medium (see Note 9). Add DMSO, as needed, to get 0.5% in each final concentration and complete with FETAX medium to the appropriate volume.

An example of a concentration range preparation is shown in Table 1.

Table 1
Example of standard range preparation

Concentration identification	Final concentration in FETAX medium (mg/L)	Compound stock solution 10 g/L (µL)	DMSO (µL)	Complete with FETAX medium to (mL)
1	0	0	160	32
2	1	4	196	40
3	5	16	144	32
4	10	32	128	32
5	25	80	80	32
6	50	160	0	32

4. Concentration range is kept at around 4°C during the 96-h test period. But stock solution prepared in DMSO is kept at room temperature to avoid freezing.

3.2.2. Egg Seeding and Treatment (T0 + 4–5 h)

1. Deliver 8 mL of each concentration in a 50-mm sterile vented Petri dish previously labeled (concentration and compound name) under a laminar flow microbiological safety cabinet. If compound range has been refrigerated, let it at least 1 h 30 min at room temperature before adding the eggs. Low temperature is toxic for egg development and induces malformations. In case of a FETAX test conducted with a metabolic activation system (MAS), it should be added simultaneously with the compound (see Note 10).

2. Fill a 50-mm sterile vented Petri dish with 8 mL of culture medium without test compound as control culture.

3. Using MORIA thin forceps, pick over the eggs which have their pigmented pole up (animal pole), a regular spherical shape and a homogeneous cellular division (Fig. 2) under a binocular stereomicroscope placed under the laminar flow microbiological safety cabinet (*see* **Note 11**). Unfertilized eggs are totally white without pigmentation. Add 20 midblastula stage selected eggs in each Petri dish previously filled with test compound or control solution ensuring that they are at room temperature.

4. Maintain egg cultures in Petri dishes with the cover on and keep them at room temperature (around 20°C) in dark light under the laminar flow microbiological safety cabinet for 96 h.

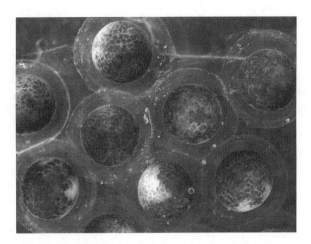

Fig. 2. Mid-blastula stage eggs.

3.2.3. Culture Monitoring (T 24 h to T 72 h)

FETAX medium with or without tested compound is changed daily under the laminar flow microbiological safety cabinet. Light can be switch on during this operation.

1. Add 8 mL of each compound final concentration prepared at T0 or culture medium in new 50-mm sterile vented Petri dishes previously labeled.

2. Keep those Petri dishes at least 1 h 30 min at room temperature to ensure that FETAX medium is at room temperature (around 20°C) before adding eggs.

3. Transfer the living larvae in the new Petri dishes under binocular stereomicroscope, at 24 h using MORIA thin forceps, as the eggs are a little sticky and at 48 h and 72 h, with a transfer polyethylene 2 mL Pasteur pipet with the thin end cut, as larvae have swimming capability.

4. Switch the light off and keep the culture in dark light under the laminar flow microbiological safety cabinet.

5. Report daily on an observation sheet the number of dead larvae and compound's precipitates for each culture (see Note 12).

3.2.4. Culture End (T 96 h): Larva Examination

Follow the different steps described below for each concentration and each larva:

1. Check that all larvae swim and if not report it on a developmental parameter sheet on which malformations will be recorded too.

2. Write down the precipitates, if any, and the number of dead larvae on the observation sheet, then remove them from the Petri dishes.

Table 2
Malformation types

General malformations		Specific malformations	
–	No swimming	Blisters	Ventral fin
			Dorsal fin
Pigmentation	No pigmentation		
	Abnormal pigmentation	Cranium	Acephaly
			Macrocephaly
Axis	Stunted larvae		Microcephaly
	Skeletal kinking		
	Wavy tail	Face	Abnormally flattened
–	Hemorrhage	Nares	Malpositioned
Oedema	Cardiac	Mouth	Small
	Abdominal		Incomplete development
	Facial		
	Cephalic	Eyes	Absent
	Optic		Malpositioned
			Irregular shape
Gut	Miscoiling		Cyclopia
Other(s)			Incomplete separation
			Abnormal pigmentation
			Failure of the choroid
			Abn pigmented optic nerves
		Heart	Enlarged
			Malpositioned
			Underdeveloped

Specific malformations are considered more severe than general ones *Abn* abnormally, *sl* slight, *mo* moderate, *se* severe, *uni* unilateral, *bi* bilateral

3. Euthanize larvae by putting them into 0.06% MS-222 solution (lethal dose) in a 50-mm Petri dish.

4. Measure only each straight larva from the head to the tail end with the measurement system (MFK2, Leitz) and report the value on the developmental parameter sheet. Do not measure larvae with axis malformations as it would not be relevant.

5. Examine each larva under a binocular stereomicroscope to identify developmental malformation described in the Table 2 and by leaning on the *Atlas of abnormalities* (5).

   Figures 3 and 4 show examples of normal and abnormal larvae.

6. After examination, eliminate larvae according to your internal rules concerning biological samples.

3.3. Result Analysis   Once FETAX technical part is completed, a teratogenic index (TI) based on mortality and the number of abnormal embryos is

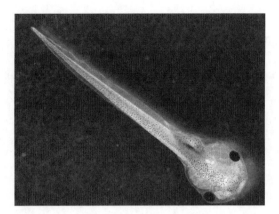

Fig. 3. Normal larva.

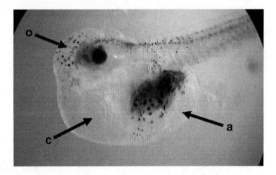

Fig. 4. Abnormal larva. *a* abdominal oedema, *c* cardiac oedema, *o* optic oedema.

calculated, larva length is analyzed with statistical tools, and finally, malformation type ratio is determined. FETAX test is then concluded positive or negative which means the compound presents or not a teratogenic potential according to this result analysis.

3.3.1. Statistical Analysis of Larva Length

Larva length is a parameter that gives information about the embryotoxic effect of the compound. A statistical analysis is applied to ensure that length differences observed between treated larvae and control ones are significant.

1. Using statistical software, enter concentration and individual length values to perform a Normality test.

2. First case: If the test is "Normal," make a Bartlett test following by a Dunnett test whether the Bartlett test is accepted; otherwise, if the Bartlett test is not accepted, perform a Kruskal–Wallis test. Second case: If the test is "not Normal" perform a Kruskal–Wallis test.

3. A compound is considered embryotoxic if a significant length difference is concluded according to the statistical tests. But it is important to check if this statistical difference is biologically relevant based on the dose-length effect relationship observed.

4. Determine the minimum concentration inhibiting growth (MCIG) which is the concentration that reduces significantly the larva length.

3.3.2. Calculation of the Teratogenic Index

The conclusion of the test is based on the value of the TI calculated as the ratio of the embryo lethal concentration 50% (EmLC50) vs. the concentration inducing 50% of malformed larvae (EmMC50) among the living ones.

1. Calculate the percentage of mortality and of malformed embryos for each concentration tested.

2. Enter these data in graph-pad Prism® software or similar.

3. Apply a nonregression linear model to establish two curves: (a) Mortality percentage as a function of concentration and (b) malformation percentage as a function of concentration.

4. Choose the appropriate function to determine the EmLC50 (x-value) that induces 50% of mortality on the curve [mortality = f(concentration)] and EmMC50 (x- value) that induces 50% of malformed embryos on the curve [malformed embryo = f (concentration)]. If the software does not give exactly the 50% value, select the closest one.

5. Determine the TI = (EmLC50)/(EmMC50).

3.3.3. Malformation Parameters

1. Create a table to gather for each concentration the number of malformed embryos, the percentage of malformed embryos among the living larvae and the percentage of malformed embryos among the living larvae for each malformation type.

2. Create an histogram malformation percentage as a function of malformation type to visualize the compound effect.

3. Evaluate the malformation severity taking into account that axis, pigmentation, hemorrhage, oedema, and gut malformations are general malformations, whereas blisters, cranium, face, nares, mouth, eyes, and heart malformations are specific ones.

Specific malformations are considered more severe than general ones.

3.4. Interpretation

1. Prior to the interpretation, FETAX assay has to be validated according to acceptance quality criteria based on control results (see Note 13).

2. The interpretation is done first with the TI. According to Sanofi-aventis historical data obtained with reference and in-house compounds, we have stated that a FETAX test is concluded positive when the TI value is higher or equal to 1.2 and negative whether the TI value is lower or equal to 1.0. When the TI value is between 1.0 and 1.2 the length parameter, mortality and types of malformations have to be considered to

conclude the test positive or negative based on the decision tree (Fig. 5).

Sometimes, the TI cannot be calculated because EmLC50 and/or EmMC50 are not reached. However, a conclusion is generally possible according to the decision tree (Fig. 6). If not, a second assay is recommended with concentration range modifications.

An example of interpretation is shown in Table 3 with nicotine tested as a reference compound. It was concluded positive due

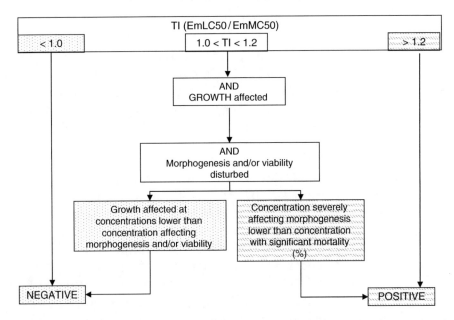

Fig. 5. Decision tree with teratogenic index (TI). Modified growth is appreciated with larva length measurement.

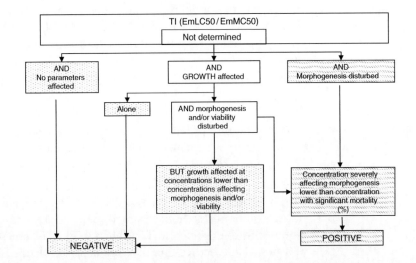

Fig. 6. Decision tree without teratogenic index (TI). Modified growth is appreciated with larva length measurement.

Table 3
Example of nicotine tested in FETAX test

Dose		Number of eggs in culture	Mortality	Number of malformed embryos	Length ± SD	
(mg/L)	(µM)		Number (%)	Number (%)	(mm)	Number of embryos measured
0	0	20	0 (0)	0	9.5 ± 0.24	20
2.5	12	20	1 (5)	0	9.4 ± 0.16*	20
10	47	20	0 (0)	2 (10.0)	9.3 ± 0.15*	18
40	189	20	2 (10)	7 (38.9)	9.2 ± 0.18**	12
160	757	20	8 (40)	12 (100.0)	9.0 ± 0.12**	7
320	1514	20	20 (100)	–	–	–
EmLC50 (mg/L)	210.1			MCIG (mg/L)	2.5	
EmMC50 (mg/L)	59.8			NOEC (mg/L)	ND	
TI	3.51					

EmLC50: embryo lethal concentration 50% EmMC50: concentration inducing 50% of malformed embryos. *TI*, teratogenic index (EmLC50/EmMC50); *MCIG*, minimum concentration inhibiting growth; *NOEC*, no observable effect concentration; *ND*, not determined; –, not done. A Dunnett test was applied to length parameter. $*p < 0.05$; $**p < 0.001$

to a TI value of 3.51, thus meaning that nicotine presented a teratogenic potential under the experimental conditions used.

3. Apart from FETAX interpretation, the No Observable Effect Concentration (NOEC) can be determined to provide complementary information regarding the minimum concentration that is safe to *Xenopus* eggs (see Note 14).

4. Notes

1. Each *Xenopus* can be injected with hCG once every 3 months three times maximum. It is recommended to have in-house 40 females and 16 males to ensure a good turn-over.

2. The main pathology *X. laevis* can suffer from is the Red Leg Disease which is a bacteria septicemia. Further information regarding this disease can be found on the Web site http://www.xlaevis.com.

   The problem is that when the clinical signs are observed the disease is at an advanced stage and then only a few frogs will survive. An antibiotic treatment exists, but its effects can interfere with FETAX results. The only efficient solution to get ride of the Red Leg Disease is to euthanize contaminated frogs.

When a *Xenopus* frog is found dead due to the Red Leg Disease, the tank is placed in quarantine to observe the others *Xenopus* during 1 month. If no Red Leg Disease symptoms appear, over this period frogs can be used to perform FETAX test.

3. *Xenopus* aquatic housing system uses a four-stage filtration system to provide a recirculating clean water. However, different kinds of tanks can be used under several conditions, such as: 3–4 L of water at room temperature per *Xenopus*, an air circulation system into water, a turnover of the tank water at least once every 2 weeks or a recirculating filtered water system and environmental enrichment devices as plastic pipes to provide hiding places.

4. *Xenopus* are very sensitive to chloride ions that are toxic for them and for egg development. Therefore, a key point is to use chloride ion-free water in the tank to get the best conditions for FETAX test success.

5. Another method to obtain fertilized eggs is to perform a natural mating. On the previous evening (T0 – 18 h), once hCG injection has been performed, one male and two females are left together in a tank overnight. At T0, eggs are collected to be selected at the mid-blastula stage to perform the test. However, the main limit of the natural fertilization is that eggs are not fertilized at the same time depending on how the sperm is spread by the male in the tank. So it is difficult to obtain a large amount of eggs at a mid-blastula stage at the same time to perform an assay. On the other hand, the advantage of the natural fertilization is that the male is not sacrificed. Therefore, it can be used once every 3 months, three times maximum.

6. The hCG injection is recommended but not mandatory for *Xenopus* male.

7. Development stage series is available on http://www.xenbase.org in the chapter "Anatomy and Development stages."

8. If not known, determine compound solubility in DMSO and FETAX since compounds are more often dissolved in DMSO and diluted at 1/200 in FETAX medium (final DMSO percent is 0.5% maximum) or directly dissolved in FETAX medium. Other vehicles or buffers can be used, but they have to be tested to verify that they are free of toxic effect on *Xenopus* egg development. In any case, avoid vehicles with chloride ions that are toxic for *Xenopus* embryos.

9. Do not make a cascade range to avoid dilution errors.

10. In the lab, MAS is not included in the method as the results obtained without MAS were satisfying so far even if it is

known that *X. laevis* eggs have a poor metabolic potential. However, information can be found in an interlaboratory validation (6, 7) and in optimization studies (8, 9). This validation and MAS model improvement studies showed that several parameters have to be well controlled to reduce variability between assays in order to obtain relevant data.

11. Eggs attributed to a compound have to be selected from the same female laying.

12. Sometimes, precipitates appear throughout the study even if at first the compound was soluble. It could be due to the refrigerate storage and/or if the compound is not stable in solution.

13. FETAX assay is accepted when control larva mortality and malformed control embryos rate are equal or lower than 10%, and control larva length is in accordance with historical data.

14. The NOEC is the tested concentration that induces neither mortality nor malformation or lower than 10% and does not involve larva length modification compared to historical data range.

References

1. ASTM. (1998) Standard guide for conducting the frog embryo teratogenesis assay – *Xenopus*. Designation E 1439-98. In *Annual book of ASTM standards*, Vol 11.5. American Society for Testing and Materials, Philadelphia, pp. 825–836.

2. Bantle, J.A., Finch R.A., Burton, D.T., Fort, D.J., Dawson, D.A., Linder, G., Rayburn, J.R., Hull, M., Kumsher-King, M., Gaudet-Hull, A.M., and Turley, S.D. (1996) FETAX interlaboratory validation study: Phase III – Part 1 testing. *J. Appl. Toxicol.* 16(6), 517–528.

3. Sipe, C.W., and Saha, M.S. (2007) The use of microarray technology in non mammalian vertebrate systems. In *Microarrays: Volume II: Applications and Data Analysis. Methods in Molecular Biology.* Vol 382 (Rampal, J.B., ed.), Humana, Totowa, NJ, pp. 1–16.

4. Vallée, M., Aiba, K., Piao, Y., Palin, M.F., Ko, M.S., and Sirard, M.A. (2008) Comparative analysis of oocyte transcript profiles reveals a high degree of conservation among species. *Reproduction* 135(4), 439–448.

5. Bantle, J.A., Dumont, J.N., Finch, R.A., Linder G., and Fort, D.J. (1998) *Atlas of abnormalities, a guide for the performance of FETAX*, 2nd ed. Oklahoma State University, Stillwater, OK.

6. Fort, D.J., Stover, E.L., Bantle, J.A., Rayburn, J.R., Hull, M.A., Finch, R.A., Burton, D.T., Turley, S.D., Dawson, D.A., Linder, G., Buchwalter, D., Dumont, J.N., Kumsher-King, M., and Gaudet-Hull, A.M. (1998) Phase III interlaboratory study of FETAX, Part 2: interlaboratory validation of an exogenous metabolic activation system for frog embryo teratogenesis assay-*Xenopus* (FETAX). *Drug Chem. Toxicol.* 21(1), 1–14.

7. Bantle, J.A., Finch, R.A., Fort, D.J., Stover, E.L., Hull, M., Kumsher-King, M., and Gaudet-Hull, A.M. (1999) Phase III interlaboratory study of FETAX. Part 3. FETAX Validation using 12 compounds with and without an exogenous metabolic activation system. *J. Appl. Toxicol.* 19, 447–472.

8. Fort, D.J., Rogers, R.L., Stover, E.L., and Finch, R.A. (2001) Optimization of an exogenous metabolic activation system for FETAX. I. Post-isolation rat liver microsome mixtures. *Drug Chem. Toxicol.* 24(2), 103–115.

9. Fort, D.J., Rogers, R.L., Paul, R.R., Stover, E.L., and Finch, R.A. (2001) Optimization of an exogenous metabolic activation system for FETAX. II. Preliminary evaluation. *Drug Chem. Toxicol.* 24(2), 117–127.

Chapter 16

Evaluation of Embryotoxicity Using the Zebrafish Model

Lisa Truong, Stacey L. Harper, and Robert L. Tanguay

Abstract

The embryonic zebrafish model offers the power of whole-animal investigations (e.g., intact organism, functional homeostatic feedback mechanisms, and intercellular signaling) with the convenience of cell culture (e.g., cost- and time-efficient, minimal infrastructure, small quantities of nanomaterial solutions required). The model system overcomes many of the current limitations in rapid to high-throughput screening of drugs/compounds and casts a broad net to evaluate integrated system effects rapidly. Additionally, it is an ideal platform to follow up with targeted studies aimed at the mechanisms of toxic action. Exposures are carried out in 96-well plates so minimal solution volumes are required for the assessments. Numerous morphological, developmental, and behavioral endpoints can be evaluated non-invasively due to the transparent nature of the embryos.

Key words: Zebrafish, Development, Embryos, *In vivo*, Vertebrate, Rapid screening

1. Introduction

Numerous biological models can be employed for toxicity evaluations. *In vitro* techniques, such as cell culture systems, are often preferred because they are both cost and time efficient. While these studies are useful, direct translation to whole organisms and human health is often difficult to infer. *In vivo* studies can provide improved prediction of biological response in intact systems but often require extensive facilities and infrastructure (1). Zebrafish (*Danio rerio*) offer a number of practical advantages as a model organism that overcomes these limitations, making these vertebrates highly amenable for toxicologically relevant research. Zebrafish can be employed as a powerful *in vivo* model system to assess biological interactions and are an outstanding platform

Jean-Charles Gautier (ed.), *Drug Safety Evaluation: Methods and Protocols*, Methods in Molecular Biology, vol. 691,
DOI 10.1007/978-1-60761-849-2_16, © Springer Science+Business Media, LLC 2011

to detail the mechanisms by which substances elicit specific biological responses. A remarkable similarity in cellular structure, signaling processes, anatomy, and physiology exists among zebrafish and other high-order vertebrates, particularly early in development (2–6). Current estimates indicate that over 90% of the human open reading frames are homologous to genes in fish (7). Thus, investigations using this model system can reveal subtle interactions that are likely to be conserved across species.

Features of the zebrafish's biology are favorable for adapting this model system to high-throughput assays. Female zebrafish are able to produce hundreds of eggs weekly, so large sample sizes are easily achieved, allowing for statistically powerful dose–response studies. This abundant supply of embryos also makes it possible to assess simultaneously the toxicity of a large number of substances in a short period. The vertebrate's rapid developmental progression compared to that of other mammals makes it an ideal model for high-throughput screening (8). For example, neuronal plate formation occurs at 10 h postfertilization (hpf), followed by organogenesis at 24 hpf, which compared to that in a rat occurs at 9.5 days and 5–6 days, respectively. The first heartbeat occurs at 30 hpf for the zebrafish and 10.2 days for rats (9).

Zebrafish embryos can be individually exposed in wells of a multi-well plate so the required volume needed for the model is small; thus, only limited amounts of materials are needed to assess an entire suite of biological interactions and responses. Early developmental life stages are often uniquely sensitive to environmental insult, due in part to the enormous changes in cellular differentiation, proliferation, and migration required to form multiple cell types, tissues, and organs (2, 5, 6, 10). Since development is highly coordinated, requiring specific cell-to-cell communications, if exposure to a substance during that critical period perturbed these interactions, development would be expected to be disrupted. Embryos are waterborne-exposed to a chemical using a continuous method in which 24 embryos are exposed per concentration in individual wells of a multi-well plate from 8 to 120 hpf. Exposure until 120 hpf is the ideal duration for a developmental toxicity testing; primarily due to the vertebrate model's ability to obtain its nutrients from its yolk sac until 5 days, which will not introduce new confounding factors. Perturbed development can manifest as morphological malformations, behavioral abnormalities, or death of the embryos. Zebrafish embryos develop externally and are optically transparent, so it is possible to resolve individual cells *in vivo* throughout the duration of an exposure using simple microscopic techniques, and numerous effects can be assessed noninvasively over the course of development.

2. Materials

2.1. Zebrafish Husbandry

1. Fish water: 0.3 g/L Instant Ocean salts (Aquatic Ecosystems, Apopka, FL) in reverse osmosis (RO) water.
2. Incubator set at $28 \pm 0.1°C$.
3. Fish food: crushed TetraMin® Tropical Flake or live *Artemia* from INVE (Salt Lake City, UT).

2.2. Dechorination

1. Compound stereo microscope for viewing embryos.
2. 90-mm glass petri dish.
3. 50 mg/mL pronase (Sigma-Aldrich) in RO water. Measure 50 mg of pronase into a 1.5-mL microcentrifuge tube and fill it with 1 mL of RO water. Aliquot 50 μL into a 1.5-mL microcentrifuge tube and place it in a freezer box, then immediately place the box in the freezer. This will make 20 1.5-mL microcentrifuge tubes that can be stored for up to 4 months. Aliquots can be thawed just prior to use.
4. Timer.

2.3. Exposure

1. Multi-well plates.
2. 8 or 12 multichannel pipettes.
3. 50-mL reagent reservoir.
4. Wide-bore Pasteur pipette.

2.4. Assessment

1. Anesthesia: 4 mg/mL of 3-aminobenzoate ethyl ester methanesulfonate salt (tricaine, Sigma-Aldrich) in RO water, pH adjusted to 7.0 with 0.1 M Tris–HCl, pH 9.0.
2. Methyl cellulose: 10 mg/mL of methyl cellulose (Sigma-Aldrich) (see Note 1).

3. Methods

3.1. Zebrafish Husbandry

1. Rear adult zebrafish *Danio rerio* in standard laboratory conditions of 28°C with a pH of 7 ± 0.2 on a 14-h light/10-h dark photoperiod (11).
2. House zebrafish in 2.0-L polycarbonate tanks with re-circulating water system. Keep adult zebrafish in groups to allow for large quantities of embryos to be collected. Group spawning also helps to increase genetic diversity.
3. Feed the fish twice daily with either crushed or live fish food.
4. Spawning: place male and female zebrafish into spawning baskets in polycarbonate tanks the afternoon before the

embryos are needed. Zebrafish will typically spawn when the lights come on after the 10-h dark period.

5. The following morning, newly fertilized eggs are collected, rinsed several times in system water, and placed into fresh fish water in a 150-mm plastic petri dish.

6. Remove the embryos that are unfertilized or necrotic prior to placing the petri dish into the incubator to keep the embryos warm until they reach 6 hpf (Fig. 1) (8).

7. Remove embryos that are not of the same stage as the majority prior to experimental use (see Note 2).

3.2. Dechorination

1. To avoid barrier effects potentially posed by the chorion (Figure 1a), all embryos should be dechorionated at 6 hpf using a modified version of Westerfields (2000) (11) protocol for pronase enzyme degradation (Figure 1b).

2. Place 6-hpf embryos into a 90-mm glass petri dish with 25 mL of fish water (see Note 3). Up to 1,200 embryos can be processed in a single dish using this method.

3. Add 50 μL of 50 mg/mL pronase to the center of the dish and continuously swirl gently to mix the solution.

4. Set a timer for 7 min and continuously swirl the embryos while occasionally observing the petri dish under the microscope to check for embryos without chorions, chorion pieces in the solution, and "deflated" chorions.

5. When 7 min have passed, or when the above are observed, remove the pronase solution by diluting the solution with fresh fish water, slowly decanting over the edge of the petri dish continuously for 1 min, then repeat this procedure for a total of 10 min (see Note 4).

6. After the rinse, allow the embryos to recover in the petri dish in an incubator (or in a room at 28°C) until 8 hpf (see Note 5).

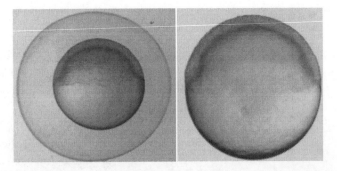

Fig. 1. Zebrafish embryos at 6-h postfertilization (hpf). Six hpf embryos (**a**) with chorion (**b**) after using pronase to enzymatically remove the chorion.

3.3. Exposure

3.3.1. Waterborne Exposure

1. Chemicals should be dissolved in fish water if possible (see Note 6). In the case that this is not possible, the solvent of choice for exposure utilizing the embryonic zebrafish is dimethyl sulfoxide (DMSO) (see Note 7).

2. Pour each test solution into a 50-mL reagent reservoir, which will fit a multichannel pipette.

3. For each exposure concentration tested, use a multichannel pipette to fill 24 individual wells in a multi-well plate with 100 μL of chemical solution. Seven concentrations and one control group can be tested using two 96-well plates.

4. At 8 hpf, transfer viable, appropriately developing embryos into individual wells of a multi-well plate using a wide-bore glass pipette (see Note 8).

5. Incubate at 28°C until 24 hpf, then perform assessments.

3.3.2. Microinjection Exposure

1. If direct delivery of a chemical is necessary to ensure accurate dose delivery, embryos should be microinjected at 8 hpf (see Note 9).

2. Align 8-hpf embryos in troughs embedded in a 1% agarose plate filled with fish water as described by *The Zebrafish Book* (9, 11).

3. Inject each embryo with 2.3 nL of the desired chemical concentration or the appropriate vehicle control directly into the yolk.

4. Place each embryo into individual wells of a 96-well plate, each filled with 100 μL of fish water. When directly delivering a chemical into the yolk sac, any concentration above 0.1% DMSO caused developmental defects not attributed to the chemical. If a chemical requires a solvent, two sets of serial dilutions should be made. Make the first serial dilution with 100% DMSO, at a 100 times higher concentration than the final concentration desired (see Note 10). For the second set of serial dilutions, from the 100% DMSO serial dilution, make a 1:10 dilution from the first serial dilution. Make sure to have an appropriate control for each chemical, which includes the correct percentage of solvent used in each solution.

5. Incubate at 28°C until first assessment at 24 hpf.

3.4. Assessment

1. At 24 hpf, embryos are assessed for viability, developmental progression, and spontaneous movements (earliest behavior in zebrafish). Developmental progression is considered perturbed if the zebrafish development is more than 12 h delayed compared to control animals. Spontaneous movements are assessed over a 2-min period and are considered perturbed if there is a lack of embryonic contractions and/or movement.

2. At 120 hpf, larval morphology (body axis, eye, snout, jaw, otic vesicle, notochord, heart, brain, somite, fin, yolk sac, trunk, circulation, pigment, and swim bladder; Fig. 2) is evaluated and recorded and behavioral endpoints (motility and tactile response) are thoroughly evaluated *in vivo*. Test for behavioral endpoints and then anesthetize the animals for thorough

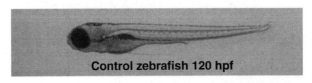

Control zebrafish 120 hpf

1. 120 hr mortality – dies between 24 and 120 hours post fertilization (hpf)

2. 24 hr mortality – dies before 24 hpf

3. 24 hr sp. Mov – no spontaneous movement at 24 hpf

4. 24 hr dev prog – delayed development

5. 24 hr notochord – notochord malformation (wavy notochord)

6. axis – curved or bent axis in either direction

7. brain – brain malformations or necrosis

8. caudal fin – malformed or missing

9. circulation – no circulation or blood flow

10. eye – eyes malformed, missing or smaller/larger than normal

11. heart – heart malformation, pericardial edema (fluid around the heart)

12. jaw – malformed

13. otic – malformed or missing

14. pectoral fin – malformed or missing

15. pigmentation – lack of pigmentation, overpigmentation

16. snout – shortened or malformed

17. somite – malformed or disorganized, missing somites

18. swim bladder inflate – failure of swim bladder to inflate

19. touch response – not responsive to touch at 120 hpf

20. trunk – short trunk, malformed or missing

21. YSE – yolk sacedema, swelling around the yolk sac

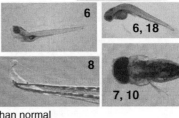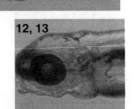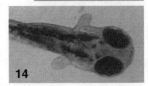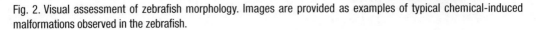

Fig. 2. Visual assessment of zebrafish morphology. Images are provided as examples of typical chemical-induced malformations observed in the zebrafish.

morphological analysis. At the end of the assessments, the zebrafish are euthanized with tricaine.

3. Evaluations are completed in a binary notation (present or not present) (see Note 11). Control and chemical-exposed groups are statistically compared using Fisher's Exact test at $p < 0.05$ with SigmaStat software for each endpoint evaluated (Fig. 2).

4. Notes

1. Methyl cellulose is unique in that it "melts" when cold and solidifies when hot. It dissolves best in cold water; however, it is best to disperse the powder form in warm water and then continue to mix while chilling. An alternate to methyl cellulose is Protoslo® (Carolina Biological Supply Company, Burlington, NC).

2. Eggs can sometimes be laid and fertilized at different times in a group spawn; therefore, always remove embryos that are developing more rapidly or significantly slower prior to using them for an experiment. As an alternate, male and female pairs can be set up in several divided tanks, and the dividers can be removed at the same time. The resulting stage-matched embryos can then be pooled prior to random embryo selection.

3. Do not bleach embryos if their chorions are to be removed by pronase digestion. Bleaching modifies the chorion, rendering the pronase treatment completely ineffective. In addition, when dechorinating embryos, it is essential to use glass petri dishes. Dechorinated embryos will stick to the bottom of plastic dishes and will be severely damaged during the procedure.

4. The newly dechorionated embryos are very delicate. Water should be administered with a gentle flow and not directly onto the embryos. Some of the embryos will not be out of their chorion even once the 10-min rinsing period is done. More will emerge during the recovery period.

5. Once an embryo is dechorionated, do not bleach the embryos.

6. Chemicals or drugs that are thought to be inactive until metabolized to an active form may be pre-exposed to induce an active conformation prior to waterborne exposures.

7. The Tanguay Laboratory at Oregon State University has demonstrated that an embryo elicited no developmental deformities at 1% DMSO when waterborne-exposed (1, 12, 13).

8. Be sure to allow the embryo to fall to the bottom of the wide-bore Pasteur pipette prior to touching the solution in the wells. If an embryo disintegrates when it reaches the solution, make sure to replace the solution and place a new embryo in the well.

9. All methods discussed involve continuous waterborne exposure, but if no analytical method is available to determine biological uptake, an alternative is to directly deliver the chemical into the animal through microinjection. Because embryos are transparent, tissue dose and distribution can also be determined using fluorescently labeled materials and laser scanning confocal microscopy.

10. Make sure to vortex each microcentrifuge tube prior to the next dilution to ensure it is a homogenous solution.

11. If more than two animals in the control group die, then the experiment is not valid and will need to be repeated. Test chemicals may have specific targets in humans, but this target may not be completely conserved structurally in other vertebrate models. The structural differences between vertebrates and humans can result in either false negatives or false positives. For example, if a drug is designed to target a human-specific structure that is not well-conserved in zebrafish, upon exposure, the drug would not influence the zebrafish target. The effects observed when this occurs are considered false negatives. Vice versa, a false positive can also occur when effects observed due to a drug impacting a specific target are expressed only in zebrafish, but this target is not structurally conserved in humans. Another consideration is that chemical toxicity may be dependent on metabolic activity. False negatives and false positives may also occur if the metabolic activity in the zebrafish embryo is distinct from human metabolic activity. It is possible to use exogenous mammalian metabolic activation system to reduce false positives and false negatives (14).

Acknowledgments

The authors would like to thank the Sinhubber Aquatic Research Laboratory and the Environmental Health Sciences Center at Oregon State University where much of the protocols were developed. This work was supported by EPA STAR grant RD-833320 and NIEHS grants ES03850 and ES07060.

References

1. Akimenko, M.A., Johnson, S.L., et al. (1995) Differential induction of four msx homeobox genes during fin development and regeneration in zebrafish. *Development* **121(2)**, 347–357.

2. Aparicio, S., Chapman, J., et al. (2002) Whole-genome shotgun assembly and analysis of the genome of Fugu rubripes. *Science* **297(5585)**, 1301–1310.

3. Blechinger, S.R., Warren Jr., J.T., et al. (2002) Developmental toxicology of cadmium in living embryos of a stable transgenic zebrafish line. *Environ. Health. Perspect.* **110(10)**, 1041–1046.

4. Busquet, F., Nagel, R., et al. (2008) Development of a new screening assay to identify proteratogenic substances using zebrafish danio rerio embryo combined with an exogenous mammalian metabolic activation system (mDarT). *Toxicol. Sci.* **104(1)**, 177–188.

5. Harper, S.L., Dahl, J.L., et al. (2008) Proactively designing nanomaterials to enhance performance and minimize hazard. *Int. J. Nanotechnology* **5(1)**, 124–142.

6. Henken, D.B., Rasooly, R.S., et al. (2003) Recent papers on zebrafish and other aquarium fish models. *Zebrafish* **1**, 305–311.

7. Kimmel, C.B., Ballard, W.W., et al. (1995) Stages of embryonic development of the zebrafish. *Dev. Dyn.* **203(3)**, 253–310.

8. Levin, E.D., Swain, H.A., et al. (2004) Developmental chlorpyrifos effects on hatchling zebrafish swimming behavior. *Neurotoxicol. Teratol.* **26(6)**, 719–723.

9. Rasooly, R.S., Henken, D., et al. (2003) Genetic and genomic tools for zebrafish research: the NIH zebrafish initiative. *Dev. Dyn.* **228(3)**, 490–496.

10. Rubinstein, A.L. (2003) Zebrafish: from disease modeling to drug discovery. *Curr. Opin. Drug Discov. Devel.* **6(2)**, 218–223.

11. Spitsbergen, J., Kent, M. (2003) The state of the art of the zebrafish model for toxicology and toxicologic pathology research – advantages and current limitations. *Toxicological Pathology* **31**, 62–87.

12. Usenko, C.Y., Harper, S.L., et al. (2007) *In vivo* evaluation of carbon fullerene toxicity using embryonic zebrafish. *Carbon* **45**, 1891–1898.

13. Usenko, C.Y., Harper, S.L., et al. (2008) Exposure to fullerene C60 elicits an oxidative stress response in embryonic zebrafish. *Toxicol. Appl. Pharmacol.* **(229)**, 44–55.

14. Westerfield, M. (1995) The Zebrafish Book. Eugene, University of Oregon Press.

Part VII

Chemical Protein Adducts

Chapter 17

Protocols of *In Vitro* Protein Covalent Binding Studies in Liver

Jean-François Lévesque, Stephen H. Day, and Allen N. Jones

Abstract

Xenobiotics, including therapeutic agents, can produce a variety of beneficial, as well as adverse, effects in mammals. One potential source of drug-mediated toxicity stems from metabolic activation of the parent compound, typically catalyzed by one or more members of the cytochrome P450 family of enzymes. The resulting electrophile, if not quenched by low molecular weight endogenous nucleophiles, can form covalent adducts to cellular proteins, potentially resulting in enzyme inactivation, cell death, or formation of an immunogenic species. The toxicological consequences of exposure to such reactive intermediates range from mild inflammation to organ failure, anaphylaxis, and death. At Merck Research Laboratories, the potential of drug candidates to bind covalently to proteins is evaluated at the lead optimization stage of drug discovery by incubating a radiolabeled analog of the compound in question with liver microsomal preparations (under oxidative conditions) or whole cells (full cellular metabolic capability), typically derived from rat and human liver. A semi-automated method based on the Brandel Harvester technique then is used to measure the formation of covalent adducts of the test compound to liver proteins. This assay is viewed as an important component of drug discovery programs, since the findings are employed to guide specific efforts to abrogate bioactivation issues through informed structural modification of lead compounds.

Key words: Covalent protein binding, Bioactivation, Reactive intermediate, Idiosyncratic toxicity, Drug metabolism, Hepatocytes, Microsomes, Radiolabeled compound, Cytochrome P450

1. Introduction

Covalent binding (CB) of chemically reactive metabolites to cellular proteins has been recognized as one mechanism by which xenobiotics can exert their toxic manifestations (reviews: (1–7); examples: (8–12)). The process of "metabolic activation," which typically (although not exclusively) is mediated by one or more isoforms of the cytochrome P450 family of monooxygenases, results in the formation of a reactive electrophilic species which,

Jean-Charles Gautier (ed.), *Drug Safety Evaluation: Methods and Protocols*, Methods in Molecular Biology, vol. 691,
DOI 10.1007/978-1-60761-849-2_17, © Springer Science+Business Media, LLC 2011

in turn, may be quenched by low molecular weight endogenous nucleophiles (e.g., water and glutathione). However, should the reactive intermediate modify key structural or functional proteins, cellular toxicity and organ failure can result, while modification of non-critical proteins or other cellular components may elicit an immune response (12). From a drug development perspective, these adverse effects are of particular concern in that they may be idiosyncratic in nature and not become evident until late in the development process (Phase II and III, or even post-marketing) when extensive resources already have been committed to the project. The inability to predict accurately which drug structures will be subject to metabolic activation, together with our limited understanding of the molecular mechanisms of xenobiotic-mediated toxicity, has led to the implementation at Merck Research Laboratories of a paradigm whereby compounds are evaluated for their metabolic activation potential early in the drug development process. With the benefit of information on bioactivation pathways at the lead optimization stage, efforts can be made to abrogate this potential liability through informed structural modification of lead compounds.

The ability to assay drug candidates using a consistent screening paradigm in rat and human liver microsomal preparations (assessing primarily oxidative metabolism) and hepatocytes (for assessing all routes of metabolism) provides a basis by which their propensity to undergo metabolic activation can be compared, and the potential liability can be weighed in terms of the overall drug development program. The procedure utilizes commercially available rat and human liver microsomes and hepatocytes, although preparations from other species and organs can be substituted if needed. The procedure also requires that a radiolabeled version of the compound to be studied be made available, typically utilizing carbon-14 or tritium. The radiolabeled compound of interest is incubated in triplicate in a 48- or 96-well plate along with suitable controls, blanks, and nucleophilic "trapping agents," as required. After quenching the reaction, the proteins in each well are precipitated, isolated, solubilized, and counted in a liquid scintillation counter, and the amount of drug-related material bound to the proteins is calculated (13). If a tritiated tracer is used, a parallel experiment is run to assay for tritium loss in the form of tritiated water, since metabolic activation at the labeled site would lead to loss of the label and an underestimation of the amount of CB.

A targeted acceptable level of CB of 50 pmol-eq/(mg protein at 1 h) was chosen, since this value provides a conservative factor of 20 below the level at which hepatic toxicity is observed for several known hepatotoxins that form reactive metabolites, while still being a factor of 10 above normal background during liquid scintillation counting procedures to afford a suitable dynamic range. It should be emphasized, however, that the value of 50 pmol-eq/mg protein is not viewed as an absolute "threshold" above which compounds are not progressed into development, since a decision on the latter requires that *all* of the known attributes and liabilities of the drug candidate in question are taken into consideration in assessing the risk/benefit ratio (12).

2. Materials

Water is doubly distilled or deionized; HPLC grade is satisfactory. All solvents are of HPLC grade.

2.1. Test Compounds

1. Unlabeled test compounds, 3–5 mg (see Note 1).
2. ^{3}H or ^{14}C radiolabeled analogs of the test compounds, typically 50–100 µCi (see Note 1). Appropriate radiation safety procedures need to be followed.

2.2. In Vitro Microsomal Covalent Binding Assay

2.2.1. In Vitro Microsomal Incubations

1. Potassium phosphate buffer (125 mM, pH 7.4). Store at 4°C.
2. Rat and human liver microsome solutions from pooled donors, stored at –80°C until needed (BD Gentest, Woburn, MA). Protein concentration: 20 mg/mL.
3. Fresh 5 mM NADPH solution prepared in phosphate buffer.
4. Non-sterile polypropylene square-well 96-well plate with 2-mL capacity (product #140504; Beckman Coulter, Mississauga, Canada).
5. Incubator: A Thermomixer R from Eppendorf (Westbury, NY) equipped with a thermoblock for microplates.

2.2.2. Filtering and Washing of Microsomal Proteins

1. Semi-automated 48-well harvesting system from Brandel (Gaithersburg, MD) equipped with a 4×12 aspiration probe, a 3×16 filter grid, and a vacuum pump.
2. Whatman GF/B filter papers from Brandel.
3. Protein washing solution: ~1.5 L of 80:20 methanol:water.
4. Harvester storage solution: ~1 L of 20:80 methanol:water.

2.2.3. Sample Transfer to Scintillation Vials and Scintillation Counting

1. 48-sample manual deposit system from Brandel (see Note 2).
2. Racks for liquid scintillation counter (LSC) vials (18-sample format) and 7-mL LSC vials appropriate for the LSC being used.
3. 7.5% sodium dodecyl sulfate (SDS, Sigma–Aldrich, St-Louis, MO) w/v in water.

4. Rotary incubator shaker (e.g., Innova 4000 from New Brunswick Scientific, Edison, NJ).

5. Ultima Gold scintillant from Perkin Elmer (Boston, MA).

6. Multi-purpose LSC compatible with the deposit system used.

2.3. In Vitro Hepatocyte Covalent Binding Assay

2.3.1. Hepatocyte Thawing

1. Cryopreserved rat and human hepatocytes (Celsis, Chicago, IL) kept in liquid nitrogen (see Note 3).

2. Thawing of cryopreserved hepatocytes:

   (a) Gibco ice-cold hepatocytes wash medium (HWM) (Invitrogen, Carlsbad, CA). Store at 4°C.

   (b) 50-mL conical tubes (one for each vial being thawed)

   (c) Percoll sterile solution (GE Healthcare, Uppsala, Sweden). Store at 4°C.

   (d) Phosphate-buffered saline (PBS) 10× pH 7.4 (Mediatech; Herriden, VA). Store at 4°C.

3. Sterile 9.55 g/L Krebs–Henseleit solution pH 7.4 containing 2.5 mM $CaCl_2$, 25 mM sodium bicarbonate, and 12.5 mM Hepes (all reagents are from Sigma–Aldrich; St-Louis, MO). Store at 4°C.

4. Trypan Blue 0.4% (Invitrogen; Carlsbad, CA).

5. Hemacytometer.

2.3.2. Hepatocyte Incubations

1. Sterile 48-well cell culture plate with lid (Costar #3548, Corning, NY).

2. Gas tank of 95:5 O_2:CO_2.

3. Incubator (see Subheading 2.2.1).

2.3.3. In Vitro Hepatocyte Covalent Binding Sample Processing

1. See Subheadings 2.2.2 and 2.2.3.

2.4. Monitoring of Tritium Release

1. See Subheadings 2.2.1 and 2.3.2.

2.4.1. In Vitro Microsomal and Hepatocyte Incubations

2.4.2. Solid Phase Extraction Method

1. Waters brand Oasis® HLB extraction cartridge, 60 mg (3 mL) (Milford, MA). Eight required.

2. Waters extraction manifold with a tube holder and eight 16×100 mm glass tubes.

3. 7-mL scintillation vials.

2.4.3. HPLC-Radiometric Method

1. Eppendorf 5810 R bench-top centrifuge allowing centrifugation of 96-well deep-well plates (Eppendorf).

2. [^{3}H]H$_2$O standard: 2.5 nCi/mL [^{3}H]H$_2$O (American Radiolabeled Chemicals, St. Louis, MO) in 1 mL of 75:25 water:acetonitrile.

3. Test compound standard: 2.5 μM (~250 nCi/mL) of compound in 1 mL of 75:25 water:acetonitrile.

4. HPLC-PDA-Radiometric system:

   (a) Waters 2795 high-pressure liquid chromatograph (HPLC) equipped with a Waters 2996 photodiode-array (PDA) detector and a YMC ODS-A 4.6 × 150 mm (3 μm) reverse phase column (Waters, Milford, MA) kept at 50°C. Injection volume: 50 μL.

   (b) Mobile phase: 0.1% v/v formic acid in water (A) and 0.1% v/v formic acid in acetonitrile (B); 1 mL/min flow rate.

   (c) The input of the PDA detector is connected to a Perkin Elmer 150 TR Radiometric detector. Radiometric parameters: 500 μL flow cell, 6 s update time, analog output of 80,000, and 3:1 ratio between scintillation cocktail and HPLC flow rates. Scintillation cocktail: Flow-Scint II from Perkin Elmer.

3. Methods

3.1. Test Compound Stock Solution Preparation

1. For ^{3}H labeled compounds: Prepare 0.5 mL of a 1 mM stock solution of unlabeled compound in acetonitrile to which is added ~50 μCi tracer in a minimum volume of solvent (see Notes 1 and 4–6). An aliquot of the solution should be counted in a LSC to verify the amount of radioactivity present.

2. For ^{14}C labeled compounds: Prepare 0.5 mL of a 1 mM solution with ≥0.025 μCi/μL radioactivity (12.5 μCi/ 0.5 mL). Depending on the specific activity of the tracer, no dilution with unlabeled compound may be necessary. It is advisable to confirm the solution activity by counting an aliquot in a LSC, especially if any dilution was performed (see Notes 1 and 4–6).

3.2. In Vitro Microsomal Covalent Binding Assay

The *in vitro* microsomal CB assay can be performed in the presence of sub-cellular fractions from various species and with different co-factors. As previously described, each compound of interest is typically incubated in triplicate with both rat and human liver microsomal proteins in the presence and absence of NADPH as a

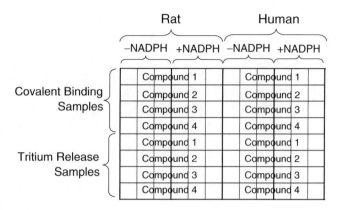

Fig. 1. Suggested incubation layout in 96-well plate format.

co-factor, to assess the implication of oxidative metabolism in reactive intermediate formation (13) (see Notes 7 and 8). Thus a total of 12 wells are required for each compound when tested in both species. A suggested layout is shown in Fig. 1 (see Note 9). In this figure, one row of wells, labeled Compound 1, would be used for the positive control and the second to fourth row would be used for test compounds (see Notes 4 and 8).

3.2.1. In Vitro Microsomal Incubations

1. 1 In a 96-well plate with 2-mL capacity, add 148 μL of potassium phosphate buffer, 2 μL of 1 mM (~0.1 μCi/μL) compound stock solution, and 10 μL of microsome solution (20 mg/mL) to six wells per compound for each species. To the first three wells, an additional 40 μL of potassium phosphate buffer is added; these will be the –NADPH controls, the other three will be +NADPH samples.

2. Pre-incubate the 96-well plate in a water bath at 37°C for 5 min.

3. Start the reaction by adding 40 μL of pre-warmed (5 min at 37°C) NADPH 5 mM solution to all of the +NADPH sample wells. Ensure that the incubations are well mixed by shaking the plate at 1,000 rpm in a plate mixer.

4. Incubate the plate at 37°C in a water bath for 60 min.

5. Quench in two steps (necessary to maximize protein precipitation) as follows. First, quench the incubations using 300 μL of room-temperature acetone and vortex the plate thoroughly (~1,200 rpm for 30 s). Then, add an additional 500 μL of acetone and vortex again (~1,000 rpm for 30 s), taking care to avoid splashing.

3.2.2. Filtering and Washing of Microsomal Proteins

1. Place a Whatman GF/B filter mat in the Brandel harvester and connect to the wash solvent bottle (80:20 methanol:water).

2. Turn on the vacuum pump.

3. Into a clean reservoir (e.g., an empty 96-well plate), deliver enough wash solvent and aspirate to fill the lines with 80:20 methanol:water.

4. Aspirate samples from the 96-well incubation plate while simultaneously delivering wash solvent (this typically takes <5 s). Move the probe up and down during aspiration to dislodge protein from the sides and bottom of the wells. Significant protein will remain in the well if this is not performed carefully. When the proteins are loaded, the flow rate may be reduced. Care should be taken not to overflow any of the wells with solvent (see Note 10).

5. Wait for about 15 s or more for all wash solvent to be pulled through the filter.

6. Repeat steps 4 and 5 three times. A total of about 1.5 L of solvent should be used for the entire assay (including line filling).

7. Turn off the vacuum pump.

8. Remove the filter mat and set it aside.

9. Dispose of the radioactive waste solvent.

10. A new filter should be placed in the harvester and the lines should be filled with 80:20 methanol:water when the instrument is not in use. Also, the clamps should be released to prevent deforming the o-rings.

3.2.3. Sample Transfer to Scintillation Vials and Scintillation Counting

1. Place three LSC racks in the rack holder of the Brandel manual deposit system.

2. Place 48 vials (7-mL) in the racks, leaving the first and last positions in each rack empty.

3. Operation of the manual deposit system:

   (a) Place the filter mat on the flat holder with a guide post at each end. There should be only one possible orientation. Position everything so that the mat has the same orientation (in relation to you) as when on the harvester (see Note 11).

   (b) Slide the other flat holder over the guide posts, sandwiching the filter mat in between.

   (c) Pass this apparatus through the "squeezer" a couple of times. This helps separate the individual filters from the mat.

   (d) Place the apparatus on the 48 vials prepared in step 2.

   (e) Using the "stamper," stamp all the filters into the vials in one swift firm motion (see Note 12).

4. Ensure that the filters are lying relatively flat at the bottom of the scintillation vials, as opposed to standing on end. Use the back of a Pasteur pipet to gently tap them down if necessary.

5. Standards and blanks are prepared in triplicate in vials containing blank filters obtained by rinsing a mat with 80:20 methanol:water on the harvester and stamping.

   (a) "Maximum" controls: Add 2 µL of stock solution of each compound tested. These will give the initial counts in the incubations.

   (b) Blank. These will serve as zero protein controls and give background.

6. Add 1 mL of 7.5% SDS to each vial (all vials should be included). Cap all the vials tightly and carefully, and place them on a rotary shaker overnight at 55°C and 200 rpm. Vigorous shaking is important to help ensure contact of the entire filter with the SDS solution.

7. The following day, after the vials cool down, 5 mL of scintillant is added to each vial, capped, and shaken vigorously by hand.

8. Allow it to sit for about 1 h prior to scintillation counting to allow any chemiluminescence generated by the mixing process to die down.

3.2.4. Calculation of In Vitro Microsomal Covalent Binding Results

1. Since 1-h incubations are performed in a 200-µL incubation volume containing 10 µM of test compound (~1,000 nCi/mL) and 1 mg/mL of protein, the maximum amount of protein labeling that could be observed would represent 10,000 pmol-eq/(mg protein at 1 h) (see Notes 13 and 14).

2. Scintillation counting results for "Maximum" controls, which contains the initial levels of radioactivity added to the incubation mixture, represent 10,000 pmol-eq/(mg protein at 1 h) of CB. However, 85% of filtered proteins are recovered using this procedure, which may lead to an underestimation of CB. We must, therefore, adjust the Maximum control so that it takes into account a 15% loss of signal. The CB of test compounds to microsomal proteins is determined by calculating the relative amount of radioactivity recovered in the protein pellet trapped on the filter mat (P) of the harvester vs. the "Maximum" controls (M). Counts in the blank samples (B) must be subtracted for all samples, as indicated in Eq. 1. Results obtained for the Merck in-house positive control, [^{14}C]L-746530 (11), as well as for other compounds known to cause protein labeling are presented in Table 1.

$$\text{Microsomal CB} = 10,000 \times \left[\frac{(P - B)}{((0.85 \times M) - B)}\right] \quad (1)$$

$$\text{Units: pmol} - \text{eq}/(\text{mg protein at 1 h})$$

Table 1
In vitro liver microsomal covalent binding results for reference compounds, including [¹⁴C]L-746530, the Merck in-house positive control

Compounds	Rat		Human	
	−NADPH pmol-eq/ (mg at 1 h)	+NADPH pmol-eq/ (mg at 1 h)	−NADPH pmol-eq/ (mg at 1 h)	+NADPH pmol-eq/(mg at 1 h)
[¹⁴C]Accolate	15.8 ± 0.5	59 ± 5	12.7 ± 0.4	75 ± 3
[¹⁴C]Acetaminophen	6 ± 1	108 ± 1	28 ± 7	184 ± 7
[¹⁴C]Diazepam	<5	378 ± 9	<5	107 ± 21
[¹⁴C]Tamoxiphen	11 ± 1	408 ± 8	11 ± 6	106 ± 5
[¹⁴C]L-746530	101 ± 4	$2,039 \pm 110$	64 ± 1	$1,002 \pm 28$

Equation 1. Calculation of *in vitro* microsomal CB, where *P* represents the counts for the protein pellet trapped on the filter mat, *M* the counts from the Maximum control, and *B* the counts in blank samples.

3.3. Hepatocyte In Vitro Covalent Binding Assay

The hepatocyte *in vitro* CB assay is generally used to assess bioactivation issues for compounds undergoing a combination of Phase I and Phase II metabolism. It helps to put into perspective the bioactivation of drug candidates via oxidative metabolism vs. other metabolic pathways such as glucuronidation and sulfation. This assay is also used to evaluate potential CB issues associated with the formation of acyl-glucuronide or acyl-CoA metabolites (14–16). Natural trapping agents such as reduced glutathione that are present in hepatocytes may trap soft electrophilic reactive metabolites, leading to lower levels of CB than that observed in the microsomal assay (16).

3.3.1. Hepatocyte Thawing

1. Remove cryovials from liquid nitrogen storage and immediately thaw them in a 37°C water bath with gentle mixing. Make sure all ice crystals are gone before proceeding.

2. Transfer the contents of each vial into separate 50-mL conical tubes on ice and, very slowly, add ~50 mL of ice-cold HWM to the cells and gently mix by hand between additions.

3. Pelletize the cells by centrifugation at 500 rpm for 3 min. Aspirate the supernatants and resuspend the cell pellets in 20 mL of ice-cold HWM.

4. Add 10 mL of 90:10 ice-cold isotonic Percoll:PBS solution (30% Percoll final concentration).

5. Centrifuge the cells at 800 rpm for 4 min, wash the cells in Krebs–Henseleit–Hepes buffer (~50 mL) once, and then resuspend the cells in ~10 mL of Krebs–Henseleit–Hepes buffer.

6. Determine cell viability and fix cell concentration by Trypan blue exclusion counting on the hemacytometer (mix 1 vol. of cells with 1 vol. of Trypan blue 0.4%, and transfer 10 μL to the hemacytometer to count). Cell viability should be >80%.

7. Dilute the hepatocyte suspension in Krebs–Henseleit–Hepes buffer to a concentration of 1×10^6 cells/mL.

3.3.2. Hepatocyte Incubations

1. Add 0.25 mL of 1×10^6 cells/mL to the selected wells of a 48-well plate.

2. Pre-incubate the plate with the lid on for 20 min in an incubator set at 300 rpm, 37°C, and under 95:5 O_2:CO_2 atmosphere (see Note 15).

3. Add 2.5 μL of 1 mM (~0.1 μCi/μL) compound stock solution to the appropriate wells ($n = 3$ per compound, per species), which will give a final concentration of 10 μM (~1,000 nCi/mL). It is important to keep the amount of organic solvent in the incubation mixture to ≤1% v/v (14). Also prepare $n = 3$ blank wells per compound and per species, containing 0.25 mL of 1×10^6 cells/mL, which will be used later for the preparation of t=2 min control samples, as described at step 6.

4. Incubate with the lid and the incubator covers on for 2 h at 300 rpm, 37°C, and under 95:5 O_2:CO_2 atmosphere.

5. Add 2.5 μL of compound stock solution to the blank wells prepared previously, and place the 48-well plate back in the incubator for ~2 min. These samples will be compared to those incubated for 2 h to assess the implication of metabolism in the CB of tested compounds to liver proteins.

6. Quench incubations by adding 500 μL of room-temperature acetone and mix the content of each well by pipetting and dispensing the liquid multiple times. Then, transfer the homogenous samples to the top 48 wells of a 96-well deep-well plate (see Note 16).

3.3.3. Hepatocyte In Vitro Covalent Binding Sample Processing

1. Harvest and wash the hepatocyte proteins as described in Subheading 3.2.2.

2. Transfer the filtered proteins to scintillation vials, solubilize the proteins, and measure radioactivity by scintillation counting as described in Subheading 3.2.3.

3. Prepare the following controls and blanks in triplicate in vials containing blank filters (obtained by rinsing a mat with 80:20

methanol:water on the harvester and stamping) and process as indicated in step 2:

(a) "Maximum" control: 2.5 μL of stock solution of each compound tested. These will give the initial counts in the incubations.

(b) Blank: These will serve as zero protein controls and give background.

3.3.4. Calculation of In Vitro Hepatocyte Covalent Binding Results

1. For this assay, CB is also calculated on a per mg incubated protein basis. Since 2-h incubations are performed in a 250-μL incubation volume containing 10 μM of test compound and 1×10^6 cells/mL (protein content equivalent to 1.7 mg/mL), the maximal amount of protein labeling that could be observed would represent 5,882 pmol-eq/(mg protein at 2 h) (see Note 17).

2. Scintillation counting results for "Maximum" controls, which contain the initial levels of radioactivity added to the incubation mixture, represent 5,882 pmol-eq/(mg protein at 2 h) of CB. However, 85% of filtered proteins are recovered using this procedure, which may lead to an underestimation of CB. We must, therefore, adjust the Maximum control so that it takes into account a 15% loss of signal. The CB of test compounds to hepatocyte proteins is determined by calculating the relative amount of radioactivity recovered in the protein pellet trapped on the filter mat of the harvester (P) vs. the "Maximum" controls (M). Counts in the blank samples (B) must be subtracted for all samples, as indicated in Eq. 2. Results obtained for the Merck in-house positive control, [^{14}C]L-746530 (11), as well as for [^{14}C]Accolate and [^{14}C]Diazepam are presented in Table 2.

$$\text{Hepatocyte CB} = 5,882 \times \left[\frac{(P - B)}{((0.85 \times M) - B)} \right] \tag{2}$$

Units: pmol − eq/(mg protein at 2 h or 2 min)

Equation 2. Calculation of the *in vitro* hepatocyte CB, where P represents the counts for the protein pellet trapped on the filter mat, M the counts of the Maximum control, and B the counts in blank samples.

3.4. Monitoring of Tritium Release

Additional incubations are routinely performed for tritiated compounds to monitor the metabolic lability of the site of tritiation in both microsomal and hepatocyte assays by measuring the formation of tritiated water. This is important to consider in the interpretation of CB results since loss of the radiolabel could lead to underestimation of the *in vitro* protein labeling. It is preferable

Table 2
***In vitro* hepatocyte covalent binding for [¹⁴C]Accolate, [¹⁴C]Diazepam, and [¹⁴C] L-746530, a Merck in-house reference compound**

Compounds	Rat		Human	
	2 min pmol-eq/ (mg at 2 min)	120 min pmol-eq/ (mg at 2 h)	2 min pmol-eq/ (mg at 2 min)	120 min pmol-eq/ (mg at 2 h)
[¹⁴C]Accolate	9 ± 3	33 ± 5	3.3 ± 0.6	34 ± 2
[¹⁴C]Diazepam	<5	58 ± 12	<5	<5
[¹⁴C]L-746530	110 ± 33	$1,008 \pm 162$	64 ± 38	614 ± 191

for the tritium loss, measured as tritiated water, to be less than 1% of the total radiolabeled incubated material.

Both analytical approaches used for this assay rely on the retention of the test compound material and its metabolites on the stationary phase of a solid phase extraction (SPE) cartridge or a HPLC column, and the elution of tritiated water in the SPE flow-through or the HPLC solvent front. Tritium release is confirmed by monitoring the disappearance of putative tritiated water in the collected flow-through or solvent front fraction upon sample evaporation.

3.4.1. In Vitro Microsomal and Hepatocyte Incubations

In parallel with both *in vitro* microsomal and hepatocyte CB assays, a second sample set is prepared under identical conditions (see Subheadings 3.2.1 and 3.3.2) up to the point of ending the incubation. Instead of quenching with four volumes of acetone, five volumes of ice-cold water are added for the SPE procedure, while the HPLC procedure quenches with one volume of acetonitrile (for compatibility with the HPLC eluant). As depicted in Fig. 1, these incubations are generally performed in the bottom half of the 96-well plate for the microsomal assay, whereas extra wells are used in the 48-well incubation plate for the hepatocyte assay. Blank incubations may also be prepared as controls (see Note 18).

3.4.2. SPE Method

1. Cartridge preparation: While the incubation is underway, condition the Oasis® cartridges by adding 1 mL of methanol to each and drawing it through, then equilibrate by adding 1 mL of water and drawing it through.

2. Stop the incubations by adding 5 vol. of ice-cold water (1 mL) and vortexing, and putting the reaction mixtures on ice for 10 min.

3. Vortex the incubations and transfer 50 μL from each tube to a scintillation vial. Add 4 mL of scintillation cocktail and analyze the samples by LSC (set 1, original samples).

4. Load 1 mL from each well onto an individual cartridge, and collect the filtrate.

5. Transfer 400 μL of each filtrate to a liquid scintillation vial. Add 4 mL of scintillation cocktail and analyze the samples by LSC (set 2).

6. Transfer 500 μL of each filtrate to individual glass tubes and dry under nitrogen. Reconstitute the residue in 500 μL of water and mix well. Transfer 400 μL to a scintillation vial, add 4 mL of scintillation cocktail and analyze by LSC (set 3).

7. Calculation of % tritium loss is given by Eq. 3.

$$\% \, \text{Tritium loss} = \frac{\left[\dfrac{S2}{400} - \dfrac{S3}{500} \right]}{\left[\dfrac{S1}{50} \right]} \tag{3}$$

Equation 3. Calculation of % tritium loss using SPE method, where $S1 = \text{dpm}$ for each original sample (set 1), $S2 = \text{dpm}$ of the corresponding sample in the SPE filtrate (set 2), and $S3 = \text{dpm}$ of the corresponding sample in evaporated and reconstituted SPE filtrate (set 3).

3.4.3. HPLC-Radiometric Method

1. Centrifuge samples for 10 min at 16000 rcf at room temperature and dilute the supernatants with one volume of water (see Note 19).

2. Prepare the following standards and controls in HPLC vials containing supernatant of blank incubations processed as indicated in step 1:

   (a) Compound standard: Add 2.5 μM (250 nCi/mL) of each test compound in separate HPLC vials (this takes into account the fourfold dilution factor).

   (b) [^{3}H]H$_2$O standard: Add 2.5 nCi/mL of [^{3}H]H$_2$O into a blank sample, which represents 1% of the incubated material.

   (c) Blank sample.

3. Analyze incubations and controls using an HPLC-Radiometric detection system equipped with a reverse phase column (see Subheading 2.4.3 for details). The mobile phase is typically 0.1% formic acid in water (A) and 0.1% formic acid in acetonitrile (B), with a gradient of 10–90% B over 18 min, followed by isocratic at 90% B for 2 min.

4. Post-injection, process all samples and integrate all peaks in the chromatographic traces from the Radiometric detector. Report the relative amount of the solvent front peak (SFP) vs. total

peak area as a percentage (% SFP wet), as well as the SFP area (W) (see Note 20).

5. In cases where a peak in the solvent front is detected:

   (a) Evaporate the samples of interest to dryness (e.g., +NADPH microsomal incubation or $t = 120$-min hepatocyte incubation) and selected control samples (e.g., [^{3}H] H$_2$O 2.5 nCi/mL standard) under a nitrogen stream.

   (b) Reconstitute in 75:25 acetonitrile:water, and reanalyze by HPLC-Radiometric detection. Integrate and note the SFP area (D). Disappearance of the SFP should be observed if tritiated water is present in the samples. Presence of peaks in the solvent front post-evaporation would be indicative of the formation of polar metabolites, but not [^{3}H]H$_2$O.

6. Report as a percentage the proportion of the SFP area lost upon evaporation, as determined using HPLC-Radiometric detection (Eq. 4).

$$\% \text{ Tritium loss} = \% \text{SFP Wet} \times \left[\frac{W - D}{W} \right] \qquad (4)$$

Equation 4. Calculation of % tritium loss using HPLC-Radiometric method, where % SFP wet is the % of the SFP area relative to total area in the original sample, W is the SFP area in the original sample, and D is the SFP area in the evaporated sample.

4. Notes

1. The chemical and radiochemical purity of the compounds needs to be very high. Chemical impurities present in sufficient amounts can cause CYP inhibition. This could reduce metabolism and the concomitant formation of potential reactive intermediates, leading to false-negative CB results. Radiochemical purity should be >98.5% with no more than 0.5% of any one impurity. Should the impurity be more reactive than the compound of interest, it would lead to protein labeling and potentially false-positive results. For example, a 1% radioimpurity that binds 100% to microsomal proteins would lead to 117 pmol-eq/(mg 1 h) of labeling.

2. This contains a paper tray assembly to hold the filter, a paper tray carriage with punches to punch out the discs, and an aluminum holder for three LSC racks, each holding 18 vials (7-mL). This system takes the filter paper sheets from the harvester, punches out the samples as discs, and deposits them directly into the scintillation vials. Different brands of counters

use slightly different vial configurations and counter racks, so it is critical that the harvester and deposit system match the LSC that will be used (Beckman, Packard, LKB, Wallac, Perkin Elmer) to simplify the transfer and avoid loss of material. LSC sample racks and vials need to be appropriate for the counter being used.

3. Approximately 2×10^6 viable cells are needed to conduct hepatocyte *in vitro* CB for one compound in one species, according to the method described in Subheading 3.3.1. The use of human hepatocytes from multiple donors ($\geq n = 3$ donors) is preferable to minimize donor-to-donor variability and the potential impact on enzyme activity. Some vendors will recommend variations of this thawing procedure, which should therefore be followed.

4. Different commercially available radiolabeled compounds can be used as positive controls. In addition to [^{14}C]tamoxiphen (Toronto Research Chemicals; Toronto, Canada) and [^{14}C] diazepam (Amersham Biosciences; Piscataway, NJ), compounds such as [^{14}C]naphthalene and [^{14}C]imipramine could also be used (American Radiolabeled Chemicals Inc; St. Louis, MO). *In vitro* microsomal CB results for the later two compounds were previously published (13).

5. In general, the high specific activity of tritiated compounds (Ci/mmol) means the mass contribution is usually negligible. So for tritiated compounds, a 1-mM stock solution of cold material is prepared to which is added the minimum volume of tritiated compound required to generate a 0.1 μCi/μL solution. For ^{14}C labeled material, the specific activity (mCi/mmol) is generally too low to make a 1-mM solution with 0.1 μCi/μL radioactivity. Therefore, the solution is prepared at 1 mM concentration and at least 0.025 μCi/μL, which will give a limit of detection of approximately 10 pmol-eq/ (mg 1 h).

6. The solvent used to prepare stock solutions must have minimal impact on P450 enzymatic activity at levels ≤1% v/v in the incubation mixture. Typically ethanol or acetonitrile is used, whereas dimethylsulfoxide (DMSO), for example, should be avoided (17).

7. Incubates done in absence of NADPH are used to assess the potential of compounds to cause protein labeling even in the absence of a co-factor. In addition, it is used to evaluate potential nonspecific binding of the radiolabeled material to the harvester filter mat.

8. Parallel incubations are often performed in the presence of a chemical agent, such as reduced glutathione, cyanide, semicarbazide or methoxylamine, to trap reactive species

potentially formed during microsomal incubations. The microsomal incubations are performed in the presence of NADPH as described in Subheading 3.2.1 except that three additional wells containing mM concentrations of trapping agents are prepared. For example, 5 mM reduced glutathione (GSH; soft nucleophile), 1 mM NaCN (hard nucleophile), or 1 mM semicarbazide or methoxylamine (aldehyde trapping agents) is typically used (12). Trapping of reactive metabolites would lead to decreased CB of the tested compound to microsomal proteins, and to the concomitant formation of a trapping agent adduct with the radioactive molecule, which can often be detected by HPLC-Radiometric-MS/MS detection. Identification of the site of trapping agent addition to the molecule is indicative of the potential reactive species formed, and helps pharmaceutical scientists to solve bioactivation issues at the drug discovery stage (11, 12, 16, 18). The use of a trapping agent (three wells per compound per species) will reduce by one the number of compounds that can be included in each assay.

9. Because of the large number of samples in these assays, it is imperative to plan their location in advance and maintain a consistent layout and a consistent pattern of reagent addition. The procedure can be automated using a liquid handling system such as those marketed by Biomek, Tecan, and Hamilton, which helps reduce operator fatigue and run-to-run variation.

10. There should not be any protein remaining in the plate after this washing step.

11. Occasionally some proteins will stick to the "stamper" using this technique. To avoid this, the filter mat can be placed protein side down in step 3. Switching the top and bottom LSC racks after step 3e will restore the proper orientation.

12. The mapping of samples will differ between the original layout in a 96-well plate (4 rows × 12 columns format) and the final mapping on the filter mat of the Brandel harvester (3 rows × 16 columns format). During processing on the harvester, the parallel arrangement of the plate is converted to a linear arrangement, as depicted in Fig. 2.

13. While it is possible to determine the percent protein recovery in each sample, experience has shown that the results can be variable due to the difficulty in accurately and reproducibly making the measurement. The average recovery has been about 85%; therefore, this value is used as an estimation for the amount of protein recovered.

14. Maximal CB in microsomes for a 200-μL incubation with 1 mg/mL liver microsomal proteins, and 10 μM of incubated

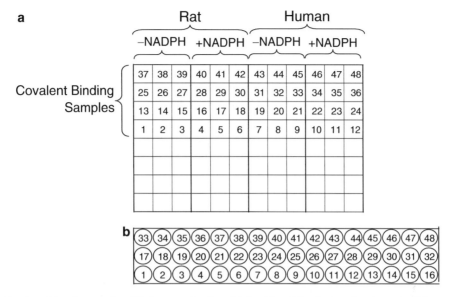

Fig. 2. Mapping of *in vitro* covalent binding samples from (**a**) the 96-well incubation plate (4 × 12) to (**b**) the Brandel Harvester filter mat (3 × 16) with filtered protein facing upward.

material would be of 10,000 pmol-eq/(mg at 1 h), as shown in Eq. 5.

$$\text{Maximal microsomal CB} = \left[\frac{(200 \times 10^{-6}\,\text{L})(10 \times 10^6\,\text{pmol/L})}{(200 \times 10^{-3}\,\text{mL})\,(1\,\text{mg/mL})} \right] \quad (5)$$

$$= 10,000\,\text{pmol} - \text{eq/(mg at 1h)}$$

Equation 5. Maximal extent of CB of a test compound to microsomal proteins in experimental conditions as described in Subheading 3.2.

15. The following experimental set-up helps to monitor the gas flow during the hepatocyte incubations: Make two holes in a rubber cap and insert a short and a long plastic pipet. Install the rubber cap on the top of a 1-L Erlenmeyer flask half filled with water, with the long pipet beneath the water surface and the short one above it. Connect the long pipet to the gas tank, and the short pipet to the incubator. During incubations, ensure that a gentle flow of bubbles is observed in the Erlenmeyer flask.

16. It is suggested to use a similar format to that presented in Fig. 1, where microsomal –NADPH and +NADPH samples would be substituted with hepatocyte $t = 2$ min and 120-min incubations, respectively. Also, it is important to minimize residual protein in the bottom of the incubation wells.

17. Maximal CB in hepatocytes for a 250-μL incubation with 1×10^6 cells/mL, 10 μM of incubated material, and a 1.7 mg

protein content per million cells would be of 5,882 pmol-eq/ (mg at 2 h), as detailed in Eq. 6.

$$\text{Maximal hepatocyte CB} = \left[\frac{(250\times10^{-6}\,\text{L})(10\times10^{6}\,\text{pmol/L})}{(250\times10^{-3}\,\text{mL})\,(1\times10^{6}\,\text{cells/mL})\,(1.7\,\text{mg}/10^{6}\,\text{cells})}\right] (6)$$

$$= 5,882\,\text{pmol} - \text{eq}/(\text{mg at 2 h})$$

Equation 6. Maximal extent of CB of a test compound to hepatocytes under the experimental conditions described in Subheading 3.3.

18. Incubations can also be performed with [6β-³H]testosterone (50 μM) as a positive control in the tritium release assay. In both microsomal and hepatocyte incubation conditions, conversion of [6β-³H]testosterone to 6β-OH-testosterone, and concomitant formation of [³H]H$_2$O are observed (19).

19. Since hepatocyte incubations are performed in a flat-bottom 48-well plate, it is suggested that the quenched samples be transferred into a 96-well deep-well plate prior to centrifugation. It is important to minimize residual proteins in the bottom of the incubation wells.

20. The HPLC-Radiometric trace is also used to evaluate the metabolic stability of ³H and ¹⁴C labeled compounds. The peak area of the parent compound is compared between the +NADPH and the −NADPH samples for microsomal incubations, and between t=120 and 2 min for hepatocyte incubations. Metabolic stability is reported as % of parent remaining after microsomal or hepatocyte incubations. Results obtained are used to put into perspective CB results. Follow-up analysis by HPLC-Radiometric-MS/MS is often required to characterize *in vitro* metabolites formed. Special care is made to monitor metabolically mediated molecular cleavages which would lead to the release of a non-radiolabeled portion of the molecule containing substructures known to form reactive intermediates (e.g., thiophene ring).

Acknowledgments

The authors would like to acknowledge Amandine Chefson, Varsha Didolkar, Mireille Gaudreault, Robert Houle, Deborah Nicoll-Griffith, Thomas Baillie, and Dennis Dean for their contribution to this chapter. We also thank Dongping Fan, from the Merck Labeled Compound Synthesis group, for the synthesis and purification of [¹⁴C]Accolate.

References

1. Baillie, T.A. (2008) Metabolism and toxicity of drugs. Two decades of progress in industrial drug metabolism. *Chem. Res. Toxicol.* **21**, 129–137.

2. Baillie, T.A. (2006) Future of toxicology – metabolic activation and drug design: challenges and opportunities in chemical toxicology. *Chem. Res. Toxicol.* **19**, 889–893.

3. Erve, J.C.L. (2006) Chemical toxicology: reactive intermediates and their role in pharmacology and toxicology. *Expert Opin. Drug Metab. Toxicol.* **2**, 923–946.

4. Guengerich, F.P. (2006) Cytochrome P450s and other enzymes in drug metabolism and toxicity. *AAPS J.* **8**, E101–E111.

5. Williams, D.P. (2006) Toxicophores: investigations in drug safety. *Toxicology* **226**, 1–11.

6. Kalgutkar, A.S., Gardner, I., Obach, R.S., Shaffer, C.L., Callegari, E., Henne, K.R., Mutlib, A.R., Dalvie, D.K., Lee, J.S., Nakai, Y., O'Donnell, J.P., Boer, J., and Harriman, S.P. (2005) A comprehensive listing of bioactivation pathways of organic functional groups. *Curr. Drug Metab.* **6**, 161–225.

7. Williams, D.P. and Parks, B.K. (2003) Idiosyncratic toxicity: the role of toxicophores and bioactivation. *Drug Discov. Today* **8**, 1044–1050.

8. Zhang, D., Krishna, R., Wang, L., Zeng, J., Mitroka, J., Dai, R., Narasimhan, N., Reeves, R.R., Srinivas, N.R., and Klunk, L.J. (2005) Metabolism, pharmacokinetics, and protein covalent binding of radiolabeled Maxipost (BMS-204352) in humans. *Drug Metab. Dispos.* **33**, 83–93.

9. Damsten, M.C., Commandeur, J.N.M., Fidder, A., Hulst, A.G., Touw, D., Noort, D., Nico P. E., and Vermeulen, N.P.E. (2007) Liquid chromatography/tandem mass spectrometry detection of covalent binding of acetaminophen to human serum albumin. *Drug Metab. Dispos.* **35**, 1408–1417.

10. Kang, P., Dalvie, D., Smith, E., Zhou, S., and Deese, A. (2007) Identification of a novel glutathione conjugate of flutamide in incubations with human liver microsomes. *Drug Metab. Dispos.* **35**, 1081–1088.

11. Chauret, N., Nicoll-Griffith, D., Friesen, R., Li, C., Trimble, L., Dube, D., Fortin, R., Girard, Y., and Yergey, J. (1995) Microsomal metabolism of the 5-lipoxygenase inhibitors L-746,530 and L-739,010 to reactive intermediates that covalently bind to protein: the role of the 6,8-Doxabicyclo[3.2.1]Octanyl Moiety. *Drug Metab. Dispos.* **23**, 1325–1334.

12. Evans, D.C., Watt, A.P., Nicoll-Griffith, D.A., and Baillie, T.A. (2004) Drug-protein adducts: an industry perspective on minimizing the potential for drug bioactivation in drug discovery and development. *Chem. Res. Toxicol.* **17**, 3–16.

13. Day, S.H., Mao, A., White, R., Schulz-Utermoehl, T., Miller, R., and Beconi, M.G. (2005) A semi-automated method for measuring the potential for protein covalent binding in drug discovery. *J. Pharmacol. Toxicol. Methods* **52**, 278–285.

14. Benet, L.Z., Spahn-Langguth, H., Iwakawa, S., Volland, C., Mizuma, T., Mayer, S., Mutschler, E., and Lin, E.T. (1993) Predictability of the covalent binding of acidic drugs in man. *Life Sci.* **53**, PL141–PL146.

15. Olsen, J., Li, C., Bjørnsdottir, I., Sidenius, U., Hansen, S.H., and Benet, L.Z. (2005) *In vitro* and *in vivo* studies on acyl-coenzyme A-dependent bioactivation of zomepirac in rats. *Chem. Res. Toxicol.* **18**, 1729–1736

16. Lévesque, J.-F., Day, S., Chauret, N., Seto, C., Trimble, L., Bateman, K., Silva, J., Berthelette, C., Lachance, N., Boyd, M., Li, L., Sturino, C., Wang, Z., Zamboni, R., Young, R., and Nicoll-Griffith, D. (2007) Metabolic activation of indole-containing prostaglandin D2 receptor 1 antagonists: impacts of glutathione trapping and glucuronide conjugation on covalent binding. *Bioorg. Med. Chem. Lett.* **17**, 3038–3043.

17. Chauret, N., Gauthier, A., and Nicoll-Griffith, D.A. (1998) Effect of common organic solvent on *in vitro* cytochrome P450-mediated metabolic activities in human liver microsomes. *Drug Metab. Dispos.* **26**, 1–4.

18. Kalgutkar, A.S. and Soglia, J.R. (2005) Minimising the potential for metabolic activation in drug discovery. *Expert Opin. Drug Metab. Toxicol.* **1**, 91–142.

19. Di Marco, A., Marcucci, I., Verdirame, M., Pérez, J., Sanchez, M., Peláez, F., Chaudhary, A., and Laufer, R. (2005) Development and validation of a high-throughput radiometric CYP3A4/5 Inhibition assay using tritiated testosterone. *Drug Metab. Dispos.* **33**, 349–358.

Chapter 18

Utilization of MALDI-TOF to Determine Chemical-Protein Adduct Formation *In Vitro*

Ashley A. Fisher, Matthew T. Labenski, Terrence J. Monks, and Serrine S. Lau

Abstract

Biological reactive intermediates can be created via metabolism of xenobiotics during the process of chemical elimination. They can also be formed as by-products of cellular metabolism, which produces reactive oxygen and nitrogen species. These reactive intermediates tend to be electrophilic in nature, which enables them to interact with tissue macromolecules, disrupting cellular signaling processes and often producing acute and chronic toxicities. Quinones are a well-known class of electrophilic species. Many natural products contain quinones as active constituents, and the quinone moiety exists in a number of chemotherapeutic agents. Quinones are also frequently formed as electrophilic metabolites from a variety of xeno- and endobiotics. Hydroquinone (HQ) is present in the environment from various sources, and it is also a known metabolite of benzene. HQ is converted in the body to 1,4-benzoquinone, which subsequently gives rise to hematotoxic and nephrotoxic quinone–thioether metabolites. The toxicity of these metabolites is dependent upon their ability to arylate proteins and to produce oxidative stress. Protein tertiary structure and protein amino acid sequence combine to determine which proteins are targets of these electrophilic quinone–thioether metabolites. We have used cytochrome *c* and model peptides to view adduction profiles of quinone–thioether metabolites, and have determined by MALDI-TOF analysis that these electrophiles target specific residues within these model systems.

Key words: BQ, MALDI-TOF, NAC-BQ, Post-translational modifications, Protein adduction, Quinone–thioether

1. Introduction

Protein adduction, or chemical-mediated post-translational modifications, typically refers to protein covalent binding by electrophilic xenobiotics and/or their metabolites. Such reactive electrophilic intermediates are frequently formed during the process of chemical elimination, from xenobiotics, such as therapeutic

Jean-Charles Gautier (ed.), *Drug Safety Evaluation: Methods and Protocols*, Methods in Molecular Biology, vol. 691,
DOI 10.1007/978-1-60761-849-2_18, © Springer Science+Business Media, LLC 2011

drugs and environmental contaminants. Since many xenobiotics are lipophilic in nature, the body seeks ways in which to convert them into more water soluble metabolites to facilitate renal excretion. It is during this metabolic conversion that reactive intermediates are inadvertently generated. Biological reactive intermediates can also be formed during normal cellular metabolism (1). For example, advanced glycation endproducts (AGEs) are formed from the reaction of reducing sugars with amino groups of proteins, resulting in the formation of reactive dicarbonyl compounds, such as methylglyoxal (2, 3). Additionally, reactive intermediates formed as by-products of cellular metabolism include superoxide anion, hydroxyl radical, and nitric oxide. The generation of these reactive intermediates can result in the subsequent formation of additional endogenous electrophiles, such as 4-hydroxynonenal (4, 5). Because these reactive intermediates tend to be electrophilic in nature, they can interact with a variety of tissue macromolecules, initiating processes that may produce acute tissue injury or chronic disease (1). Many of these reactive intermediates are known to modify specific thiols on sensor proteins, such as glutathione S-transferase zeta and thioredoxin, and thus inactivate the proteins (6, 7). However, other reactive intermediates can modify proteins on amino acid residues distant from their catalytic site, thereby promoting a toxicological response by interfering with critical protein–protein interactions and disrupting cellular signaling pathways (8, 9).

Quinones represent an extensive class of electrophilic xenobiotics that can form covalent adducts with proteins, and can produce toxicological effects via such adduction. Quinones are also capable of redox cycling, and consequently producing reactive oxygen species (10) and subsequent oxidative stress (11–13). 1,4-Benzoquinone (BQ) is a reactive electrophile formed via the metabolism of benzene (a low molecular weight hydrocarbon and an environmental pollutant) to HQ, or from HQ directly. Because of the electrophilic nature of BQ, several GSH molecules can be sequentially conjugated to BQ via the free cysteinyl sulfhydryl present in GSH (10, 14–16). This conjugation results in the formation of conjugates with varying degrees of GSH including mono-, bis-, tris-, and tetra-substituted GSH conjugates of HQ (17). Subsequent metabolism of these conjugates via the mercapturic acid pathway ultimately yields the corresponding N-acetylcysteine conjugates, such as 2-(N-acetylcystein-S-yl)hydroquinone (NAC-HQ). These quinone–thioether metabolites cause extensive renal proximal tubular cell necrosis and effects are mediated via their ability to generate ROS and their protein-arylation capabilities (18–20). Although the compounds studied represent metabolites of known environmental toxicants, the quinone moiety also exists as the pharmacophore in many chemotherapeutic drugs. In this instance, the ability of these drugs to covalently bind to tissue macromolecules is a desired property of these cytotoxicants. In contrast, the covalent binding of electrophilic drug metabolites is also of importance to the pharmaceutical industry because reactive drug metabolites may contribute to unwanted drug-induced toxicities. Thus, the pharmaceutical industry often assays for the ability of candidate drugs to undergo protein covalent binding as an index of reactive intermediate formation, which can ultimately assist in the further development of otherwise attractive drug candidates (9).

We herein describe MALDI-TOF based approaches to identify amino acid residues within peptides and proteins that are selectively adducted by reactive electrophilic quinone–thioethers. In order to decrease the analytical complexity inherent in the use of these compounds during mass spectral analysis, we utilized the mono-substituted NAC-HQ metabolite to investigate the adduction profile following reaction of this compound with several model peptides and proteins.

2. Materials

2.1. Sample Preparation

1. 1,4 BQ, *N*-1, and silver oxide (Aldrich, Milwaukee, WI).
2. HPLC-grade solvents including acetonitrile, acetic acid, methanol, and trifluoroacetic acid (TFA) (EMD Chemicals).
3. Shimadzu HPLC system (LC-10AS) with a UV–Vis spectrophotometric detector (280 nm) and an Ultrasphere ODS C18 column (5 μm packing, 10 mm × 25 cm, Beckman–Coulter).
4. 0.2 μm syringe filter (Whatman).
5. Rotovapor (Buchi) used in combination with a water aspirator pump (Cole–Parmer) for rotary evaporation during compound preparation.

2.2. Peptide Reaction

1. Ac-GAKKAG-OH (Ac-Gly-Ala-Lys-Lys-Ala-Gly-OH) can be purchased from American Peptide Inc, Sunnyvale, CA. Ac-QADGCAGPAG-OH (Ac-Gln-Ala-Asp-Gly-Cys-Ala-Gly-Pro-Ala-Gly) and Ac-QGADDEDDAG-OH (Ac-Gln-Gly-Ala-Asp-Asp-Glu-Asp-Asp-Ala-Gly-OH) can be purchased from Global Peptide, Fort Collins, CO. These custom peptides are >95% HPLC purity as characterized by HPLC and MS. The peptides come as lyophilized powders and are stored at –20°C immediately upon arrival.
2. Peptide reaction buffer(s): 10 mM Tris–HCl (Sigma) pH 7.5 and/or 50 mM ammonium acetate (Fisher Scientific), pH 6.
3. C18 packed tips (ZipTip) (Millipore, Inc).
4. Wetting solution: 100% acetonitrile (EMD chemicals).

5. Equilibration solution: 0.1% TFA in Milli-Q water (EMD chemicals).

6. Wash solution: 0.1% TFA in Milli-Q water (EMD Chemicals).

7. Elution solution: 0.1% TFA/50% acetonitrile (EMD Chemicals). These ZipTip solutions can be stored at room temperature and are stable for long periods of time.

8. A Shimadzu HPLC system (LC-10AS) with a UV–Vis spectrophotometric detector (280 nm) and an Ultrasphere ODS C18 column (5 μm packing, 10 mm×25 cm, Beckman–Coulter).

9. α-Cyano-4-hydroxycinnamic acid (CHCA): 50% acetonitrile, 0.1% TFA in deionized water.

10. CHCA matrix (Sigma) and Voyager MALDI-TOF sample plate laser etched stainless steel, 100-position (Applied Biosystems).

2.3. Protein Reaction

1. Cytochrome *c* reaction buffer: 10 mM Tris–HCl (Sigma), pH 7.5, used with horse heart cytochrome *c* (Sigma).

2. Microcon 3,000 Da molecular weight cut-off centrifugal filter (Millipore).

3. 3,5-Dimethoxy-4-hydroxycinnamic acid (sinapinic acid): 30–50% acetonitrile, 0.1% TFA in deionized water.

4. 3,5-Dimethoxy-4-hydroxycinnamic acid (sinapinic acid) (ACROS organics) and Voyager MALDI-TOF sample plate laser etched stainless steel, 100-position (Applied Biosystems).

3. Methods

The basic scope of this chapter is to determine an electrophile-specific adduction profile using MALDI-TOF (matrix-assisted laser desorption ionization-time of flight) analysis. By using quinones as our model electrophile and multiple *in vitro* reaction targets, including peptides and proteins, we should be able to identify the resulting quinone adduction profile on whole proteins, as well as determine the potential amino acid targets of these compounds with the use of small peptides. This will also help guide us in any quinone-specific post adduction chemistry that may be occurring.

MALDI ionization is used for the analysis of biomolecules, including peptides and proteins, where the matrix assists in desorption and ionization of the analyte. After the analyte is mixed with the appropriate matrix and spotted on the sample plate, the laser is used for ionization of the analyte. The ions are then separated based upon the time it takes for them to traverse the flight tube to the detector. This is referred to as a time-of-flight mass analyzer (21, 22). By using MALDI-TOF analysis as our primary tool, we can achieve a projected quinone adduction profile on specified proteins and peptides, as well as determine accurate mass modifications of these compounds.

3.1. Preparation of Compounds for In Vitro Reaction

1. *N*-Acetylcysteine (NAC) is dissolved in 1% acetic acid in water (~25 ml). BQ is dissolved in a mixture of 50% acetonitrile:water (~60 ml). NAC is added dropwise to the BQ solution.

2. The mixture is stirred for 15 min and the solution is extracted twice with three volumes of ethyl acetate to remove residual BQ and HQ formed by reduction. The solution is rotary evaporated down to 10–15 ml and the aqueous phase is lyophilized (see Note 1) (17).

3. The resulting product is purified by HPLC after dissolving it in 1% acetic acid in water (200 mg/ml) and injecting aliquots (100 μl). The sample elutes isocratically at 10 min using acetic acid:methanol:water (1:20:80 v/v.), at a flow rate of 3.0 ml/min, over 35 min and monitored at 280 nm.

4. These compounds must be in their oxidized forms in order for them to adduct nucleophilic protein residues, and so we manually oxidize them from the HQ conjugate to the BQ conjugate. NAC-HQ is dissolved in deionized distilled water with 0.1% TFA at a concentration of 50 mg/ml. Approximately 5 mg of silver is added and the solution is vortexed for 1 min. The solution is filtered through a 0.2 μm syringe filter.

5. The solution is then purified by HPLC. The mobile phase is acetic acid:methanol:water (1:10:90 v/v.) Aliquots of oxidized 2-(*N*-acetylcystein-*S*-yl)benzoquinone (NAC-BQ) (50 μl) are injected into the HPLC system and separated isocratically at 3.0 ml/min.

6. The product elutes at 12.4 min. The yellow product is then reanalyzed by HPLC using the previously described method and gives rise to a single UV-absorbing peak (see Note 2).

3.2. Reaction of Compounds with Peptides to Determine Amino Acid Targets and Accurate Adduct Masses

1. N-terminal protected peptides are used to ensure that the compound will not bind to the peptide N-terminus. Different peptides are used with various amino acid targets to differentiate among likely targets of these compounds. Examples include: (1) Ac-GAKKAG-OH (Ac-Gly-Ala-Lys-Lys-Ala-Gly-OH), (2) Ac-QGADDEDDAG-OH (Ac-Gln-Gly-Ala-Asp-Asp-Glu-Asp-Asp-Ala-Gly-OH), and (3) Ac-QADGCAGPAG-OH (Ac-Gln-Ala-Asp-Gly-Cys-Ala-Gly-Pro-Ala-Gly). These peptides are used to determine specificity of different amino acids (Lys and Cys) towards our quinone–thioether compounds. Specific residues within these peptides, including Lys and Cys,

have been shown to be targets of various other electrophiles
(4, 23). Additionally, residues with less nucleophilic regions,
such as carboxy groups, may also be targets, so we have
included a peptide with several Asp and Glu residues.

2. The peptides are dissolved in various buffers. The solubility of
the peptides is sequence dependent and involves hydropho-
bicity and hydrogen bonding. These selected peptides will
solubilize readily in water; however, if the peptide is extremely
acidic, the pH can be raised to increase solubility and if the
peptide is extremely basic, the pH can be lowered to increase
solubility. Peptides (1) and (2) from above are likely soluble
in any aqueous solvent regardless of pH, because they contain
a high charge distribution. Peptide (3) contains a Cys residue
and these residues are susceptible to oxidation and polymerization, so it can be dissolved in a solvent system that is slightly
acidic. A small amount of dithiothreitol (DTT), reducing
agent, can be added to increase stability of these residues.
Because we are using these peptides for protein adduction
studies, the solvents we use here may be considerably different than many suggested solvents for these types of peptides.

3. These buffer conditions can vary greatly depending upon the
compound in use for protein adduction reactions. Dissolve
peptide (1) in 10 mM Tris–HCl pH 7.5, peptide (2) in
50 mM ammonium acetate pH 6, and peptide (3) in water
(see Note 3).

4. Following solubilization of these peptides, they are aliquoted
for storage and use. They can be stored at –20°C and can be
thawed for individual use. Each aliquot will contain 100 μg.
One aliquot can be divided into a control sample and a treated
sample. The treated sample will be reacted with NAC-BQ at
a 1:10 molar ratio of peptide:NAC-BQ. NAC-BQ will be
weighed out and added as a dry powder to the solubilized
peptide and reacted for 30 min to 1 h at room temperature.

5. Following the reaction, the excess NAC-BQ is removed.
Because of the small molecular weight of the peptides, only
C18 packed tips (ZipTip) can be used for NAC-BQ removal
or HPLC analysis can also be done to remove the excess
compound.

6. The C18 packed tips are typically used for desalting and con-
centrating peptides or small proteins before MALDI-TOF
analysis. These C18 pipette tips can hold up to 10 μl of volume,
but 5 μl can be used as to not waste too much sample. First,
ensure the final sample solution has a pH <4, so add 0.5 μl
TFA to the 5 μl sample volume. Depress the pipettor plunger
to a dead stop and aspirate wetting solution into the tip.
Dispense to waste and repeat. Aspirate equilibration solution.

Dispense to waste and repeat. Bind peptides to C18 pipette tip by aspirating and dispensing the sample seven to ten cycles for maximum binding. Aspirate wash solution into tip and dispense to waste and repeat once. In order to elute the peptides, dispense 1–4 µl of elution solution into a clean vial using a standard pipette tip. Aspirate and dispense eluant through C18 pipette tip at least three times without introducing air into the sample.

7. HPLC analysis can be performed to remove excess NAC-BQ from peptide reactions. Aliquots of NAC-BQ reacted peptides (100 µg) were injected into the HPLC system and the sample was eluted with a linear gradient of trifluoroacetic acid:acetonitrile:water (0.1:1:98.9 to 0.1:40:59.9 v/v) at a flow rate of 3 ml/min over 35 min. These aliquots are collected in glass vials, lyophilized to dryness, and can be stored at –20°C until ready for use. Typically, the aliquots are then dissolved in deionized, distilled water and used for MALDI-TOF analysis.

8. The reacted and purified peptide sample(s) is free of any salts or excess NAC-BQ that would interfere with MALDI-TOF analysis. The NAC-BQ adduct will still remain on the peptide.

9. For MALDI-TOF analysis, a matrix solution will be mixed with the peptide solution at a 1:1(v/v) ratio. The peptide solution that is mixed with matrix will be pure based on the above procedures using C18 tips or HPLC for purification. Ideal final protein concentration for peptides and proteins is 0.1–10 µM. For peptides and proteins of less than 10 kDa, CHCA is used as the matrix. This matrix can then be premixed with the peptide solution in a small Eppendorf tube (see Note 4). It is important that neither the matrix nor the peptide precipitates when the two solutions are mixed. The mixture (1–2 µl) can then be applied to the sample support (MALDI-TOF plate) and the sample is allowed to air evaporate. The dried sample is quite stable and can be stored at room temperature for several days to several weeks. An example of a MALDI-TOF spectrum following this type of reaction is shown in Fig. 1.

3.3. Reaction of Compounds with Pure Protein for Whole Protein Analysis to Determine Adduct Profile

1. This purified compound (NAC-BQ) can also be used in a reaction with pure cytochrome *c* from horse heart to determine adduction profile by NAC-BQ on cytochrome *c* and any resulting post-adduction chemistry as a result of NAC-BQ adduction. The data generated from peptide studies with NAC-BQ can be used as a guide to project the correct amino-acid targets and mass modifications.

2. Horse heart cytochrome *c* (1 mg) is dissolved in 10 mM Tris–HCl, pH 7.5 (see Note 5). The cytochrome *c* solution

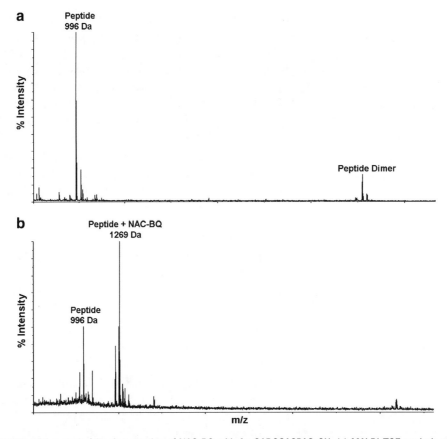

Fig. 1. MALDI-TOF analysis following reaction of NAC-BQ with Ac-QADGCAGPAG-OH. (**a**) MALDI-TOF analysis of control peptide in 10 mM Tris–HCl, pH 7.5. (**b**) The peptide was reacted with BQ at a ratio of 1:10 for 30 min at room temperature while rotating. At the end of the 30 min incubation, the sample was then HPLC-purified to remove excess NAC-BQ and lyophilized to dryness. The sample was then reconstituted in 10 mM Tris–HCl, pH 7.5. The resulting MALDI-TOF spectrum shows addition of NAC-BQ to the cysteine residue on the peptide, corresponding to one addition of NAC-BQ at 1,269 *m/z*.

is aliquoted (100 μl) prior to NAC-BQ reaction for use as a control sample.

3. The cytochrome *c* solution is reacted with dry NAC-BQ at a 1:10 molar ratio at room temperature for 30 min to 1 h (see Note 6).

4. The mixture is filtered once through a Microcon 3,000 Da molecular weight cut-off centrifugal filter for 20 min at 13,000 × *g* to remove excess NAC-BQ. The reaction mixture is then washed with 1 ml of 10 mM Tris–HCl, pH 7.5, and centrifuged as above.

5. Once completed, the filter is turned upside down in a new filter tube and centrifuged for 2 min at 2,000 × *g* to collect the remaining protein solution that was on the filter. Measure the volume to determine the protein concentration, as all of the NAC-BQ-reacted protein and the native protein should

remain on top of the filter because these have a mass of greater than 3,000 Da. The unreacted NAC-BQ should pass through the filter as it has a molecular mass of 269 Da. By collecting the solution remaining on the filter, this will be the solution containing the reacted protein and will be used for further analysis.

6. When using high salt buffers or any type of denaturing agent, the protein will need to be further purified using C18 packed tips. The protocol for using these tips with proteins is the same as described previously with the peptide.

7. For MALDI-TOF analysis, a matrix solution will be mixed with the protein solution at a 1:1(v/v) ratio. Ideal final protein concentration for peptides and proteins is 0.1–10 μM. For proteins of greater than 10 kDa, sinapinic acid is used as the matrix. This matrix can then be premixed with the protein solution in a small Eppendorf tube (see Note 4). It is important that neither the matrix nor the protein precipitates when the two solutions are mixed. The mixture (1–2 μl) can then be applied to the sample support (MALDI-TOF plate) and the sample is allowed to air evaporate. The dried sample is quite stable and can be stored at room temperature for several days to several weeks. An example of a MALDI-TOF spectrum following this type of reaction is shown in Fig. 2.

3.4. Detailed Program Method and Laser Use for Pure Protein/ Peptides (22)

1. MALDI-TOF spectra are taken on Applied Biosystems Voyager DE-STR instrument with a 2-m flight path in the positive ion mode. The instrument is equipped with a nitrogen laser operating at 337 nm.

2. Open the Voyager Control Panel and click the load/eject button to load the sample plate (see Note 7).

3. Load a standard instrument setting file (.bic). Peptide spectra can be acquired in reflectron mode (for higher resolution) over the mass range 700–5,000 Da. Choose a file that corresponds to this setting. Additionally, this setting should include the appropriate matrix for peptide use which corresponds to α-cyano-hydroxycinnamic acid. Whole protein spectra can be acquired in linear mode over the mass range 8,000–40,000 Da and the matrix was selected as sinapinic acid for this whole protein acquisition (21) (see Note 8).

4. Save the parameters and manually turn on the high voltage and let it warm for 30 min.

5. Set the laser intensity to 1,300–1,500, set the desired sample position, and begin acquisition (see Note 9).

6. A good peak should correspond to signal intensity roughly between 5,000 and 40,000 (see Note 10).

7. The spectra can be sequentially stacked when analyzing peptide and whole protein samples.

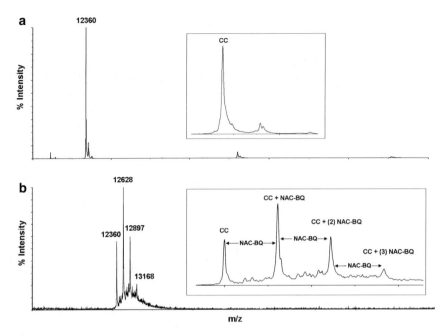

Fig. 2. MALDI-TOF whole protein spectra for cytochrome *c* reacted with NAC-BQ. (**a**) Control spectrum of cytochrome *c* in 10 mM Tris–HCl pH 7.5, where the peak at 12,360 *m/z* indicates native cytochrome *c*. (**b**) Cytochrome *c* was incubated in 10 mM Tris–HCl pH 7.5 and then reacted with a 1:10 molar ratio of NAC-BQ. The excess NAC-BQ was removed using Microcon 3,000 Da molecular weight cut-off centrifugal filters. The resulting MALDI-TOF spectrum shows several additions of 268 Da to cytochrome *c*, corresponding to one addition at 12,628 *m/z*, two additions at 12,897 *m/z*, and three additions at 13,168 *m/z*. The insets in (**a**) and (**b**) are magnified regions of each spectrum. Reproduced from (24) with permission from American Chemical Society.

8. Internal and external calibration can be applied to samples. Internal calibration standards typically include cytochrome *c*, bovine trypsin, and carbonic anhydrase. These standards should bracket the mass range of interest and should be of similar intensities as the samples (see Note 11). External calibration can also be applied to samples. This type of file can be acquired using a protein mixture (cytochrome *c* and myoglobin) and saved for use with real samples. Typically, these standards are spotted nearby the sample positions and applied to the actual samples. This calibration file must be created and saved in Data Explorer. Then, existing calibration files can be manually applied to real samples with each acquisition (see Note 12).

9. The Data Explorer Software program is used to analyze all MALDI-TOF spectra (see Note 13).

10. Keep the sample plate covered and protected at all times. Finger prints and scratches will interfere with good data acquisition.

11. Clean the sample plate after all sample positions have been filled and analyzed (see Note 14).

4. Notes

1. NAC-HQ is weighed after lyophilization and stored in glass vials at −20°C. This compound is also stable at room temperature.

2. NAC-BQ is weighed and stored in glass vials at −20°C, although it will be stable for long periods of time at room temperature.

3. We found that Lys residues adduct NAC-BQ more efficiently when in a neutral to basic pH, such as 10 mM Tris–HCl, pH 7.5. Subjecting Lys residues to a neutral/basic pH, they are more nucleophilic, priming them for higher reaction efficiency with NAC-BQ. Glu residues adduct NAC-BQ when in a more acidic pH, such as 50 mM ammonium acetate, pH 6.0. This environment seems to stabilize a resonance structure that becomes protonated at a low pH and thus enables this residue to bind NAC-BQ via Michael addition (24). Cys residues adduct NAC-BQ in water much better than in a buffered system. Ideally, peptides containing Cys residues should be used with a mild reducing agent or kept at a lower pH because of disulfide formation. We observe that disulfide formation does occur; however, it is much more prevalent in basic conditions and seems to be not as probable in water. Additionally, we still are able to form NAC-BQ adducts on Cys residues using water as a solvent system, so we avoid using any buffering system. Furthermore, DTT and other reducing agents, interfere with NAC-BQ adduction because they likely scavenge the electrophilic compound and prevent it from binding to the Cys residue.

4. The matrix solution is usually made with a concentration of 20 mg/ml; however, it is good practice to make small volumes and try to use fresh matrix solutions whenever possible. The matrix solutions are saturated solutions. Following addition of the solvents to the matrix, the solution is vortexed and then allowed to settle for a few minutes and use the top matrix solution layer, free of undissolved matrix.

5. A buffering system is used that consists of 10 mM Tris–HCl, pH 7.5 and NAC-BQ adduct formation is much more efficient in this buffer than in water. This is likely because many of the NAC-BQ-adducts form on Lys residues and these residues are more nucleophilic in buffered systems.

6. The reaction can proceed for longer than 1 h; however, it has been shown that the *N*-acetylcysteine bond to the BQ ring is not stable in high salt or high pH conditions for periods of time exceeding 6 h. Therefore, sample preparation

time is critical for accurate adduct mass analysis. When the NAC-BQ compound is stable, it will form adducts with a mass of 268 Da. Following NAC-BQ adduction and thioether bond elimination due to microenvironment instability, the resulting adduct mass will be 105 Da. This mass is indicative of the BQ ring (24).

7. Multiple sample plate configurations may be stored in the computer, but only select the configuration that corresponds to the plate being loaded so that the positions can be navigated based on plate configuration.

8. The instrument can be set to incorporate a much broader range of masses from 1,000 to 100,000 Da. Because cytochrome *c* is being analyzed, a program is used that narrows the mass range window closer to the actual mass of cytochrome *c*.

9. The laser intensity becomes saturated at 1,800 and is higher for these samples at these concentrations. The laser intensity used is dependent upon the instrument laser, in addition to the type and concentration of sample being analyzed.

10. In order to optimize the acquisition, the laser intensity can be raised or lowered, and the laser position with the sample can be moved to a more desirable location.

11. In order to avoid overloading the signal with the calibration standards, work with the dilution factor of the standards.

12. External calibration is not as good as internal calibration; however, the closer the standard is to the sample spot, the better the calibration and less the error.

13. Basic features of Data Explorer include peak detection and peak labeling, graphics, resolution, baseline correction, noise reduction and smoothing, and calibration options.

14. Wash the sample plate with methanol and deionized water (v/v 1:1) and rinse well with deionized water. If sample or matrix residue persists, apply 0.1% detergent solution to sample plate and use a soft tooth brush to scrub the plate. Rinse well with deionized water. Allow the plate to dry completely before applying any samples.

Acknowledgments

This work was supported by GM070890 (SSL) and ES07091 (AAF). The authors acknowledge the support of the P30 ES06694 Southwest Environmental Health Sciences Center, in particular the Arizona Proteomics Consortium (APC). Special thanks go to Dr. George Tsaprailis, Director of the APC.

References

1. Monks, T.J. (2006) Introduction. *Drug Metab Rev* **38**, 599–600.

2. Brouwers, O., Teerlink, T., van Bezu, J., Barto, R., Stehouwer, C., and Schalkwijk, C. (2007) Methylglyoxal and methylglyoxal-arginine adducts do not directly inhibit endothelial nitric oxide synthase. *Ann. N. Y. Acad. Sci.* **1126**, 231–234.

3. Kankova, K. (2008) Diabetic threesome (hyperglycaemia, renal function and nutrition) and advanced glycation end products: evidence for the multiple-hit agent?, *Proc. Nutr. Soc.* **67**, 60–74.

4. Carbone, D.L., Doorn, J.A., Kiebler, Z., and Petersen, D.R. (2005) Cysteine modification by lipid peroxidation products inhibits protein disulfide isomerase. *Chem. Res. Toxicol.* **18**, 1324–1331.

5. Sampey, B.P., Carbone, D.L., Doorn, J.A., Drechsel, D.A., and Petersen, D.R. (2007) 4-Hydroxy-2-nonenal adduction of extracellular signal-regulated kinase (Erk) and the inhibition of hepatocyte Erk-Est-like protein-1-activating protein-1 signal transduction. *Mol. Pharmacol.* **71**, 871–883.

6. Anderson, W.B., Board, P.G., and Anders, M.W. (2004) Glutathione transferase zeta-catalyzed bioactivation of dichloroacetic acid: reaction of glyoxylate with amino acid nucleophiles. *Chem. Res. Toxicol.* **17**, 650–662.

7. Go, Y.M., Halvey, P.J., Hansen, J.M., Reed, M., Pohl, J., and Jones, D.P. (2007) Reactive aldehyde modification of thioredoxin-1 activates early steps of inflammation and cell adhesion. *Am. J. Pathol.* **171**, 1670–1681.

8. Luo, J., Hill, B.G., Gu, Y., Cai, J., Srivastava, S., Bhatnagar, A., and Prabhu, S.D. (2007) Mechanisms of acrolein-induced myocardial dysfunction: implications for environmental and endogenous aldehyde exposure. *Am. J. Physiol. Heart. Circ. Physiol.* **293**, H3673–3684.

9. Baillie, T.A. (2006) Future of toxicology-metabolic activation and drug design: challenges and opportunities in chemical toxicology. *Chem. Res. Toxicol.* **19**, 889–893.

10. Ross, D. (2000) The role of metabolism and specific metabolites in benzene-induced toxicity: evidence and issues. *J. Toxicol. Environ. Health* A **61**, 357–372.

11. Pagano, G. (2002) Redox-modulated xenobiotic action and ROS formation: a mirror or a window? *Hum. Exp. Toxicol.* **21**, 77–81.

12. Bolton, J.L., Trush, M.A., Penning, T.M., Dryhurst, G., and Monks, T.J. (2000) Role of quinones in toxicology. *Chem. Res. Toxicol.* **13**, 135–160.

13. Verrax, J., Delvaux, M., Beghein, N., Taper, H., Gallez, B., and Buc Calderon, P. (2005) Enhancement of quinone redox cycling by ascorbate induces a caspase-3 independent cell death in human leukaemia cells. An *in vitro* comparative study. *Free Radic. Res.* **39**, 649–657.

14. Ruiz-Ramos, R., Cebrian, M.E., and Garrido, E. (2005) Benzoquinone activates the ERK/MAPK signaling pathway via ROS production in HL-60 cells. *Toxicology* **209**, 279–287.

15. Person, M.D., Mason, D.E., Liebler, D.C., Monks, T.J., and Lau, S.S. (2005) Alkylation of cytochrome c by (glutathion-S-yl)-1,4-benzoquinone and iodoacetamide demonstrates compound-dependent site specificity. *Chem. Res. Toxicol.* **18**, 41–50.

16. Lindsey, R.H., Jr., Bender, R.P., and Osheroff, N. (2005) Effects of benzene metabolites on DNA cleavage mediated by human topoisomerase II alpha: 1,4-hydroquinone is a topoisomerase II poison. *Chem. Res. Toxicol.* **18**, 761–770.

17. Lau, S.S., Hill, B.A., Highet, R.J., and Monks, T.J. (1988) Sequential oxidation and glutathione addition to 1,4-benzoquinone: correlation of toxicity with increased glutathione substitution. *Mol. Pharmacol.* **34**, 829–836.

18. Peters, M.M., Jones, T.W., Monks, T.J., and Lau, S.S. (1997) Cytotoxicity and cell-proliferation induced by the nephrocarcinogen hydroquinone and its nephrotoxic metabolite 2,3,5-(tris-glutathion-S-yl)hydroquinone. *Carcinogenesis* **18**, 2393–2401.

19. Kleiner, H.E., Jones, T.W., Monks, T.J., and Lau, S.S. (1998) Immunochemical analysis of quinol–thioether-derived covalent protein adducts in rodent species sensitive and resistant to quinol–thioether-mediated nephrotoxicity. *Chem. Res. Toxicol.* **11**, 1291–1300.

20. Yoon, H.S., Monks, T.J., Walker, C.L., and Lau, S.S. (2001) Transformation of kidney epithelial cells by a quinol thioether via inactivation of the tuberous sclerosis-2 tumor suppressor gene. *Mol. Carcinog.* **31**, 37–45.

21. Kussmann, M., Lassing, U., Sturmer, C.A., Przybylski, M., and Roepstorff, P. (1997) Matrix-assisted laser desorption/ionization mass spectrometric peptide mapping of the neural cell adhesion protein neurolin purified by sodium dodecyl sulfate polyacrylamide gel

electrophoresis or acidic precipitation. *J. Mass Spectrom.* **32**, 483–493.

22. Voyager. (2004) Voyager Biospectrometry Workstation Training, Applied Biosystems, Forester City, CA.

23. Stewart, B.J., Doorn, J.A., and Petersen, D.R. (2007) Residue-specific adduction of tubulin by 4-hydroxynonenal and 4-oxononenal causes cross-linking and inhibits polymerization. *Chem. Res. Toxicol.* **20**, 1111–1119.

24. Fisher, A.A., Labenski, M.T., Malladi, S., Gokhale, V., Bowen, M.E., Milleron, R.S., Bratton, S.B., Monks, T.J., and Lau, S.S. (2007) Quinone electrophiles selectively adduct "electrophile binding motifs" within cytochrome c. *Biochemistry* **46**, 11090–11100.

Chapter 19

Utilization of LC-MS/MS Analyses to Identify Site-Specific Chemical Protein Adducts *In Vitro*

Ashley A. Fisher, Matthew T. Labenski, Terrence J. Monks, and Serrine S. Lau

Abstract

Biologically reactive intermediates are formed following metabolism of xenobiotics, and during normal oxidative metabolism. These reactive species are electrophilic in nature and are capable of forming stable adducts with target proteins. These covalent protein modifications can initiate processes that lead to acute tissue injury or chronic disease. Recent advancements in mass spectrometry techniques and data analysis has permitted a more detailed investigation of site-specific protein modifications by reactive electrophiles. Knowledge from such analyses will assist in providing a better understanding of how specific classes of electrophiles produce toxicity and disease progression via site-selective protein-specific covalent modification. Hydroquinone (HQ) is a known environmental toxicant, and its quinone–thioether metabolites, formed via the intermediate generation of 1,4-benzoquinone (1,4-BQ), elicit their toxic response via the covalent modification of target proteins and the generation of reactive oxygen species. We have utilized a model protein, cytochrome *c*, to guide us in identifying 1,4-BQ- and 1,4-BQ-thioether derived site-specific protein modifications. LC-MS/MS analyses reveals that these modifications occur selectively on lysine and glutamic acid residues of the target protein, and that these modifications occur within identifiable "electrophile binding motifs" within the protein. These motifs are found within lysine-rich regions of the protein and appear to be target sites of 1,4-BQ-thioether adduction. These residues also appear to dictate the nature of post-adduction chemistry and the final structure of the adduct. This model system will provide critical insight for *in vivo* adduct hunting following exposure to 1,4-BQ-thioethers, but the general approaches can also be extended to the identification of protein adducts derived from other classes of reactive electrophiles.

Key words: Cytochrome *c*, 1,4-Benzoquinone, LC-MS/MS, 2-(*N*-acetylcystein-*S*-yl)-1,4-benzoquinone, Post-translational modifications, Trypsin solution digest

1. Introduction

Metabolism of xenobiotics leads to formation of a variety of reactive intermediates. Similar reactive intermediates can be formed as by-products of cellular metabolism, including reactive oxygen

Jean-Charles Gautier (ed.), *Drug Safety Evaluation: Methods and Protocols*, Methods in Molecular Biology, vol. 691,
DOI 10.1007/978-1-60761-849-2_19, © Springer Science+Business Media, LLC 2011

and nitrogen species, as well as reactive dicarbonyl degradation products, such as methylglyoxal (1). Additionally, many of these reactive intermediates damage cellular membranes, resulting in lipid peroxidation, which results in the formation of several α,β-unsaturated aldehydes, including 4-hydoxynonenal (4-HNE) (2). Many reactive aldehydes are generated endogenously during glycation, amino acid oxidation, and lipid peroxidation, and contribute to disease progression, including diabetes and atherosclerosis (3, 4). The majority of reactive intermediates are electrophilic in nature, which allow them to adduct nucleophilic residues within target proteins. α,β-Unsaturated aldehydes form stable covalent adducts with cysteine, histidine, and lysine residues (2, 5, 6). Other reactive electrophiles, such as quinones, produce toxic effects as a result of covalent protein adduction and the generation of reactive oxygen species. It is important to note that these two effects of quinone are not mutually exclusive, since protein-bound quinones can remain redox active. Quinones form protein adducts with nucleophilic residues within target proteins, including lysine, cysteine, and histidine residues (7–10). Because reactive electrophiles are capable of forming covalent adducts with proteins, they may subsequently alter the structure and function of target proteins. Such functional alterations may include interference with protein–protein interactions and subcellular protein localization, and disruption of cellular signaling pathways.

To assess the impact of electrophile-derived covalent protein adducts on protein structure and function, electrophiles with known toxicity were utilized. Hydroquinone (HQ), and its thioether metabolites, produce renal proximal tubular cell necrosis and are nephrocarcinogenic in rats. The adverse effects of these chemicals are in part a consequence of their oxidation to the corresponding electrophile 1,4-benzoquinone (1,4-BQ), the electrophilic nature of which facilitates conjugation with glutathione (GSH) via the nucleophilic cysteine free sulfhydryl (10–13). The subsequent metabolism of 1,4-BQ-GSH conjugates via the mercapturic acid pathway results in the eventual formation of 2-(*N*-acetylcystein-*S*-yl)hydroquinone (NAC-HQ), which upon oxidation gives rise to 2-(*N*-acetylcystein-*S*-yl)-1,4-benzoquinone (NAC-BQ) (14).

Cytochrome *c* has been studied as a model protein to characterize NAC-BQ-mediated site-specific covalent adduction. We have determined that specific motifs within target proteins ("electrophile binding motifs") predispose these proteins to chemical adduction. We have chemically reacted NAC-BQ with cytochrome *c*, purified the protein adduct solution, and subsequently utilized LC-MS/MS and data analysis to identify the specific sites at which amino acid modifications occur. The analysis also reveals insights into the resulting post-adduction chemistry. This model system will provide critical insight for *in vivo* adduct hunting following exposure to 1,4-BQ-thioethers, but the general approaches can also be extended to the identification of protein adducts derived from other classes of reactive electrophiles.

2. Materials

2.1. Single Protein Reacted with Chemical in Solution

2.1.1. Single Protein Reaction

1. NAC-BQ synthesized and purified (see Chapter 18).

2. Cytochrome *c* reaction buffer: 10 mM Tris–HCl, pH 7.5 used with horse heart cytochrome *c* (Sigma). Store cytochrome *c* at −20°C in a dessicator.

3. Microcon 3,000 Da molecular weight cut-off centrifugal filter (Millipore).

4. Voyager MALDI-TOF sample plate laser etched stainless steel, 100-position (Applied Biosystems).

2.1.2. LC-MS/MS Sample Preparation

1. pH-indicator strips (EMD chemicals).

2. Digestion buffer(s): 50 mM Tris–HCl, pH 7.5 or 50–100 mM NH_4HCO_3, pH 8.0.

3. 2 M DTT stock solution: 154.3 mg DTT (Sigma) in 500 μl deionized distilled water (see Note 1).

4. 10 mM DTT solution for reduction: 5 μl 2 M DTT in 1 ml of 0.1 M NH_4HCO_3 (Sigma).

5. 55 mM Iodoacetamide (Sigma) stock solution: 10 mg in 1 ml 0.1 M NH_4HCO_3.

6. Trypsin modified sequencing grade (Promega): 20 μg lyophilized powder. Store at −20°C. Dilute to 0.1 μg/μl and can be stored in solution at −20°C for several weeks.

2.1.3. LC-MS/MS Analysis

1. ThermoFinnigan LTQ mass spectrometer (San Jose, CA) equipped with a Michrom Paradigm MS4 HPLC, a SpectraSystems AS3000 autosampler, and a nanoelectrospray source.

3. Methods

3.1. Single Protein Reacted with Chemical in Solution

Purified quinone–thioether compounds, including NAC-BQ, can be used in a reaction with pure cytochrome *c* from horse heart to determine site-specific adductions by these compounds, specifically, NAC-BQ on cytochrome *c* (see Note 2). Furthermore, this will guide us in identifying target residues and any resulting post-adduction chemistry as a result of NAC-BQ adduction.

*3.1.1. Chemical Reaction
with Single Protein*

1. Horse heart cytochrome c (1 mg) is dissolved in 10 mM Tris–HCl pH 7.5 (1 ml) (see Note 3). The cytochrome c solution is aliquoted (100 μl) prior to NAC-BQ reaction for use as a control sample.

2. The cytochrome c solution is reacted with dry NAC-BQ at a 1:10 molar ratio at room temperature for 30 min to 1 h (see Note 4).

3. The mixture is filtered once through a Microcon 3,000 Da molecular weight cut-off centrifugal filter for 20 min at $13,000 \times g$ to remove excess NAC-BQ. The reaction mixture is then washed with 1 ml of 10 mM Tris–HCl, pH 7.5, and centrifuged as above (see Note 5).

4. Once complete, the filter is turned upside down in a new filter tube and centrifuged for 2 min at $2,000 \times g$ to collect the remaining protein solution that was on the filter. Measure the volume to determine the protein concentration, as all of the NAC-BQ-reacted protein and the native protein should remain on top of the filter because these have a mass of greater than 3,000 Da. The unreacted NAC-BQ should pass through the filter as it has a molecular mass of 269 Da. By collecting the solution remaining on the filter, this will be the solution containing the reacted protein and will be used for further analysis (see Note 6).

5. The control cytochrome c solution and the NAC-BQ-reacted cytochrome c solution will be spotted on the MALDI target plate to determine the adduction profile before proceeding forward with LC-MS/MS analysis (described in detail in Chapter 18).

*3.1.2. Solution Digest
of Single Protein Samples*

1. Use both control and NAC-BQ-adducted samples and treat them equally throughout. Because these samples are approximately 1 mg/ml, it is sufficient to take 10 μl from these to proceed with the following steps. This will provide approximately 10 μg of protein for each sample (see Note 7).

2. Most successful proteins digests conducted using trypsin as the proteolytic enzyme occur using 50 mM Tris–HCl, pH 7.5 or 50–100 mM NH_4HCO_3 as the buffering system. These buffers are usually in the pH range of 7.4–8.0. This is ideal for trypsin digestion to occur (see Note 8).

3. The samples described here are in 10 mM Tris–HCl pH 7.5 buffering system, so in this case, the buffering system should be sufficient. However, in the event where the proteins of interest are in different buffering systems, it is important to spike in NH_4HCO_3 or Tris–HCl pH 7.5 to a final concentration of 50 mM Tris–HCl pH 7.5 or 50–100 mM NH_4HCO_3 pH 8. Try to keep the volume as low as possible in this step, so use small amounts of buffer when possible.

4. For proteins that have disulfide bonds, a reduction/alkylation process will be necessary prior to trypsin digestion. These reduction/alkylation steps need to take place in the dark (see Note 9).

5. Add 40 μl of 10 mM DTT stock solution to both control and treated samples and incubate at 56°C for 45 min.

6. Remove samples from heat and allow cooling to room temperature.

7. Make a 55 mM Iodoacetamide stock solution and add 40 μl of this stock solution to both control and treated samples. Incubate at room temperature for 30 min.

8. The ratio of trypsin to sample should be 1:50 to 1:20 (1 mg trypsin to every 50–20 mg protein). Add the appropriate amount of trypsin to control and treated samples. Gently flick the tubes to mix.

9. Place the samples in 37°C water bath for 2 h and after 2 h, add an additional amount of trypsin to each sample, equal to the first amount added.

10. Continue to incubate at 37°C for 17–18 h to ensure complete digestion (see Note 10).

11. Trypsin digestion reaction can be stopped by freezing samples at −20°C, or 4 μl of glacial acetic acid can be added.

12. Reduce the volume of the samples to approximately 10 μl by vacuum concentration.

3.2. LC-MS/MS Analysis

1. LC-MS/MS analyses of protein digests are carried out using a linear quadrupole ion trap ThermoFinnigan LTQ mass spectrometer (San Jose, CA) equipped with a Michrom Paradigm MS4 HPLC, a SpectraSystems AS3000 autosampler, and a nanoelectrospray source (15). Peptides are eluted from a 15 cm pulled tip capillary column (100 μm I.D.× 360 μm O.D; 3–5 μm tip opening) packed with 7 cm Vydac C18 (Hesperia, CA) material (5 μm, 300 Å pore size), using a gradient of 0–65% solvent B (98% methanol/2% water/0.5% formic acid/0.01% trifluoroacetic acid) over a 60-min period at a flow rate of 350 nl/min. The LTQ electrospray positive mode spray voltage is set at 1.6 kV, and the capillary temperature at 180°C.

2. Dependent data scanning is performed by the Xcalibur v 1.4 software (16) with a default charge of 2, an isolation width of 1.5 amu, an activation amplitude of 35%, activation time of 30 ms, and a minimal signal of 100 ion counts. Global dependent data settings are as follows, reject mass width of 1.5 amu, dynamic exclusion enabled, exclusion mass width of 1.5 amu, repeat count of 1, repeat duration of 1 min, and exclusion

duration of 5 min. Scan event series includes one full scan with mass range 350–2,000 Da, followed by three dependent MS/MS scans of the most intense ion.

3.3. Data Analysis

1. Database Searching: Tandem MS spectra of peptides are analyzed with TurboSEQUEST™ v3.1, a program that allows the correlation of experimental tandem MS data with theoretical spectra generated from known protein sequences (17). The peak list (dta files) for the search is generated by Bioworks 3.1. Parent peptide mass error tolerance is set at 1.5 amu and fragment ion mass tolerance is set at 0.5 amu during the search. The criteria used for preliminary positive peptide identification are the same as previously described, namely peptide precursor ions with a +1 charge having an Xcorr > 1.0, +2 Xcorr > 2.5, and +3 Xcorr > 3.5. A dCn score > 0.08 and a fragment ion ratio of experimental/theoretical >50% were also used as filtering criteria for reliable matched peptide identification (18).

2. All matched peptides are confirmed by visual examination of the spectra. All spectra are searched against current ipiRAT v3.22 database from EMBL (see Note 11). Tandem MS spectra of peptides are also analyzed with X!Tandem (http://www.thegpm.org; version 2007.01.01.1), which is similar to Sequest, and correlates the MS/MS spectra with amino acid sequences in a user-specified NCBI database (19, 20). X!Tandem is set up to search a subset of the ipi.RAT.v3.31 database also assuming trypsin. Sequest is set up to search the ipi.RAT.v3.31.fasta database assuming the digestion enzyme trypsin. Sequest and X!Tandem are searched with a fragment ion mass tolerance of 0.50 Da and a parent ion tolerance of 1.5 Da. Modifications including +105 (BQ), and +268 (NAC-BQ), at Lys, Arg, and Glu are specified in Sequest and X!Tandem as variable modifications (see Note 12).

3. P-Mod software is used to confirm X!Tandem and Sequest data, including the identification of spectra displaying characteristics of 1,4-BQ or NAC-BQ adductions. This program is extremely beneficial when using pure proteins and can provide reliable data without use of additional programs; however, having multiple routes to find the same data is preferred. The protein sequence of cytochrome c, CYC_HORSE P00004, is obtained from the NCBI database (http://www.ncbi.nlm.nih.gov). P-Mod is an algorithm that screens data files for MS/MS spectra corresponding to peptide sequences in a search list. Modification of the primary peptide sequence shifts the peptide mass, which may be experimentally observed as a difference between the measured mass of the modified peptide precursor ion (adjusted for charge state) and the predicted mass of the unmodified peptide. The mass shift also will be observed in the m/z values of fragment ions containing the modified

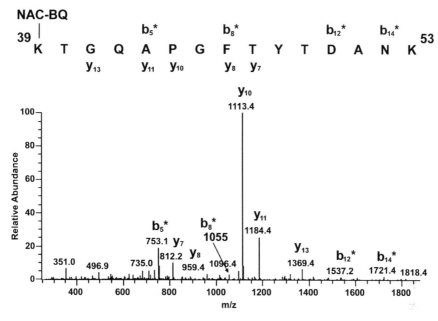

NAC-BQ

39   b₅*   b₈*   b₁₂*   b₁₄*   53
K T G Q A P G F T Y T D A N K

y₁₃   y₁₁ y₁₀   y₈ y₇

Fig. 1. LC-MS/MS spectra of the NAC-BQ modified cytochrome *c* peptide. The LC-MS/MS raw data was analyzed by Sequest, X!Tandem, and P-Mod, followed by manual validation. The peptide [39]KTGCQAPGFTYTDANK[53] was identified with a 268-Da adduct on K[39].

amino acid. Scores with *P*-values greater than 0.01 were discarded as false positives (*21*). Upon collision-induced dissociation (CID) of the peptides, b- and y-ion fragments are generated: the b-ion series represents cleavage of the peptide bond with charge retention on the N-terminal piece, and y-ions result from cleavage of the amide bonds with charge retention on the C-terminal piece (*22*). Manual validation of MS/MS spectra was then used to confirm peptide sequence and adduct mass location. Peptides identified as being adducted by both X!Tandem, Sequest, and P-Mod were then manually validated using the program IonGen (*7*). IonGen generates theoretical b- and y-ions for user-specified peptides containing an adduct. This program facilitates faster, more accurate validation of adducted peptides. Only adducted peptides identified from X!Tandem, P-Mod, and IonGen, are used. Figure 1 shows a NAC-BQ-modified peptide from cytochrome *c*.

4. Notes

1. The 2 M DTT stock solution can be stored at –20°C for 4 weeks or can be made fresh for each use.

2. Alternative pure proteins can be used to study these site-specific quinone–thioether modifications; however, cytochrome *c* was

used here because its small size and structural characterization is ideal for mass spectral analysis.

3. A buffering system is used that consists of 10 mM Tris–HCl, pH 7.5, and NAC-BQ adduct formation is much more efficient in this buffer than in water. This is likely because many of the NAC-BQ-adducts form on Lys residues and these residues are more nucleophilic in buffered systems. NH_4HCO_3 (0.1 M, pH 8.0) is used by other researchers doing proteomics work because this is the ideal buffer for trypsin digestion; however, because of the high salt concentration in addition to the high pH of this buffer, the N-acetylcysteine bond to the benzoquinone ring is not stable in these conditions for periods of time exceeding 6 h. This compound degradation results in adduction profiles that may not be accurate, and may also inhibit certain residues, including Cys, as being target residues for modifications by these compounds.

4. The reaction can proceed for longer than 1 h; however, because these quinol–thioether compounds are not stable in high salt or high pH conditions for periods of time exceeding 6 h, it is safe to keep the reaction under 1 h and the adduction efficiency will be sufficient. Therefore, sample preparation time is critical for accurate adduct mass analysis. When the NAC-BQ compound is stable, it will form adducts with a mass of 268 Da. Following NAC-BQ adduction and thioether bond elimination due to microenvironment instability, the resulting adduct mass will be 105 Da. This mass is indicative of the benzoquinone ring (7).

5. This centrifugation procedure can be modified depending upon whether it is conducted at room temperature or 4°C, where the centrifugation can be extended in conditions of 4°C. Additionally, to ensure complete removal of excess NAC-BQ, the reaction mixture can be washed repeatedly with buffer and further centrifugation can be conducted.

6. Alternative methods can be used to remove excess NAC-BQ, including dialysis and HPLC purification; however, the method used here seems to minimize sample preparation time which is critical for use with quinol–thioether adduction studies.

7. It is important to make sure that all samples are free of detergents before proceeding with trypsin digestion and this can be achieved by protein precipitation methods.

8. Additional enzymes can be used for protein digestion, including chymotrypsin, endoproteinase Asp-N, and Glu-C, all of which have specific pH ranges where they work best. Trypsin is the most common choice for proteomic procedures, so this is described here.

9. Reduction steps improve digestion efficiency by preventing disulfide formation, which helps the protein to be unfolded, exposing more tryptic sites for digestion. In cases like cytochrome c, reduction is not necessary, as there are no free cysteine residues present in the protein. The reduction and alkylation steps in this case can be skipped.

10. As stated previously, the quinone–thioether compounds have been found to be unstable in basic conditions, as well as conditions with high pH. As a result, when using compounds of this nature, the digestion procedure needs to be limited to approximately 3 h, which will minimize quinone–thioether compound exposure to the basic buffering system necessary for trypsin digestion. Efficient digestion can be accomplished in 3 h, especially when using a small pure protein such as cytochrome c.

11. Because cytochrome c used here is a pure protein, data analysis can be done against the cytochrome c database rather than the entire rat database. The trypsin is sequencing grade and there should not be much interference.

12. Again, as stated previously, the sample preparation can influence the adduction profile of these quinone–thioether compounds. Additionally, results have indicated that the microenvironment of the protein can also influence the adduction profile of these quinone–thioether compounds. As a result, after NAC-BQ adduction to cytochrome c, regions of the protein with higher pKa have directed the post-adduction chemistry from a full NAC-BQ adduct (268-Da adduct) to a 1,4-BQ adduct (105-Da adduct), indicating elimination of the thioether bond under these types of conditions (7). Also, additional modifications can be searched depending upon the residues of interest. Typically, cysteine is a target for modification; however, in the case of cytochrome c, there are no free cysteines, and as a result, this residue is not included in the modification list shown here. Modifications including oxidation of methionine residues and phosphorylation of serine or threonine residues can also be included.

Acknowledgments

This work was supported by GM070890 (SSL) and ES07091 (AAF). The authors acknowledge the support of the P30 ES06694 Southwest Environmental Health Sciences Center, in particular the Arizona Proteomics Consortium (APC). Special thanks go to Dr. George Tsaprailis, Director of the APC.

References

1. Yao, D., Taguchi, T., Matsumura, T., Pestell, R., Edelstein, D., Giardino, I., Suske, G., Rabbani, N., Thornalley, P.J., Sarthy, V.P., Hammes, H.P., and Brownlee, M. (2007) High glucose increases angiopoietin-2 transcription in microvascular endothelial cells through methylglyoxal modification of mSin3A. *J. Biol. Chem.* **282**, 31038–31045.

2. Carini, M., Aldini, G., and Facino, R.M. (2004) Mass spectrometry for detection of 4-hydroxy-trans-2-nonenal (HNE) adducts with peptides and proteins. *Mass Spectrom. Rev.* **23**, 281–305.

3. Halliwell, B. (2000) Lipid peroxidation, antioxidants and cardiovascular disease: how should we move forward? *Cardiovasc. Res.* **47**, 410–418.

4. Uchida, K., Kanematsu, M., Sakai, K., Matsuda, T., Hattori, N., Mizuno, Y., Suzuki, D., Miyata, T., Noguchi, N., Niki, E., and Osawa, T. (1998) Protein-bound acrolein: potential markers for oxidative stress. *Proc. Natl. Acad. Sci. U S A* **95**, 4882–4887.

5. Dalle-Donne, I., Carini, M., Vistoli, G., Gamberoni, L., Giustarini, D., Colombo, R., Maffei Facino, R., Rossi, R., Milzani, A., and Aldini, G. (2007) Actin Cys374 as a nucleophilic target of alpha,beta-unsaturated aldehydes. *Free Radic. Biol. Med.* **42**, 583–598.

6. Szapacs, M.E., Riggins, J.N., Zimmerman, L.J., and Liebler, D.C. (2006) Covalent adduction of human serum albumin by 4-hydroxy-2-nonenal: kinetic analysis of competing alkylation reactions. *Biochemistry* **45**, 10521–10528.

7. Fisher, A.A., Labenski, M.T., Malladi, S., Gokhale, V., Bowen, M.E., Milleron, R.S., Bratton, S.B., Monks, T.J., and Lau, S.S. (2007) Quinone electrophiles selectively adduct "electrophile binding motifs" within cytochrome c. *Biochemistry* **46**, 11090–11100.

8. Koen, Y.M., Yue, W., Galeva, N.A., Williams, T.D., and Hanzlik, R.P. (2006) Site-specific arylation of rat glutathione s-transferase A1 and A2 by bromobenzene metabolites *in vivo*. *Chem. Res. Toxicol.* **19**, 1426–1434.

9. Meier, B.W., Gomez, J.D., Zhou, A., and Thompson, J.A. (2005) Immunochemical and proteomic analysis of covalent adducts formed by quinone methide tumor promoters in mouse lung epithelial cell lines. *Chem. Res. Toxicol.* **18**, 1575–1585.

10. Person, M.D., Mason, D.E., Liebler, D.C., Monks, T.J., and Lau, S.S. (2005) Alkylation of cytochrome c by (glutathion-S-yl)-1,4-benzoquinone and iodoacetamide demonstrates compound-dependent site specificity. *Chem. Res. Toxicol.* **18**, 41–50.

11. Lindsey, R.H., Jr., Bender, R.P., and Osheroff, N. (2005) Effects of benzene metabolites on DNA cleavage mediated by human topoisomerase II alpha: 1,4-hydroquinone is a topoisomerase II poison. *Chem. Res. Toxicol.* **18**, 761–770.

12. Ross, D. (2000) The role of metabolism and specific metabolites in benzene-induced toxicity: evidence and issues. *J. Toxicol. Environ. Health A* **61**, 357–372.

13. Ruiz-Ramos, R., Cebrian, M.E., and Garrido, E. (2005) Benzoquinone activates the ERK/MAPK signaling pathway via ROS production in HL-60 cells. *Toxicology* **209**, 279–287.

14. Murty, V.S., and Penning, T.M. (1992) Characterization of mercapturic acid and glutathionyl conjugates of benzo[a]pyrene-7,8-dione by two-dimensional NMR. *Bioconjug. Chem.* **3**, 218–224.

15. Shevchenko, A., Wilm, M., Vorm, O., and Mann, M. (1996) Mass spectrometric sequencing of proteins silver-stained polyacrylamide gels. *Anal. Chem.* **68**, 850–858.

16. Andon, N.L., Hollingworth, S., Koller, A., Greenland, A.J., Yates, J.R., III, and Haynes, P.A. (2002) Proteomic characterization of wheat amyloplasts using identification of proteins by tandem mass spectrometry. *Proteomics* **2**, 1156–1168.

17. Yates, J.R., III, Eng, J.K., McCormack, A.L., and Schieltz, D. (1995) Method to correlate tandem mass spectra of modified peptides to amino acid sequences in the protein database. *Anal. Chem.* **67**, 1426–1436.

18. Cooper, B., Eckert, D., Andon, N.L., Yates, J.R., and Haynes, P.A. (2003) Investigative proteomics: identification of an unknown plant virus from infected plants using mass spectrometry. *J. Am. Soc. Mass Spectrom.* **14**, 736–741.

19. Craig, R., and Beavis, R.C. (2003) A method for reducing the time required to match protein sequences with tandem mass spectra. *Rapid Commun. Mass Spectrom.* **17**, 2310–2316.

20. Craig, R., Cortens, J.P., and Beavis, R.C. (2004) Open source system for analyzing, validating, and storing protein identification data. *J. Proteome Res.* **3**, 1234–1242.

21. Hansen, B.T., Davey, S.W., Ham, A.J., and Liebler, D.C. (2005) P-Mod: an algorithm and software to map modifications to peptide sequences using tandem MS data. *J. Proteome Res.* **4**, 358–368.

22. Standing, K.G. (2003) Peptide and protein de novo sequencing by mass spectrometry. *Curr. Opin. Struct. Biol.* **13**, 595–601.

Chapter 20

One-Dimensional Western Blotting Coupled to LC-MS/MS Analysis to Identify Chemical-Adducted Proteins in Rat Urine

Matthew T. Labenski, Ashley A. Fisher, Terrence J. Monks, and Serrine S. Lau

Abstract

The environmental toxicant hydroquinone (HQ) and its glutathione conjugates (GSHQs) cause renal cell necrosis via a combination of redox cycling and the covalent adduction of proteins within the S_3 segment of the renal proximal tubules in the outer stripe of the outer medulla (OSOM). Following administration of 2-(glutathion-S-yl)HQ (MGHQ) (400 µmol/kg, i.v., 2 h) to Long Evans (wild-type Eker) rats, Western analysis utilizing an antibody specific for quinol–thioether metabolites of HQ revealed the presence of large amounts of chemical–protein adducts in both the OSOM and urine. By aligning the Western blot film with a parallel gel stained for protein, we can isolate the adducted proteins for LC-MS/MS analysis. Subsequent database searching can identify the specific site(s) of chemical adduction within these proteins. Finally, a combination of software programs can validate the identity of the adducted peptides. The site-specific identification of covalently adducted and oxidized proteins is a prerequisite for understanding the biological significance of chemical-induced posttranslational modifications (PTMs) and their toxicological significance.

Key words: LC-MS/MS, Covalent modification, Quinones, Quinone–thioethers

1. Introduction

Hydroquinone (HQ) is an environmental toxicant found in some hair/skin products, as a food preservative in some countries, and as a byproduct of combustion, and it is a metabolite of both benzene and phenol. HQ is metabolized in the liver by CYP enzymes to 1,4-benzoquinone (1,4-BQ), followed by the reductive Michael addition of glutathione (GSH). Subsequent cycles of oxidation and

Jean-Charles Gautier (ed.), *Drug Safety Evaluation: Methods and Protocols*, Methods in Molecular Biology, vol. 691, DOI 10.1007/978-1-60761-849-2_20, © Springer Science+Business Media, LLC 2011

GSH addition result in the formation of multi-GSH substituted HQ–GSH conjugates, including 2,3,5-tris-(glutathion-*S*-yl)HQ (TGHQ), which is the most potent nephrotoxic metabolite of HQ. Upon uptake by the epithelial cells lining the S3 segment of the outer stripe of the outer medulla (OSOM), metabolites of TGHQ remain capable of redox cycling and of covalently adducting proteins, the combination of which results in proximal tubular necrosis (1). Because the dead and dying cells detach from the proximal tubule and the intracellular contents leak into the tubular lumen, the urine becomes semi-enriched of adducted proteins. Therefore, Long Evans rats treated with MGHQ were placed in metabolic cages and urine collected for a period of 2 h. Western blotting was performed on urinary proteins using an antibody specific for the quinol–thioether protein adducts (2). Because Western blot analysis revealed that urine contained more adducted proteins than tissue extracts from the OSOM (based on milligram total protein), urine was selected as the source for initially identifying protein targets of MGHQ and for searching specific amino acids within the protein that become covalently modified.

Using an antibody raised against 2-bromo-(*N*-acetylcystein-*S*-yl)HQ (BrHQ-NAC) protein adducts, we are able to align immunopositive bands from the Western blot film with protein-stained bands from gel electrophoresis to identify adducted proteins from urine of MGHQ-treated rats (3). Representative blots are shown in Fig. 1. Once these bands have been identified, they are excised from the stained gel and promptly digested with

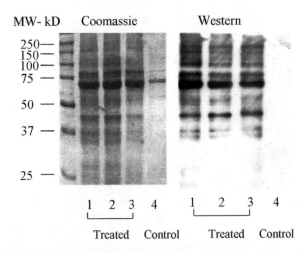

Fig. 1. Alignment of protein-stained gel with Western blot film. Parallel gels were performed; one for protein staining and the other for Western blotting. The first gel was stained for 1 h with Coomassie blue protein stain. The second gel was transferred to a PVDF membrane and then probed with an antibody specific to protein adducts that occur as a result of MGHQ treatment, anti-BrHQ-NAC. Both the stained protein gel and the Western blot film were aligned, and stained protein bands that correspond to immunopositive bands on the film were excised and digested with trypsin.

trypsin. Peptides are then extracted from the gel matrix and analyzed by tandem mass spectrometry coupled to liquid chromatography (LC-MS/MS). Analyzing the MS/MS data generated from the mass spectrometer requires at least one peptide matching program such as Sequest, X!Tandem, or MASCOT, but analysis with more than one of these programs is preferred. Such programs compare the various b and y ions generated from collision-induced dissociation of the peptide, to those predicted for known peptides from a user-specified database. A built-in feature of all of these programs is the ability to specify a mass addition on an amino acid; for example, +105 amu on Lys will prompt the program to search for native lysines as well as lysine +105 amu. This is generally used for common modifications such as oxidized methionines, but can also be used for chemical-mediated modifications such as a HQ adduct. Once the MS/MS-peptide matching software identifies a peptide as containing a chemical modification, that peptide must be validated both manually and by using supplementary software programs designed specifically for this purpose. By utilizing the above outlined strategy, it is possible to identify the specific site of the chemically mediated post-translational modification. Complementary techniques, such as computer modeling, can then be employed to determine the structural consequences of the chemical adduction, and biochemical analyses used to determine whether any functional consequences arise as a consequence of the structural modification. This technique can also be applied to more complex matrices such as tissue homogenates or cell lysates by running the sample on a 2D gel instead of the 1D gel presented in this chapter. The general work flow for these studies is shown in Fig. 2.

2. Materials

2.1. Protein Band(s) from Gel Electrophoresis (In Vivo/Complex Sample)

2.1.1. One-Dimensional SDS–Polyacrylamide Gel Electrophoresis

1. Separating buffer: 1.5 M Tris–HCl, 14 mM sodium dodecyl sulfate, pH to 8.8 with HCl. Store at room temperature.
2. Stacking buffer: 0.5 M Tris–HCl, 14 mM sodium dodecyl sulfate, pH to 6.8 with HCl. Store at room temperature.
3. 40:1 Acrylamide:Bis solution (BioRad). Store at 4°C.
4. N,N,N',N'-Tetramethylethylenediamine (TEMED) (BioRad).
5. Ammonium persulfate (Fischer Scientific).
6. 50% Sucrose solution (Sigma).
7. Running buffer: 25 mM Tris–HCl (Sigma), 192 mM glycine (Sigma), 0.1% sodium dodecyl sulfate (SDS) (Sigma), pH to 8.3 with HCl. Store at room temperature.
8. Running unit: Hoefer SE 600.

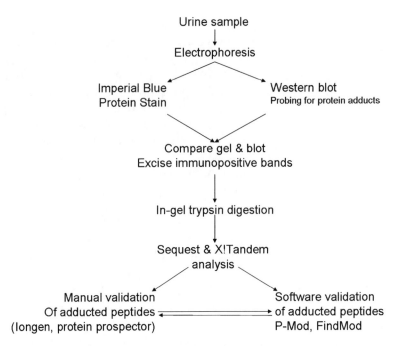

Fig. 2. General schematic for site-specific identification of immunopositive protein adducts excreted in urine of rats treated i.v. with MGHQ. Immediately after i.v. treatment with MGHQ, the Long Evans rats were placed in metabolism cages and urine was collected for 2 h. Urine was spun at 14,000 × *g* for 10 min to pellet urinary particulates. Urinary proteins were then diluted in sample buffer. Parallel gels were then run; one for Western blotting with anti-BrHQ-NAC and the other for protein staining with Imperial or Coomassive blue stain. The film from the Western blot is then aligned with the stained gel, immunopositive protein bands are excised, and the protein digested with trypsin. The peptides are then analyzed via MS/MS. Raw data from mass spectrometry are then analyzed using different peptide matching software programs searching for adducts on specific types of amino acids, i.e., +105 (HQ) on Lys, Arg, and Cys. Peptides found to be adducted are then validated manually using Iongen and Protein Prospector, and with other software programs, such as P-Mod and FindMod.

9. Glass plates: 18 × 16 cm (Hoefer).

10. Spacers: 1.5 mm (Hoefer).

11. Comb: 1.5 mm, 10 lanes (Hoefer).

12. Sample buffer: Laemmli sample buffer 2× (Bio-Rad, Hercules, CA).

2.1.2. Western Blot
for Protein Adducts

1. Polyvinylidene difluoride membrane (PVDF) (Pierce).

2. Methanol (Sigma).

3. Transfer buffer: 200 ml methanol, 700 ml MilliQ H_2O, 100 ml 10× Tris/glycine buffer (BioRad). Store at room temperature.

4. Sandwich cassette (BioRad).

5. Sponges (BioRad).

6. Filter paper (Biorad).

7. 0.02% Polyvinyl alcohol (PVA) (w/v) (Sigma). Prepare fresh with each use.

8. Tris–Saline buffer: 0.02 M Tris–HCl, 0.137 M NaCl, pH to 7.6 with HCl. Store at room temperature.

9. Block buffer: 5% non-fat milk in Tris–Saline buffer (Carnation). Prepare fresh with each use.

10. Wash buffer: 0.005% Casein, 0.154 M NaCl, 0.01 M Tris–HCl, 0.0005 M thimerosal, pH to 7.6 with HCl. Store at 4°C. Solution expires after 2 weeks.

11. Detergent buffer: use wash buffer with the addition of 0.02% sodium dodecyl sulfate (v/v) and 0.1% Triton X-100 (v/v) (Sigma). Store at 4°C. Solution expires after 2 weeks.

12. Primary antibody: generated in-house (3).

13. Secondary antibody: goat anti-rabbit IgG-HRP (Santa Cruz Biotechnology, SC-2030). Store at 4°C.

14. Electro-chemiluminescence Western Blotting Detecting Reagents (GE Health sciences). Store at 4°C.

2.1.3. Gel Staining

1. Stain: 45% deionized H_2O, 45% methanol, 10% acetic acid, 0.04% Coomassie blue G-250 (Sigma).

2. Wash: 45% deionized H_2O, 45% methanol, 10% acetic acid.

2.1.4. In-Gel Digestion Sample Preparation

1. Acetonitrile (ACN)/deionized water.

2. Digestion buffer: 100 mM NH_4HCO_3.

3. Disulfide reduction: 10 mM DTT in 100 mM NH_4HCO_3.

4. Thiol alkylation: 55 mM iodoacetamide in 100 mM NH_4HCO_3.

5. Digestion: trypsin-modified sequencing grade (Promega), 20 µg lyophilized powder. Store at –20°C. Dilute to 0.1 µg/µl.

6. Digestion quench: 2% trifluoroacetic acid (TFA).

7. Peptide extraction solutions: 30% ACN 0.1% TFA and 60% ACN 0.1%TFA.

3. Methods

In order to fully benefit from this strategy, it is essential to understand what types of metabolites are formed from the parent chemical, the relative abundance of each metabolite, which of the metabolites are capable of protein adduction, what amino acids are potential targets, and the precise molecular weight of each modified amino acid. Some of the above variables may be determined by *in vitro* studies, as outlined in the previous chapters. Once the above variables have been addressed and a full understanding of the metabolic fate of the chemical is elucidated, one can then select the most abundant or likely toxic metabolite with which to raise an antibody against. Antibodies directed at chemical adducts are generally not commercially available and, therefore, must be created in-house or from an antibody contract laboratory. These antibodies typically have a high background and unique characteristics compared to the more common antibodies generated against a protein or peptide. For these reasons, the Western blot protocol described below requires a more stringent washing procedure and the use of a chemical (polyvinyl alcohol) and a protein (5% milk) block. Such protocols will necessarily vary depending upon the nature of the raised antibody, the protocol described below being the best for the antibody generated against BrHQ-NAC, and purified against 2-(*N*-acetylcystein-*S*-yl)HQ (NAC-HQ).

The most challenging part of this protocol is exactly how the investigator interprets the enormous amount of data generated by the mass spectrometer from either a simple, 1-protein analysis, or from the analysis of a complex sample that contains multiple proteins. To address this challenge, the use of software programs capable of matching MS/MS spectra to peptides is necessary. There are a number of software programs that can perform this task, including Sequest, X!Tandem, and MASCOT. These programs use different matching algorithms, and for the most accurate and rigorous results, it is recommended that more than one program be used to analyze the same set of data. Once the data have been analyzed with these programs, and adducted peptides with reasonable scores have been identified, the data should next be validated to ensure that the identified adduct is a valid hit, and not an artifact of the analysis. There are several programs that can assist in this validation, including P-Mod and FindMod (http://ca.expasy.org/tools/findmod/). These programs will parse the raw data for the user-specified peptide and determine whether or not it is adducted. After the adducted peptide has been identified and validated, it is then reasonable to validate manually the peptide using programs such as Iongen (4) or Protein Prospector (http://prospector.ucsf.edu) to generate the theoretical ions that can be matched to the spectra of interest.

3.1. One-Dimensional SDS–Polyacrylamide Gel Electrophoresis

This section describes one-dimensional SDS–polyacrylamide gel electrophoresis (1D-GE) for the Hoeffer SE-600 system with 11×14 cm gels, but these instructions can easily be modified to fit other electrophoresis systems.

1. Thoroughly clean two 16×20 cm glass plates and two 1.5-mm thick spacers (19 mm by 16 cm) with distilled water. Dry the equipment using wipes and check that there are no visible particles or lint on the glass plates or spacers. It is of extreme importance that the glass plates be as clean as possible. Once clean, assemble the plates in the gel pouring apparatus.

2. A 10%, 1.5-mm thick gel is typically used to maximize protein load and resolution for a broad range of molecular weights, which is critical for later mass spectrometric analysis. Prepare a 10% gel by mixing 8.8 ml of 4× separating buffer with 8.813 ml of 40:1 acrylamide:bis solution (BioRad), 18.21 ml of MiliQ H_2O, 3.76 ml of 50% sucrose, 352.5 μl of 10% ammonium persulfate, and 23.5 μl of TEMED (see Note 1). Pour the separating gel, leaving a 1-cm gap between the top of the separating gel and the bottom of the comb. Gently add isobutanol to the top of the gel and let the gel polymerize for 1 h.

3. Pour off the isobutanol and dry the space between the two glass plates. Prepare a 2× stacking gel by mixing 1.5 ml of 4× stacking buffer with 1 ml of 40:1 acrylamide:bis solution (BioRad), 6.4 ml of H_2O, 100 μl of 10% ammonium persulfate, and 20 μl of TEMED (see Note 1). Pour the stacking gel and insert a 10-well comb between the two glass plates. Let the stacking gel polymerize for 30 min. Carefully remove the comb and place the gel in the gel unit. Fill the unit with running buffer making sure to wash out each well thoroughly with running buffer.

4. Dilute samples with water to normalize volume and then add sample buffer in a 1:1 ratio. For the stained gel, 300 μg of protein will be loaded per lane. For the Western blot, 150 μg of protein will be loaded per lane (see Note 2).

5. Fill the gel running apparatus to fill line with running buffer and close the lid after connecting electrodes. Connect the electrode ends to power supply and run at 25 V constant till dye front runs through the stacking gel. Increase voltage to 100 V constant through the resolving gel and stop power once the dye front is at the bottom or just run off the bottom of the gel.

6. Remove gel from glass plates into a glass container and rinse with ddH_2O 3×5 min to remove excess SDS and other contaminants that will interfere with the staining process. Remove excess H_2O from the gel-containing glass container and cover gel with Imperial Blue Gel Stain and shake lightly for 1 h. Pour excess stain off and add water down the side of the container careful not to damage the gel, and shake lightly for 10 min. Continue this process until the background is sufficiently diminished. Bands of interest can now be excised in preparation of digest and LC-MS/MS analysis.

3.2. Western Blot

1. Cut PVDF and blotting paper to a size slightly larger than the gel. Immerse PVDF membrane into 100% methanol for 1 min to activate it, and then remove from methanol and place in milliQ water for 1 min, shaking by hand to remove excess methanol. Finally, place membrane, blotting paper, and two sponges in transfer buffer until ready to use (see Notes 3 and 4).

2. Open the cassette and place the black half down in the transfer buffer with the red part toward you. Place a soaked sponge on the black part of the cassette (see Note 5). Then place blotting paper followed by the gel. Quickly place the wet PVDF membrane over the gel and immediately add a wet blotting paper on top of the membrane. Add some transfer buffer to the top of the "sandwich" to ensure it remains soaked. Now add the final sponge to the sandwich and close the cassette. Leave submerged in transfer buffer until ready.

3. Transfer: Place cassette in transfer box and quickly add transfer buffer to the box at fill line. Connect to power supply and transfer for 1.5 h at 100 V constant (see Note 6).

4. Block: Once transfer is complete, remove cassette, open, remove PVDF membrane, quickly place it in 0.02% PVA, shake by hand for 1 min, pour off, and add 5% milk to cover the membrane (see Note 7). Incubate either at room temperature for 1 h, or at 4°C overnight.

5. Primary antibody: After blocking, pour off milk solution and quickly add antibody diluted to proper concentration to the membrane and incubate at room temperature for 90 min.

6. Wash: Pour off primary antibody solution and rinse the membrane with milliQ water three times, then add the detergent buffer to cover the membrane and rotate slowly for 5 min. Pour off detergent buffer and rinse the membrane three times with milliQ water. Then add washing buffer to the membrane and incubate for 5 min rotating slowly. Repeat the washing buffer and wash one more time.

7. Secondary antibody: After the final wash, add the secondary antibody after appropriate dilution in wash buffer. Incubate for 90 min at room temperature rotating slowly. At the end of this incubation, repeat wash from step 6.

8. Developing: Pick the membrane up with tweezers from a corner and dab on opposite corner on a paper towel to remove excess wash buffer. Place on Saran wrap with the protein side up and add the mixed ECL solution (1:1, Reagent A, Reagent B) and incubate for 1 min. Lift the membrane off the wrap with tweezers by the corner and dab corner on a paper towel to remove excess ECL solution and place on a clean Saran wrap. Fold the Saran wrap over to cover the protein side and place in a membrane cassette. Develop the film.

9. Using the ladder, line up stained gel and Western blot film to determine which bands are immunopositive and thus adducted. Cut out bands that are immunopositive.

3.3. In-Gel Digest of Protein Band (1D-GE)

1. Generally, adducted proteins are low in abundance and keratin (found in skin and hair) is a major contaminant capable of suppressing the signal of the protein contained within the band. In order to avoid this, bench top, tips, and tubes must be as clean as possible. Gloves and laboratory coat should always be worn while handling the samples and it may also be necessary to wear a hair cap and work under a hood.

2. Gel bands/spots are washed with 100 µl of ddH$_2$O 2 × 10 min (see Note 8). After incubation, ddH$_2$O is removed, and 40 µl of 50% ACN is added, the tube incubated for 15 min, and removed. Then 40 µl of 100% ACN is added to the tube containing the band/spot and incubated for 15 min or until band becomes white and sticky. Remove ACN, add 40 µl of 100 mM ammonium bicarbonate, and incubate for 5 min. Then add 40 µl of 100% ACN and incubate for an additional 15 min. Pull off excess solution and dry gel pieces under vacuum centrifugation until bands are very dry (see Note 9).

3. Let samples return to room temperature after drying. Then add 40 µl of 10 mM DTT solution to each band/spot and incubate in 55°C water bath for 45 min (see Note 10). After incubation, remove from the water bath and allow samples to return to room temperature. Remove excess solution, add 40 µl of 55 mM IAA solution, and incubate at room temperature in the dark for 30 min. Remove excess solution, add 40 µl of 100 mM ammonium bicarbonate, incubate for 5 min, and then add 40 µl of 100% ACN and incubate for an additional 15 min. Pull off excess solution and dry as described above.

4. Add 40 µl of trypsin containing digestion solution and incubate on ice for 45 min (see Note 11). Remove excess trypsin containing digestion solution, add 40–60 µl of digestion buffer (without trypsin), and incubate at 37°C for 12–16 h.

5. After incubation, add 10 µl of 2% TFA to the digestion mixture to acidify reaction and thereby quenching the trypsin, and remove supernatant to a clean tube. Cover gel band/spot with 0.1% TFA in water and place the tube in a floating rack in a sonicating bath for 30 min to begin peptide extraction. Remove the supernatant and combine with previous solution. Repeat previous step by adding 30% ACN 0.1% TFA, sonicating for 30 min, and combining the supernatants. Repeat the above step for a final time with 60% ACN 1% TFA. Pool all supernatants for each sample and dry volume down to ~10 µl in preparation for mass spectrometric analysis. The samples can be stored at –20°C for short term or at –80°C for long term.

3.4. LC-MS/MS Analysis

1. LC-MS/MS analyses of protein digests are carried out using a linear quadrupole ion trap ThermoFinnigan LTQ mass spectrometer (San Jose, CA) equipped with a Michrom Paradigm MS4 HPLC, a SpectraSystems AS3000 autosampler, and a nanoelectrospray source (5).

2. Peptides are eluted from a 15-cm pulled tip capillary column (100 μm I.D.×360 μm O.D; 3–5 μm tip opening) packed with 7-cm Vydac C18 (Hesperia, CA) material (5 μm, 300 Å pore size), using a gradient of 0–65% solvent B (98% methanol/2% water/0.5% formic acid/0.01% trifluoroacetic acid) over a 60-min period at a flow rate of 350 nl/min. The LTQ electrospray positive mode spray voltage is set at 1.6 kV and the capillary temperature at 180°C.

3. Dependent data scanning is performed using the Xcalibur v 1.4 software (6) with a default charge of 2, an isolation width of 1.5 amu, an activation amplitude of 35%, an activation time of 30 ms, and a minimal signal of 100 ion counts. Global dependent data settings are as follows: reject mass width of 1.5 amu, dynamic exclusion enabled, exclusion mass width of 1.5 amu, repeat count of 1, repeat duration of 1 min, and exclusion duration of 5 min. Scan event series include one full scan with mass range 350–2,000 Da, followed by three dependent MS/MS scans of the most intense ion.

3.5. Data Analysis

1. Tandem MS spectra of peptides are analyzed with TurboSEQUEST™ v3.1 (7). The peak list (data files) for the search is generated by Bioworks 3.1. Parent peptide mass error tolerance is set at 1.5 amu and fragment ion mass tolerance is set at 0.5 amu during the search. The criteria that are used for a preliminary positive peptide identification are the same as previously described, namely, peptide precursor ions with a +1 charge having a Xcorr >1.8, +2 Xcorr > 2.5, and +3 Xcorr > 3.5. A dCn score > 0.08 and a fragment ion ratio of experimental/theoretical >50% were also used as filtering criteria for reliable matched peptide identification (8).

2. All matched peptides are confirmed by visual examination of the spectra. All spectra are searched against the ipiRAT v3.22 database from EMBL downloaded on October 06, 2006. At the time of the search, the ipiRAT protein database from EMBL contained 41,336 proteins. Tandem MS spectra of peptides are also analyzed with X!Tandem (http://www.thegpm.org; version 2007.01.01.1). X!Tandem is set up to search a subset of the ipi.RAT.v3.31 database also assuming trypsin. Sequest is set up to search the ipi.RAT.v3.31.fasta database (41,251 protein entries), assuming the digestion enzyme trypsin. Sequest and X!Tandem are searched with a fragment ion mass tolerance of 0.5 Da and a parent ion toler-

ance of 1.5 Da. Oxidation of methionine, iodoacetamide derivative of cysteine, +105 (HQ), +268 (NAC-BQ), +226 (CSHQ) at Lys, Arg, and Glu are specified in Sequest and X!Tandem as variable modifications.

4. Notes

1. Do not add APS and TEMED until right before pouring the gel as the gel will start to polymerize as soon as they are added.

2. Using the 2:1 ratio for loading protein for either the stained gel or Western blot, respectively, will ensure that immunopositive bands will be visible and comparable with the imperial blue stained gel, and that there will be enough protein present in each band for protein identification. If this experiment is run on a mini gel, protein concentrations must be adjusted to ensure good resolution.

3. It is extremely important not to let the PVDF membrane dry once it has been wet as it will interfere with the protein transfer. Drying of the membrane will appear as streaking or lines running across it. If it dries before the transfer has begun, repeat the activation step. If it dries after the transfer, it must be soaked in 1% (v/v) Tween20 in TBS for 1 h for mixing or until streaks disappear.

4. This process should be carried out about 10 min before the gel electrophoresis is completed. This step should be continuous; where once the electrophoresis is completed, the transfer should begin immediately.

5. When preparing for the transfer, everything including sponges and blotting paper must remain wet with transfer buffer and without the presence of air bubbles. Dryness and bubbles will interfere with the transfer.

6. The voltage may never actually reach the 100 V it was set to.

7. Be careful not to pour any liquid directly onto the membrane; instead, pour down the side of the container in which the membrane is contained in.

8. For all of the steps presented in Subheading 3.32, the band/spot should be submerged completely and volumes can be adjusted accordingly.

9. It is critical that the gel bands are completely dry. This usually takes around 15 min of vacuum centrifugation is obvious when the band/spot is no longer stuck to the side of the tube, and makes a "rattle" sound when shaken.

10. Both the DTT and IAA solutions and incubation of band/spots with these solutions should be protected from the light. This can be achieved by simply covering with aluminum foil.

11. If band/spot absorbs entire 40 μl of trypsin containing digestion solution, add an additional 20–40 μl.

Acknowledgments

This work was supported by GM070890 (SSL) and ES07091 (AAF). The authors acknowledge the support of the P30 ES06694 Southwest Environmental Health Sciences Center, in particular the Arizona Proteomics Consortium (APC). Our special thanks to Dr. George Tsaprailis, Director of the APC.

References

1. Lau, S. S., Monks, T. J., Everitt, J. I., Kleymenova, E., and Walker, C. L. (2001) Carcinogenicity of a nephrotoxic metabolite of the "nongenotoxic" carcinogen hydroquinone, *Chem Res Toxicol* **14**, 25–33.

2. Kleiner, H. E., Jones, T. W., Monks, T. J., and Lau, S. S. (1998) Immunochemical analysis of quinol–thioether-derived covalent protein adducts in rodent species sensitive and resistant to quinol–thioether-mediated nephrotoxicity, *Chem Res Toxicol* **11**, 1291–1300.

3. Kleiner, H. E., Rivera, M. I., Pumford, N. R., Monks, T. J., and Lau, S. S. (1998) Immunochemical detection of quinol–thioether-derived protein adducts, *Chem Res Toxicol* **11**, 1283–1290.

4. Fisher, A. A., Labenski, M. T., Malladi, S., Gokhale, V., Bowen, M. E., Milleron, R. S., Bratton, S. B., Monks, T. J., and Lau, S. S. (2007) Quinone electrophiles selectively adduct "electrophile binding motifs" within cytochrome c, *Biochemistry* **46**, 11090–11100.

5. Shevchenko, A., Wilm, M., Vorm, O., and Mann, M. (1996) Mass spectrometric sequencing of proteins silver-stained polyacrylamide gels, *Anal Chem* **68**, 850–858.

6. Andon, N. L., Hollingworth, S., Koller, A., Greenland, A. J., Yates, J. R., III, and Haynes, P. A. (2002) Proteomic characterization of wheat amyloplasts using identification of proteins by tandem mass spectrometry, *Proteomics* **2**, 1156–1168.

7. Yates, J. R., III, Eng, J. K., McCormack, A. L., and Schieltz, D. (1995) Method to correlate tandem mass spectra of modified peptides to amino acid sequences in the protein database, *Anal Chem* **67**, 1426–1436.

8. Cooper, B., Eckert, D., Andon, N. L., Yates, J. R., and Haynes, P. A. (2003) Investigative proteomics: identification of an unknown plant virus from infected plants using mass spectrometry, *J Am Soc Mass Spectrom* **14**, 736–741.

Chapter 21

Identification of Chemical-Adducted Proteins in Urine by Multi-dimensional Protein Identification Technology (LC/LC–MS/MS)

Matthew T. Labenski, Ashley A. Fisher, Terrence J. Monks, and Serrine S. Lau

Abstract

Recent technological advancements in mass spectrometry facilitate the detection of chemical-induced posttranslational modifications (PTMs) that may alter cell signaling pathways or alter the structure and function of the modified proteins. To identify such protein adducts (Kleiner et al., Chem Res Toxicol 11:1283–1290, 1998), multi-dimensional protein identification technology (MuDPIT) has been utilized. MuDPIT was first described by Link et al. as a new technique useful for protein identification from a complex mixture of proteins (Link et al., Nat Biotechnol 17:676–682, 1999). MuDPIT utilizes two different HPLC columns to further enhance peptide separation, increasing the number of peptide hits and protein coverage. The technology is extremely useful for proteomes, such as the urine proteome, samples from immunoprecipitations, and 1D gel bands resolved from a tissue homogenate or lysate. In particular, MuDPIT has enhanced the field of adduct hunting for adducted peptides, since it is more capable of identifying lesser abundant peptides, such as those that are adducted, than the more standard LC–MS/MS. The site-specific identification of covalently adducted proteins is a prerequisite for understanding the biological significance of chemical-induced PTMs and the subsequent toxicological response they elicit.

Key words: MuDPIT, Covalent modification, Quinone, Quinol–thioether

1. Introduction

A number of xenobiotics are capable of giving rise to covalently adducted proteins within the kidney. The presence of such covalently modified proteins is frequently accompanied by the development of renal toxicity. Chemicals such as mycophenolic acid (1), S-(1,1,2,2-tetrafluoroethyl)-l-cysteine (2), and glutathione (GSH) conjugates of hydroquinone (HQ) all exert their toxic

Jean-Charles Gautier (ed.), *Drug Safety Evaluation: Methods and Protocols*, Methods in Molecular Biology, vol. 691,
DOI 10.1007/978-1-60761-849-2_21, © Springer Science+Business Media, LLC 2011

effects on the kidney concomitant with the presence of covalently adducted proteins (3, 4). In addition to covalently adducting proteins within the S3 segment of the proximal tubule, GSH conjugates of HQ, including 2-(glutathion-S-yl)HQ, maintain the ability to redox cycle. The combination of these insults contributes to the ensuing cell and tissue necrosis. Moreover, because the targeted cells line the tubular lumen, dead and dying cells detach from the basement membrane and are sloughed into tubular fluid, resulting in the presence of both adducted and native proteins in tubular fluid, and ultimately in urine. Thus, urine is a perfect medium for the application of multi-dimensional protein identification technology (MuDPIT).

For any experiment generating samples that will be analyzed by mass spectroscopy, it is recommended that that sample be cleaned of any excess salt, small molecules, or other contaminants that may interfere with either protein digestion or the mass spectroscopic analysis. We have found that using a gravity-flow size exclusion column, followed by lyophilization, provides an appropriate level of sample clean-up. For experiments described herein, a solution digestion using trypsin was utilized. Following protein digestion and concentration of the peptide solution, the sample is then loaded onto the first HPLC column (strong cation exchange (SCX)) in preparation for MuDPIT analysis. MuDPIT utilizes two degrees of peptide separation, increasing the amount of peptide matches and protein coverage. In combination with data-dependent MS-MS scanning, more peptide ions are sampled and sequenced; relative to LC–MS/MS, this results in greater protein coverage per protein identified. Raw MS/MS data are analyzed using the matching correlation algorithm Sequest (5). The Sequest data output is then analyzed using Scaffold, a program that runs X!Tandem (6) on the Sequest output to validate identified peptides, and which also performs protein and peptide statistical analysis. Once modified peptides are identified, visual inspection and validation of the spectra are suggested, followed by further conformational analysis with a program such as P-Mod or FindMod. The larger the data set, the higher the likelihood of a false positive; it is, therefore, important to emphasize the use of multiple programs to validate the data.

2. Materials

2.1. Size Exclusion

1. PD-10 Desalting columns, code no. 17-0851-01 (GE Healthcare).

2.2. Solution Digest

1. Dithiothreitol (DTT), iodoacetamide, and ammonium bicarbonate (NH_4HCO_3) (Sigma).

2. 2 M DTT stock solution: 154.3 mg of DTT in 500 µl of deionized distilled water (see Note 1).

3. DTT solution for reduction: 5 µl of 2 M DTT in 1 ml of 0.1 M NH_4HCO_3.

4. Iodoacetamide stock solution: 10 mg in 1 ml of 0.1 M NH_4HCO_3.

5. Trypsin-modified sequencing grade (Promega): 20 µg of lyophilized powder. Store at –20°C. Dilute to 0.1 µg/µl and can be stored in solution at –20°C for several weeks.

2.3. MuDPIT Analysis

1. Silica tubing O.D. 363 µm, I.D. 250 µm (Polymicro, Phoenix, AZ) for strong cation exchange column.

2. Silica tubing O.D. 363 µm, I.D. 100 µm (Polymicro, Phoenix, AZ) for C18 column.

3. SCX resin, 5 µm Whatman partisphere.

4. C18 reverse phase (RP) resin, 5 µm Vydac.

5. HPLC grade methanol.

6. Compressed nitrogen tank with regulator, connected to a "bomb."

2.4. Mobile Phase

1. Mobile phase A: 10% methanol/0.5% formic acid, 0.01% TFA.

2. Mobile phase B: 98% methanol/0.5% formic acid, 0.01% TFA.

3. Mobile phase C: 10% methanol/0.5% formic acid, 0.01% TFA.

4. Mobile phase D: 500 mM ammonium acetate/10% methanol/ 0.5% formic acid, 0.01% TFA.

3. Methods

The main feature of MuDPIT is the use of two different types of HPLC separation columns; one made of strong cation exchange material and the second column composed of C18 material. Acidified peptides are loaded onto the cation exchange column, where they bind. A stepwise gradient of increasing salt steps will elute the peptides from the first column, when they will then pass into the second, C18 column. Prior to the next salt elution step, an organic gradient is run, which results in the release of peptides from the C18 column at various concentrations of the organic phase. The flow is in line with a nano-ESI source into the mass spectrometer. After the organic gradient is completed, another salt-based elution is performed, and the process is repeated as many times as necessary. Simple matrices, such as urine or a semi-enriched sample from either immunoaffinity or

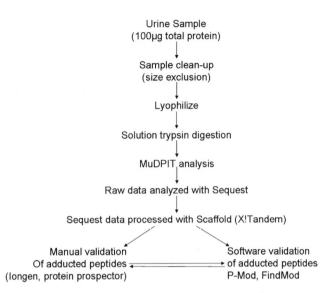

Fig. 1. General schematic for site-specific identification of quinol–thioether adducted proteins from the semi-complex urine proteome from rats treated i.v. with MGHQ. 100 µg of urinary proteins were cleaned up by passing through a size-exclusion PD-10 column, followed by lyophilizing to dryness. Protein was then reconstituted in digestion buffer and digested with trypsin. Peptides were then loaded onto the mass spectrometer for MuDPIT analysis. Raw data from the mass spectrometry was first analyzed for both adducted and native peptides with Sequest. The Sequest output was then compared and validated using Scaffold (combines X!Tandem and Peptide Profit algorithms with SEQUEST). All adducted peptides were then validated both manually using IonGen and/or protein prospector, and with other software programs (P-Mod, FindMod).

tag-affinity, are best suited for MuDPIT analyses, although there has also been much success with more complex matrices. A general work flow for this set of experiments is shown in Fig. 1.

3.1. Size Exclusion

1. Equilibrate PD-10 desalting column with 25 ml of water and discard the flow through (see Note 1).

2. Dilute protein sample to 2.5 ml and add to the column. Disregard flow through.

3. Elute protein from column by adding 3.5 ml of water to the top. Collect flow through and freeze at −20°C immediately.

4. Lyophilize sample till dry.

3.2. Solution Digestion

1. Reconstitute samples in 100 µl of 0.1 M NH_4HCO_3 (see Note 2).

2. Most successful protein digests are conducted using trypsin as the proteolytic enzyme, with 50 mM Tris–HCl or 50–100 mM NH_4HCO_3 as the buffering system. These buffers

are usually in the pH range of 7.4–8.0. This is ideal for trypsin digestion to occur (see Note 3).

3. For proteins with disulfide bonds, a reduction/alkylation process will be necessary prior to trypsin digestion. These reduction/alkylation steps need to take place in the dark (see Note 4).

4. Prepare a 2 M stock solution of DTT and dilute 5 μl of this with 1 ml of 0.1 M NH_4HCO_3. Add 40 μl of the diluted DTT solution to both control and treated samples, and incubate at 56°C for 45 min.

5. Remove samples from heat and allow to cool to room temperature.

6. Prepare a 55 mM stock solution of iodoacetamide and add 40 μl of this stock solution to both control and treated samples. Incubate at room temperature for 30 min.

7. The ratio of trypsin to sample should be 1:50–1:20 (1 mg of trypsin to every 50–20 mg of protein). Add the appropriate amount of trypsin to control and treated samples. Gently agitate the tubes to mix.

8. Place the samples in a water bath at 37°C for 2 h and then add an additional amount (equal to the first amount added) of trypsin to each sample.

9. Continue to incubate at 37°C for 17–18 h to ensure complete digestion (see Note 5).

10. Trypsin digestion reactions can be terminated by freezing samples at –20°C, or by adding 4 μl of glacial acetic acid.

11. Reduce the volume of the samples to approximately 10 μl by vacuum concentration.

3.3. MuDPIT

3.3.1. Column Preparation

1. Cut a 35-cm long piece of silica capillary tubing (O.D. 363 μm and I.D. 250 μm) (7).

2. Using an alcohol burner, burn off insulation on outside of silica tubing in the middle 1.5 cm (see Note 6).

3. Resuspend the C18 RP resin in methanol and remove supernatant. Repeat this process three more times to remove fine particles from the mixture.

4. Pull column using a Sutter Instrument Co. Model p-2000 micropipette puller, and use a ceramic cutter (LC packing international) (see Note 7).

5. The column is then packed under high pressure (700 psi) with compressed nitrogen to 7 cm in a pressurized cell (bomb) connected to a regulator (7).

6. The SCX column is prepared in the same manner as the RP column, but without a tapered tip. A frit in a zero volume union is used as a barrier for the SCX to pack against. A 100-μm

I.D. capillary packed with 7 cm of 5 μm Vydac C18 reversed phase resin, and a separate 250-μm I.D. capillary packed with 7 cm of 5 μm Partisphere strong cation exchanger resin were used for the studies described herein.

3.3.2. MuDPIT Mass Spectrometric Analysis

1. For the nano LC/LC–MS/MS, a microbore HPLC system (Paradigm MS4, Michrom, Auburn, CA) was used with two separate SCX and RP columns.

2. The trypsin-digested peptides were pooled and acidified using trifluoroacetic acid and manually injected onto the SCX column, the effluent from the column being next fed through the RP column.

3. The 12-step MuDPIT analyses were as follows. Step 1 consists of a 5-min equilibration step with 100% buffer A, followed by another equilibration step for 5 min with 25% buffer B (75% buffer A), followed by a 40-min gradient from 25% buffer B to 65% buffer B, followed by a 10-min 65% buffer B and 10 min of 100% buffer A. Chromatography steps 2–12 follow the same pattern: 15 min of the appropriate % of buffers C and D, followed by a 2-min wash with 100% buffer C, a 5-min wash with 100% A, equilibration with 25% buffer B for 5 min, followed by a gradient from 25% buffer B to 65% buffer B for 40 min, followed by a 10-min 65% buffer B and 10 min of 100% buffer A. The stepwise gradient used was as follows: 0, 25, 50, 75, 100, 150, 200, 250, 300, 400, and 500 mM ammonium acetate, respectively, for the 11 salt steps. Eluting peptides at 350 nl/min were electrosprayed into a ThermoFinnigan LCQ-Deca XP Plus ion trap mass spectrometer (ThermoFinnigan, San Jose, CA) (8) with a spray voltage of 1.6–2.3 kV. Spectra were scanned over the range 380–2,000 amu. Automated peak recognition, dynamic exclusion, and daughter ion scanning of the most intense ion were performed using the Xcalibur v1.3 software, as described previously (9, 10).

3.4. Data Analysis

3.4.1. Database Searching

1. Analyze tandem MS spectra of peptides with TurboSEQUEST™, a program that allows the correlation of experimental tandem MS data with theoretical spectra generated from known protein sequences (5). The peak list (data files) for the search is generated by Bioworks 3.1. Parent peptide mass error tolerance was set at 1.5 amu and fragment ion mass tolerance was set at 0.5 amu during the search.

2. The criteria for a preliminary positive peptide identification: peptide precursor ions with a +1 charge having a Xcorr >1.0, +2 Xcorr > 1.5, and +3 Xcorr > 2.0. A dCn score > 0.08 and a fragment ion ratio of experimental/theoretical >50% were also used as filtering criteria for reliable matched peptide identification (11). All matched peptides were confirmed by visual examination of the spectra.

3. X!Tandem (http://www.thegpm.org; version 2007.01.01.1) was used to query the ipi.RAT.v3.31 database. Sequest was selected to query the ipi.RAT.v3.31.fasta.hdr database (41,251 entries), assuming the digestion enzyme trypsin. Sequest and X!Tandem were searched with a fragment ion mass tolerance of 0.5 Da and a parent ion tolerance of 1.5 Da.

4. Modifications searched consisted of oxidation of methionine, iodoacetamide derivative of cysteine, +105 Da (HQ), +412 Da (MGHQ), +268 Da (NACHQ), +226 Da (CSHQ), and +283 Da (CysGlyHQ); at Lys, Arg, and Glu were specified in Sequest and X!Tandem as variable modifications.

3.4.2. Criteria for Protein Identification

1. Scaffold (version Scaffold-02.05.00, Proteome Software Inc., Portland, OR) was used to validate initial MS/MS-based peptide and protein identifications, which were subsequently accepted if they could be established at greater than 90.0% probability, as specified by the Peptide Prophet algorithm (12) and contained at least 1 identified peptide. Protein probabilities were assigned by the Protein Prophet algorithm (13). Proteins that contained similar peptides and that could not be differentiated based on MS/MS analysis alone were grouped to satisfy the principles of parsimony.

3.4.3. Adduct Validation

All peptides found by Scaffold to be modified by chemical adduction were confirmed with P-Mod, and then manually validated with IonGen (14). P-Mod is an algorithm that screens data files for MSMS spectra corresponding to peptide sequences in a search list (15). Modification of the primary peptide sequence shifts the peptide mass, which may be experimentally observed as a difference between the measured mass of the modified peptide precursor ion (adjusted for charge state) and the predicted mass of the unmodified peptide. The mass shift will also be observed in the m/z values of fragment ions containing the modified amino acid. Scores with p-values greater than 0.01 are discarded as false positives. Upon collision-induced dissociation (CID) of the peptides, b- and y-ion fragments are generated: the b-ion series represents cleavage of the peptide bond with charge retention on the N-terminal fragment, and y-ions result from cleavage of the amide bonds with charge retention on the C-terminal side (16). Manual validation of MS/MS spectra is then used to confirm peptide sequence and adduct mass location. IonGen generates theoretical b- and y-ions for user-specified peptides containing adduct(s) (14).

1. Generate search file by inputting sequence of adducted peptide and any other types of modifications (oxidized methionines, alkylated cysteines, etc.).

2. Input.RAW datafile into search window and run program.

3. Look for peptide containing mass addition of interest (+105 amu for BQ modification) and make sure the amino acid adducted is a chemically appropriate target amino acid.

4. Look at p-value and make sure it is below the pre-determined cutoff ($p = <0.05$).

4. Notes

1. Water was chosen in this example, but other buffers can also be used, such as ammonium bicarbonate or ammonium acetate at 10 mM. When sample is lyophilized, the buffer will be removed, leaving only pure protein in the tube.

2. It is important to make sure that all samples are free of detergents before proceeding with trypsin digestion, and this can be achieved by protein precipitation methods.

3. Additional enzymes can be used for protein digestion, including chymotrypsin, endoproteinase Asp-N, and glutamic acid-C, all of which have specific optimal pH ranges. Trypsin is the most common choice for proteomic procedures, so methodology using this enzyme is described here.

4. Reduction steps improve digestion efficiency by preventing disulfide formation, which assists in maintaining the protein in an unfolded state, exposing more tryptic sites for digestion.

5. As stated previously, the quinol–thioether conjugates are unstable in basic conditions. Consequently, when using compounds of this nature, the digestion procedure needs to be limited to approximately 3 h, to minimize quinol–thioether exposure to the basic buffering system necessary for trypsin digestion. Efficient digestion can be accomplished in less than 3 h.

6. If insulation remains present in the area of silica tubing being pulled, the laser will burn off the insulation onto the mirror, which will decrease the effectiveness of the laser.

7. This produces a column with a tapered tip that sprays directly into the mass spectrometer. The tapered tip also retains the C18 in the column.

Acknowledgments

This work was supported by GM070890 (SSL) and ES07091 (AAF). The authors acknowledge the support of the P30 ES06694 Southwest Environmental Health Sciences Center, in particular the Arizona Proteomics Consortium (APC). Our special thanks go to Dr. George Tsaprailis, Director of the APC.

References

1. Asif, A. R., Armstrong, V. W., Voland, A., Wieland, E., Oellerich, M., and Shipkova, M. (2007) Proteins identified as targets of the acyl glucuronide metabolite of mycophenolic acid in kidney tissue from mycophenolate mofetil treated rats, *Biochimie 89*, 393–402.

2. Bruschi, S. A., Lindsay, J. G., and Crabb, J. W. (1998) Mitochondrial stress protein recognition of inactivated dehydrogenases during mammalian cell death, *Proc Natl Acad Sci U S A 95*, 13413–13418.

3. Kleiner, H. E., Rivera, M. I., Pumford, N. R., Monks, T. J., and Lau, S. S. (1998) Immunochemical detection of quinol–thioether-derived protein adducts, *Chem Res Toxicol 11*, 1283–1290.

4. Kleiner, H. E., Jones, T. W., Monks, T. J., and Lau, S. S. (1998) Immunochemical analysis of quinol–thioether-derived covalent protein adducts in rodent species sensitive and resistant to quinol–thioether-mediated nephrotoxicity, *Chem Res Toxicol 11*, 1291–1300.

5. Yates, J. R., III, Eng, J. K., McCormack, A. L., and Schieltz, D. (1995) Method to correlate tandem mass spectra of modified peptides to amino acid sequences in the protein database, *Anal Chem 67*, 1426–1436.

6. Craig, R., Cortens, J. P., and Beavis, R. C. (2004) Open source system for analyzing, validating, and storing protein identification data, *J Proteome Res 3*, 1234–1242.

7. Jorde, L. B. (2005) *Encyclopedia of genetics, genomics, proteomics, and bioinformatics*, Wiley, Chichester.

8. Washburn, M. P., Wolters, D., and Yates, J. R., III. (2001) Large-scale analysis of the yeast proteome by multidimensional protein identification technology, *Nat Biotechnol 19*, 242–247.

9. Andon, N. L., Hollingworth, S., Koller, A., Greenland, A. J., Yates, J. R., III, and Haynes, P. A. (2002) Proteomic characterization of wheat amyloplasts using identification of

proteins by tandem mass spectrometry, *Proteomics 2*, 1156–1168.

10. Lantz, R. C., Lynch, B. J., Boitano, S., Poplin, G. S., Littau, S., Tsaprailis, G., and Burgess, J. L. (2007) Pulmonary biomarkers based on alterations in protein expression after exposure to arsenic, *Environ Health Perspect 115*, 586–591.

11. Cooper, B., Eckert, D., Andon, N. L., Yates, J. R., and Haynes, P. A. (2003) Investigative proteomics: identification of an unknown plant virus from infected plants using mass spectrometry, *J Am Soc Mass Spectrom 14*, 736–741.

12. Keller, A., Nesvizhskii, A. I., Kolker, E., and Aebersold, R. (2002) Empirical statistical model to estimate the accuracy of peptide identifications made by MS/MS and database search, *Anal Chem 74*, 5383–5392.

13. Nesvizhskii, A. I., Keller, A., Kolker, E., and Aebersold, R. (2003) A statistical model for identifying proteins by tandem mass spectrometry, *Anal Chem 75*, 4646–4658.

14. Fisher, A. A., Labenski, M. T., Malladi, S., Gokhale, V., Bowen, M. E., Milleron, R. S., Bratton, S. B., Monks, T. J., and Lau, S. S. (2007) Quinone electrophiles selectively adduct "electrophile binding motifs" within cytochrome c, *Biochemistry 46*, 11090–11100.

15. Hansen, B. T., Davey, S. W., Ham, A. J., and Liebler, D. C. (2005) P-Mod: an algorithm and software to map modifications to peptide sequences using tandem MS data, *J Proteome Res 4*, 358–368.

16. Standing, K. G. (2003) Peptide and protein de novo sequencing by mass spectrometry, *Curr Opin Struct Biol 13*, 595–601.

17. Link, A. J., Eng, J., Schieltz, D. M., Carmack, E., Mize, G. J., Morris, D. R., Garvik, B. M., and Yates, J. R., III. (1999) Direct analysis of protein complexes using mass spectrometry, *Nat Biotechnol 17*, 676–682.

Part VIII

Safety Biomarkers

Chapter 22

Optimization of SELDI for Biomarker Detection in Plasma

Jean-Francois Léonard, Martine Courcol, and Jean-Charles Gautier

Abstract

The surface-enhanced laser desorption ionization (SELDI) technology is a promising approach not only for the research of biomarkers in the blood of patients in clinical applications but also in preclinical studies to assess the drug-induced toxicities. The optimization of the SELDI platform is a crucial step before running plasma samples from preclinical toxicity studies. First, mass spectrometer parameters such as the laser energy and ion focus mass values should be assessed in order to obtain the highest quality of spectra. Second, the coefficient of variation of the intensity, resolution, and signal-to-noise ratio of the peaks detected in reference samples should be evaluated and used as quality control criteria. Last, a systematic evaluation of technical bias such as the spot and chip position and the bioprocessor sequence number may be achieved using the appropriate multivariate statistical analyses.

Key words: SELDI, Reference plasma, Quality control, Bias investigation

1. Introduction

The surface-enhanced laser desorption ionization (SELDI) technique combines the capture of proteins on chromatographic retention surfaces coated on Proteinchips® and time of flight (TOF) mass spectrometry (1). This technology has potential interest not only in many therapeutic areas by the detection of biomarkers in the blood of patients with pathologies, such as prostate, ovary, or colorectal cancer (2–4) but also in the case of neurodegenerative syndrome (5) or cardiovascular disease (6). The SELDI technology can also be used in the pharmaceutical industries to find potential biomarkers of toxicity in preclinical studies by investigating the modulation of proteins in the plasma of animals treated with toxicants (7, 8).

A preliminary optimization of the SELDI platform consists to define the laser energy and focus mass range values which may be

Jean-Charles Gautier (ed.), *Drug Safety Evaluation: Methods and Protocols*, Methods in Molecular Biology, vol. 691, DOI 10.1007/978-1-60761-849-2_22, © Springer Science+Business Media, LLC 2011

chosen to get the highest possible performances of the spectrometer. This optimization step should be achieved for each kind of chromatographic retention surface such as anionic (Q10), cationic (CM10), hydrophobic (H50), or immobilized metal affinity capture (IMAC) surface, and each TOF spectrometer such as PCS4000. As many parameters can influence the reproducibility and reliability of the results, each step of the experimental protocol should be checked to avoid artifacts. In addition, quality control criteria should be used (9) and investigations of potential technical bias (10) may be conducted with the appropriate statistical tests, including uni- and multivariate analyses.

2. Materials

2.1. Test System and Plasma Collection

1. Sprague–Dawley Crl:CD®(SD)IGS BR rats, 6–7 weeks old and weighing 120–250 g (Charles River).
2. 10-mL plastic syringe with a large diameter needle.
3. EDTA plastic tubes (Sarstedt) for blood collection (see Note 1).
4. Low protein-binding plastic tubes (Protein Lobind, Eppendorf) of 500 μL for plasma storage at -80°C.

2.2. SELDI Apparatus and Chromatographic Retention Surfaces

The SELDI platform is made of three main components:
1. TOF mass spectrometer for Proteinchips®, e.g., PCS4000 (BioRad).
2. Robot for Proteinchips® preparation and matrix deposit, e.g., a Freedom Evo robot (Tecan).
3. Chromatographic retention surfaces or Proteinchips® (BioRad) (see Note 2) which are disposed in a specially designed rack called bioprocessor by SELDI users.

2.3. Solutions and Compounds

1. Urea-CHAPS solution such as U9 (BioRad).
2. 0.1 M Tris–HCl solution at pH 9 (Sigma) (see Note 3).
3. Saturated sinapinic acid stock solution half-diluted in 50/50 (v/v) mix of acetonitrile (Riedel de Haen) and 1% trifluoroacetic acid (Fluka).
4. All-in-one external calibrants (BioRad).

2.4. Softwares

1. Ciphergen Express software (BioRad).
2. Gemini software (Tecan).
3. Java interface for SELDI platform specially designed for the Tecan Freedom Evo robot (Modul-Bio).
4. Excel (Microsoft), Spotfire Decision Site (Spotfire), and JMP (SAS Institute).

3. Methods

The method described here must be considered as a means to increase the probability to detect toxicity biomarkers in the plasma of rats treated with compounds. Given that the mass spectrum patterns are highly dependent on the selected laser energy and ion focus mass, it is recommended to investigate the most appropriate acquisition condition of the data before studying the drug-induced modulated m/z. The goal is to obtain high-quality mass spectra with the highest sensitivity and a correct reproducibility of the results.

Following are the sequence of events for the SELDI platform optimization (Fig. 1):

– Constitution of a pool of plasma used as reference material (see Note 4).

– Denaturation of the reference plasma samples.

– Processing of the Proteinchips® including the equilibration, the binding/washing steps, and the matrix deposit with a robot.

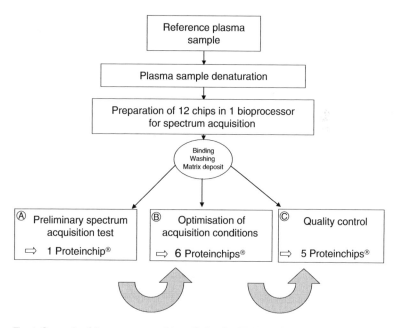

Fig. 1. Synopsis of the process used to optimize the SELDI platform. The *lower panel* of the figure shows the different steps used to assess the efficiency of the PCS4000 mass spectrometer. (**a**) One Proteinchip® allows to investigate the minimum and maximum limits of the laser energies using relevant ion focus masses (pending on peak density and/or historical data). (**b**) Then, the effects of six increasing laser energies and six focus masses are tested on a series of six Proteinchips®. (**c**) The three best acquisition conditions in term of peak intensity, resolution, and *s/n* ratio are chosen and a quality control is performed on a series of five Proteinchips®.

– Assessment of the efficiency of the PCS4000 mass spectrometer; this crucial step helps to set up the best conditions that will be used to investigate the plasma proteins with the highest possible efficiency.

3.1. Constitution of a Pool of Plasma for Quality Control and Technical Bias Investigations (Reference Plasma)

1. Carry out rat anesthesia using an isoflurane station for rodents; after laparotomy, collect the blood via the aorta by aspiration with an appropriate needle connected to a syringe (see Note 5).

2. Remove the needle and transfer the content of the syringe into EDTA tubes.

3. Mildly shake the tubes upside down.

4. Centrifuge the blood as soon as possible (within 5 min) at $2,000 \times g$ for 15 min at $+4°C$ (see Note 6).

5. Aspirate the supernatants, pool the plasma, and place on ice until aliquoting 150 μL into Protein LoBind tubes previously cooled on dry ice.

6. Store the plasma at $-80°C$ until SELDI experiments.

3.2. Denaturation of Plasma Samples

1. Thaw the aliquots of the reference pool of plasma at room temperature.

2. Immediately start sample denaturation under agitation using U9 buffer with a dilution factor of 1/2.5 for 20 min at room temperature.

3. At this step, the denatured plasmas can be stored at $-80°C$ until downstream SELDI experiments (see Note 7).

3.3. Chip Preparation

1. A total of 12 Proteinchips® (Q10 in our example) (see Note 8) are placed in a bioprocessor and equilibrated three times with 0.1 M Tris–HCl solution, pH 9 (Tris buffer), for 5 min at room temperature and under agitation.

2. Concomitantly, dilute five times the denatured plasma with the Tris buffer and aliquot it in a 96-well microplate precooled at $+4°C$ with an ice pack system (or whatever).

3. Aspirate the Tris buffer from the Proteinchips® with a robot (e.g., a Tecan Freedom Evo) and transfer 10 μL of each microplate well content onto the overall Proteinchips® spots previously filled with 90 μL of Tris buffer.

4. Carry out the binding of the anionic proteins for 45 min at room temperature under shaking.

5. Wash the chromatographic retention surfaces for 5 min under shaking with the Tris buffer to avoid nonspecific binding. Repeat the procedure three times. Perform two additional washes with MilliQ deionized water to eliminate the remaining salts.

6. Allow the Proteinchips® to dry completely for 1–1.5 h at room temperature.

3.4. Matrix Deposit

1. Perform two successive matrix deposits of 1 μL onto each spot.

2. After each sinapinic acid deposition, let the chips to dry at room temperature for 0.5 h (first deposit) and 5 h (second deposit) (see Note 9).

3.5. Preliminary Mass Spectrum Acquisition Test

The procedure described above can be used for an m/z range of 2.5–30 kDa.

1. Select one chip to carry out a rough estimation of the laser energy and focus mass ranges which can be used for the Q10 Proteinchips® according to the studied biological material.

2. Select two ion focus mass values of 4 and 16 kDa (see Note 10) and acquire the mass spectra from eight spots of the chip with increasing laser energies up to a maximum value in which more than 30% of the peaks are saturated.

3. The minimal laser energy value is determined when a dramatic decrease of the peak intensities is observed with a concomitant decrease of the peak resolutions and s/n ratios.

3.6. Optimization of the Acquisition Conditions

1. Acquire the mass spectra of reference plasmas of six Proteinchips® and within the limits of laser energy values selected above, select six increasing laser energies and six different focus mass values as shown in Table 1 (see Note 11).

2. In parallel, calibrate the PCS4000 with the all-in-one peptide and protein calibrants and perform a spot-to-spot correction to improve the mass spectra alignment.

3. Carry out an expression difference mapping (EDM) process with the Ciphergen Express software on all of the mass spectra from 2.5 to 30 kDa (see Note 12). Select the option "auto-detect peaks to cluster" and use only the first pass with an s/n ratio and a valley depth value adjusted to 3. Lastly, the minimum peak threshold must be 100% of all spectra.

4. Select a series of peaks (m/z), detected in all spectra and in all tested acquisition conditions. These m/z are considered as reference peaks in which variations of intensity, resolution, and s/n ratio may be evaluated (Fig. 2 and Table 2).

5. Export the peak information (intensity, resolution, and signal/noise ratio) in csv format and reclassify the data regarding the acquisition conditions, thanks to pivot tables with the Excel software (see Note 13).

6. For each laser energy, plot graphic representations of the Excel formatted data (see Note 14) to visualize (a) the effects of the focus mass on the peak intensity/resolution/signal-to-noise ratio and (b) the impact of each focus mass on the three main parameters of the reference peaks as shown in Figs. 3 and 4, respectively.

Table 1
Laser energy and focus mass used for the optimization of the mass spectrum acquisition condition

Spot	Chip 1			Chip 2			Chip 3			Chip 4			Chip 5			Chip 6		
	Laser energy (nJ)	Focus mass (kDa)	Partition number	Laser energy (nJ)	Focus mass (kDa)	Partition number	Laser energy (nJ)	Focus mass (kDa)	Partition number	Laser energy (nJ)	Focus mass (kDa)	Partition number	Laser energy (nJ)	Focus mass (kDa)	Partition number	Laser energy (nJ)	Focus mass (kDa)	Partition number
A–D	2,250	4	1/6	2,500	4	1/6	2,750	4	1/6	3,000	4	1/6	3,250	4	1/6	3,500	4	1/6
	2,250	6	2/6	2,500	6	2/6	2,750	6	2/6	3,000	6	2/6	3,250	6	2/6	3,500	6	2/6
	2,250	10	3/6	2,500	10	3/6	2,750	10	3/6	3,000	10	3/6	3,250	10	3/6	3,500	10	3/6
	2,250	12	4/6	2,500	12	4/6	2,750	12	4/6	3,000	12	4/6	3,250	12	4/6	3,500	12	4/6
	2,250	14	5/6	2,500	14	5/6	2,750	14	5/6	3,000	14	5/6	3,250	14	5/6	3,500	14	5/6
	2,250	16	6/6	2,500	16	6/6	2,750	16	6/6	3,000	16	6/6	3,250	16	6/6	3,500	16	6/6
E–H	2,250	4	1/6	2,250	6	1/6	2,250	10	1/6	2,250	12	1/6	2,250	14	1/6	2,250	16	1/6
	2,500	4	2/6	2,500	6	2/6	2,500	10	2/6	2,500	12	2/6	2,500	14	2/6	2,500	16	2/6
	2,750	4	3/6	2,750	6	3/6	2,750	10	3/6	2,750	12	3/6	2,750	14	3/6	2,750	16	3/6
	3,000	4	4/6	3,000	6	4/6	3,000	10	4/6	3,000	12	4/6	3,000	14	4/6	3,000	16	4/6
	3,250	4	5/6	3,250	6	5/6	3,250	10	5/6	3,250	12	5/6	3,250	14	5/6	3,250	16	5/6
	3,500	4	6/6	3,500	6	6/6	3,500	10	6/6	3,500	12	6/6	3,500	14	6/6	3,500	16	6/6

A spot partition of six allows each spot to acquire the spectra with constant laser energy and increasing focus masses (spots A–D) or vice versa (spots E–H)

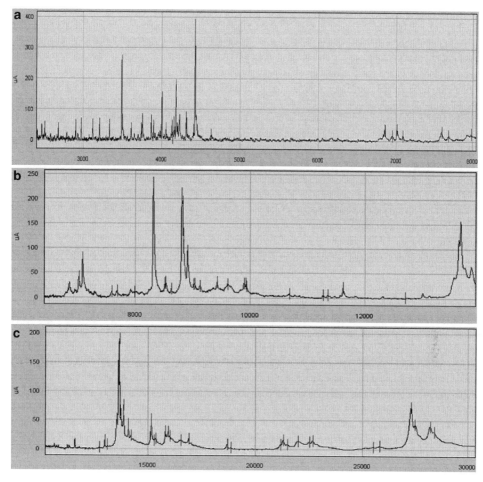

Fig. 2. Typical Q10 spectra of a reference pool of rat plasma allowing the selection of the reference peaks. The x-axis corresponds to the m/z value in Dalton and the y-axis corresponds to peak intensity in μA.

Table 2
m/z Values selected as reference peaks in our laboratory conditions

Peak ID	m/z (Da)	Peak ID	m/z (Da)
1	3,499.96	10	14,132.90
2	4,226.93	11	15,196.19
3	4,425.88	12	15,965.79
4	7,020.53	13	21,352.04
5	8,316.65	14	22,035.74
6	8,907.84	15	22,696.65
7	9,607.21	16	27,397.32
8	11,639.72	17	28,298.88
9	13,036.71	–	–

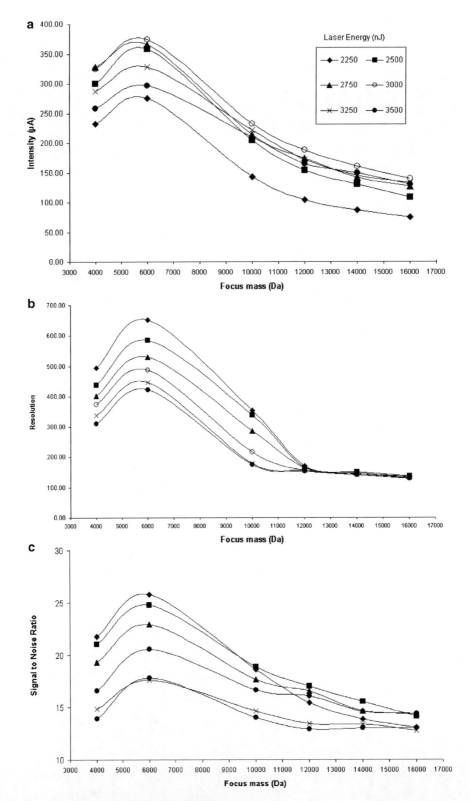

Fig. 3. Example of the effects of increasing laser energies and focus mass adjustments on the intensity (**a**), resolution (**b**), and the *s/n* ratio (**c**) of a reference peak at 4,425.88 Da.

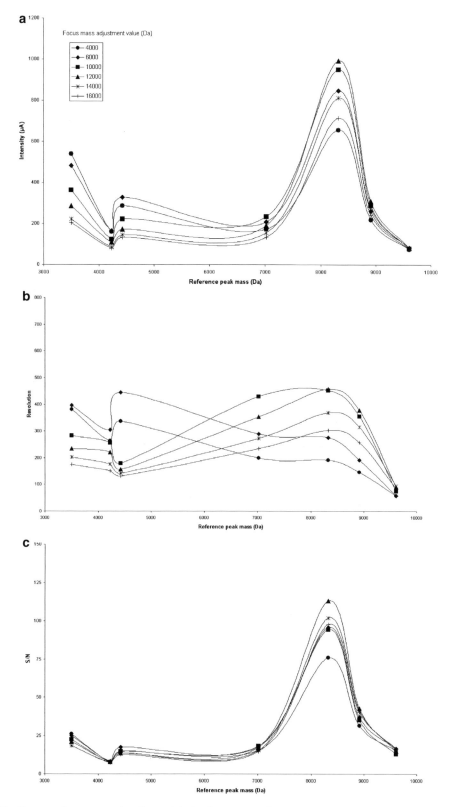

Fig. 4. The three graphs represent the effects of the ion focus mass adjustment on the intensity (**a**), resolution (**b**), and *s/n* ratio (**c**) of seven reference peaks (3,499.96, 4,226.93, 4,425.88, 7,020.53, 8,316.65, 8,907.84, and 9,607.21 Da) with a laser energy adjusted to 3,250 nJ.

7. Determine the laser energy and focus mass values with corresponding m/z ranges by a manual review of the plotted graphic representations as illustrated in Fig. 5 (see Note 15). A maximum of three acquisition protocols is recommended to avoid the generation of a huge mass of data, which may be a major issue for a rapid and efficient treatment of SELDI data in routine experiments. Therefore, the three protocols used to acquire SELDI data with Q10 Proteinchips® in our laboratory conditions are summarized in Table 3.

3.7. Quality Control

1. Using the three protocols for spectrum acquisition successively, acquire the spectra of the eight spots of the five remaining

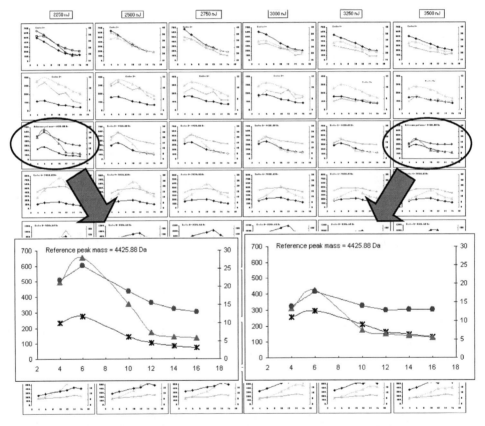

Fig. 5. Each *column* represents the data obtained for a given laser energy and each *row* corresponds to the data obtained for each reference peak. The *magnified views* give a representation of the intensity (*asterisk*), resolution (*filled triangle*), and s/n ratio (*filled circle*) when the laser energy is 2,250 nJ (**a**) or 3,500 nJ (**b**). In this example, the results show that the best acquisition condition for the reference peak at 4,426 Da is obtained when the focus mass is adjusted to 6 kDa with a laser energy of 2,500 nJ. One can observe that increasing laser energies induce a parallel decrease of the resolution and s/n ratio, whereas the effects on the peak intensity are minimal; this is the reason why a low energy should be preferentially selected knowing that a concomitant low resolution and s/n ratio may impede the further detection of plasma biomarker in SELDI plasma profiling experiments. Nevertheless, a compromise must be obtained regarding the other reference peaks and that is the reason why in our conditions the best laser energy for peaks from 2.5 to 7 kDa was 2,500 nJ with a focus mass adjusted to 6 kDa. The *x*-axis corresponds to the focus mass value in kDa. The resolution and intensity values are read on the left *y*-axis (intensity unit: μA), whereas the s/n ratio values are read on the right *y*-axis.

Table 3
Parameters of the three acquisition conditions used for plasma profiling in rats using Q10 Proteinchips® with 0.1 M Tris–HCl at pH 9

Acquisition conditions	Laser energy (nJ)	Ion focus mass (kDa)	m/z Range (kDa)
1	2,500	6	2.5–7
2	3,000	10	6–11
3	3,000	16	10–30

Proteinchips®. Perform one EDM per acquisition condition in order to get the intensity, resolution, and s/n ratio of the detected reference peaks (see Note 16).

2. For each data set of the three acquisition conditions, export the data in csv format, open the files with Excel, and using the pivot tables, calculate means and standard deviations of the intensity, resolution, and s/n ratio for each reference peak. Calculate the corresponding coefficients of variation (11).

3. Investigate the data distribution with box plot representations (12) of the three variables with Spotfire or SAS-JMP softwares (see Note 17). An example is given in Fig. 6.

4. The spot and/or chip position and/or bioprocessor sequence number (in case of large series of samples to process) are potential issues for the SELDI platform. Consequently, it is recommended to track such sources of variation using non-inferential statistics such as multivariate analyses (12, 13), which are valuable approaches for technical bias investigations.

5. For each data set (corresponding to the three acquisition conditions) and each reference peak, perform the following statistical tests on the intensity, resolution, and s/n ratio:

– Hierarchical clustering to detect aggregates regarding the spot and/or chip position in the bioprocessor and/or bioprocessor sequence number (Fig. 7).

– Principal component analysis to check abnormal clusters linked to the spot or chip position or bioprocessor sequence number. This method is also valuable to detect outliers (Fig. 8).

– Correlation matrix of all spots; check that the correlation factors are close to 1 (Fig. 9). This highly sensitive method is a valuable tool to give an alert relative to technical bias, which may be mediated by the spot position factor or by other causes of bias like robot dysfunctions, shortened laser half life laser or abnormal room temperature (13).

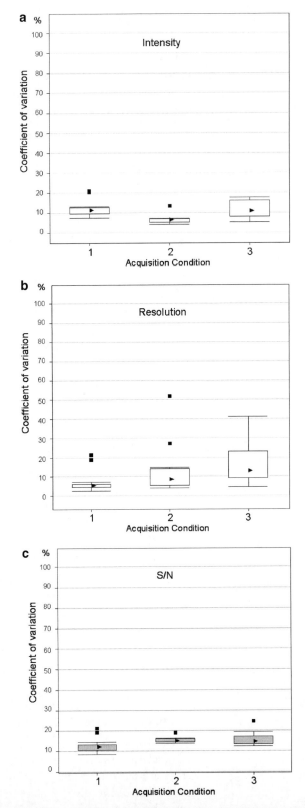

Fig. 6. The box plot representations allow a quick visualization of the data distribution by representation of the first and third quartiles with the median (*filled triangle*) and the outliers (*filled square*) calculated by Spotfire. This example gives evidence that the coefficients of variation (CV) are slightly different regarding the acquisition condition. When

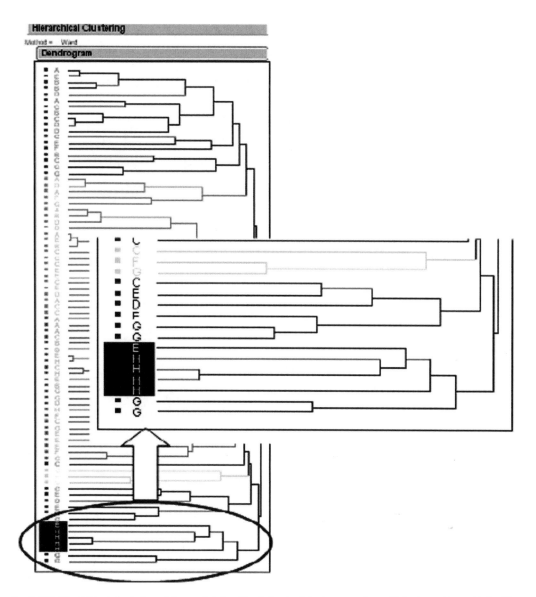

Fig. 7. The hierarchical clustering of the peak intensities helps to detect aggregates, which give evidence that a bias linked to the spot position occurs. In this example, a clustering was performed with the Ward method; the magnified view of the dendrogram shows a cluster in which a repeat of spot H appears four out of seven times. The spot position repeats among the eight clusters (corresponding to the total number of spots per chip) are investigated. If necessary, the spot-to-spot correction curve of the PCS4000 must be checked.

If the quality control performed with reference samples gives coefficients of variation equal or below 25–30% with a concomitant lack of evidence for technical bias, include the results in historical data and consider that the SELDI platform can be used to investigate potential biomarkers in the plasma of treated rats using Q10 Proteinchips®.

Fig. 6. (continued) the Tecan robot and PCS4000 parameters are well adjusted, the CV are close to 10% (see example). CVs higher than 25–30% must be considered as an alert and should trigger in-depth investigations of the SELDI platform (including PCS4000 and preparative robot) to identify the reason for such a drift. Attention must be paid especially for the laser and detector efficiencies; the correct matrix deposit step should also be checked.

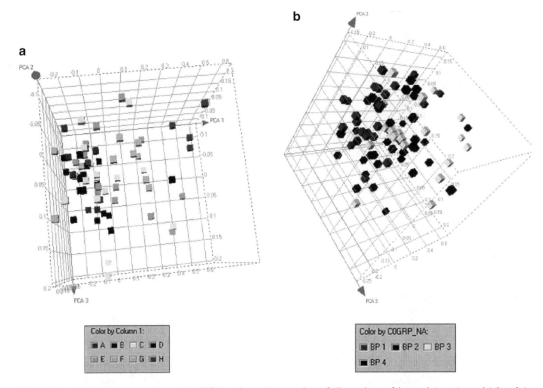

Fig. 8. The principal component analysis (PCA) reduces the number of dimensions of huge data sets and takes into account the variation of the data. This method may be helpful to detect abnormal groups of data and outliers. The figure shows 3D representation of PCA in which the effect of the spot position (**a**) or the bioprocessor number (**b**) is investigated. In these examples, no abnormal clustering was observed, leading to the conclusion that there was no evidence of technical bias due to the investigated parameters.

Grey scale maps on correlation

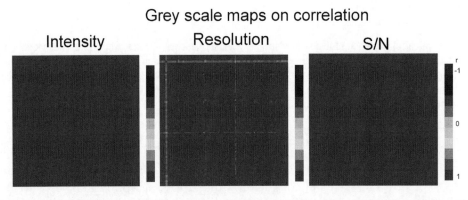

Fig. 9. Correlation matrices (*gray scale*) of the intensity, resolution, and *s/n* ratio of the overall reference peaks performed for each spot. In this example, the majority of the correlation factors (CF) are close to 1 except for one spot in which the CF range was close to 0.7, approximately. An alert is given when the correlation factors are below 0.6 and are observed in more than 10% of the spots. Our historical data matrices show that the peak resolution is the most sensitive variable; no clear explanation can be given but this may be probably due, at least in part, to the alignment issues of the Ciphergen Express software and the relatively poor resolution of the PCS4000 compared to other mass spectrometers such as MALDI TOF or ion trap equipments.

When quality control criteria are not met, additional investigations must be started to be sure that there are no hardware issues with the PCS4000 components. With the help of Biorad engineers, check the laser and/or detector and/or electronic cards efficiencies. A PCS4000 re-initialization and/or high voltage conditioning and/or TOF calibration should also be started to be sure that the mass spectrometer specifications are correct. Knowing that huge bias can be generated if the matrix is not correctly dropped onto the spots of the Proteinchips®, check the preparation of robot specifications also. Once the issues with the PCS4000 and/or the robot are solved, the optimization process should be started again.

3.8. Detection of Modulated Peaks in Plasma Samples from Study of Interest

For each SELDI profiling experiment, the plasma of the study must be randomly dispatched in the Proteinchips® spots (14). Include at least two reference plasma samples per chip and two blank spots per bioprocessor. Use the protocols of acquisition conditions previously defined and acquire the spectra.

Before analyzing the data generated with the study plasma samples, check again the variability of the SELDI platform and the lack of technical bias by analysing the reference plasma spectra; keep the same process that is previously depicted and do not change the analysis settings. If the quality criteria are met with no evidence of technical bias, include the results in historical data and carry out further analysis with the study samples to detect the differentially modulated peaks.

---

4. Notes

1. Use screw-capped EDTA tubes. Avoid tubes with glass beads and/or under vacuum as it can generate slight erythrocyte damages and a concomitant release of hemoglobin. This is to avoid interferences with the detection of the peaks of interest by the PCS4000 mass spectrometer.

2. For a better reproducibility of the results, it is recommended to use Proteinchips® from the same batch as much as possible, to avoid variations due to the manufacturing process.

3. A 0.1 M Tris – Hcl is used when Q_{10} are Processed. A pH value of 9 is considered to be optimal for peak enrichment in such chromatographic surface in our laboratory conditions.

4. Due to the species specificity of the plasma proteome, it is more convenient to use reference plasma samples taken from the same animal species used to investigate biomarkers. Commercially available (Taconic) or a home-made pool of plasma or serum (15) can be used.

5. Animals must be fasted approximately 16 h prior to the necropsy to avoid lipid overloads. For blood sampling via the abdominal aorta, a needle of large diameter (i.e., Terumo 18G) connected to a 10-mL syringe is recommended; the anesthesia must be correctly conducted to avoid heart failure during the large blood aspiration. For example, an isoflurane volatile anesthesia station for rat (TEM) is very convenient compared to other methods, e.g., pentobarbital anesthesia, which may be more difficult to monitor due to interindividual response to the anesthetic. With isoflurane, a well-trained operator can aspirate up to 7 mL of blood per animal. The obtention of plasma of good quality is a key point for SELDI profiling, and other blood sampling methods such as the tail vein puncture are not recommended, because of the high risk of hemolysis.

6. A short delay between blood sampling and centrifugation is recommended to minimize protein degradation by proteases. Other anticoagulants such as citrate may be used but lithium heparinate is an issue due to the risk of strong interferences with Proteinchips® surfaces.

7. Storage at temperature higher than –80°C is not convenient. For instance, when the tubes are thawed at room temperature after storage at –20°C, a clotting process of the denaturated plasma occurs and makes the downstream SELDI experiments quite impossible.

8. The Proteinchips® Q10 are made of cationic surface derivatized with ammonium groups. The molecular capture is based on electrostatic interactions with negatively charged proteins that bind the retention surface when the pH of the buffer is higher than the isoelectric point of the proteins of interest.

9. Automatic processing of the chips is carried out with a preparation robot. In our conditions, a Tecan Freedom Evo (low volume tubing platform) allows a correct chip preparation (washing/binding/matrix steps). The matrix deposit is a crucial point and requires the use of a high performance robot in which accuracy and reproducibility are validated. Moreover, in our laboratory conditions, a Java interface specially developed for the SELDI platform is used and contributes to performing reliable protein profiling experiments.

10. The choice of the mass range is dependent on a series of factors such as the retention surface, the biological fluid type (e.g., plasma, serum, cerebrospinal fluid, urine, saliva, and alveolar fluid), the animal species, and so forth. In our laboratory conditions, the 4–16-kDa interval corresponds to a mass range in which a high density of peaks is observed. Historical data are helpful to define the most relevant m/z range.

11. Programming different acquisition protocols is easily achieved, thanks to the spot partition available when the

PCS4000 spectrometer is monitored by the Ciphergen Express software. A laser raster allows the partition of a spot and its complete coverage; each partition gives the possibility of different conditions of mass spectrum acquisition. This is used to investigate the effects of laser energy and ion focus mass.

12. These limits correspond to the molecular weight range in which potential biomarkers may be investigated in a reliable manner considering the low resolution of the PCS4000 for the m/z higher than 30 kDa.

13. Considering the large amount of data generated in the SELDI experiments, the use of pivot table is strongly recommended to achieve easy data synthesis in Excel spreadsheets and to sort the relevant information efficiently.

14. All the graphic representations presented in this chapter are helpful to determine which laser energy and ion focus mass must be selected; of course, these parameter values strongly depend on the laboratory conditions and may be adjusted again in other SELDI platforms.

15. A global representation of the intensity, resolution, and signal-to-noise ratio of the reference peaks regarding the given laser energy is also recommended to evaluate at a glance the most appropriate acquisition condition. This approach facilitates the final choice of laser energy and focus mass values which should be selected regarding the ranges of the m/z of interest that are specific of the retention surface and the animal species studied.

16. This step implies that the routine analysis settings (baseline, filtering, and noise with appropriate calibration curve) are applied on the acquired mass spectra and that normalization of the data is performed for each mass spectrum batch.

17. A maximum value of 25–30% for the coefficients of variation is recommended for each measured variable. When the coefficients are higher than 30%, investigations must be rapidly started to determine the reason(s) of such observations. The storage of the coefficients of variation allows the constitution of historical data (11) which are helpful to track the variability of the SELDI platform.

References

1. Merchant, M., and Weinberger, S.R. (2000) Recent advancements in surface-enhanced laser desorption/ionization-time of flight-mass spectrometry. *Electrophoresis* **21**, 1164–1167.

2. Adam, B.L, Qu, Y., Davis. J., Ward, M.D., Clements, M.A., Cazares, L.H., Semmes, O.J., Schellhammer, P.F., Yasui, Y., Feng, Z., and Wright, G.L. Jr. (2002). Serum protein finger-printing coupled with a pattern-matching algorithm distinguishes prostate cancer from benign prostate hyperplasia and healthy men. *Cancer Res.* **62**, 3609–3614.

3. Petricoin, E.F., Ardekani, A.M., Hitt, B.A., Levine, P.J., Fusaro, V.A., Steinberg, S.M., Mills, G.B., Simone, C., Fishman, D.A., Kohn, E.C., and Liotta, L.A. (2002). Use of

proteomic patterns in serum to identify ovarian cancer. *Lancet* **359**, 572–577.

4. Ward, D.G., Suggett, N., Cheng, Y., Wei, W., Johnson, H., Billingham, L.J., Ismail, T., Wakelam, M.J., Johnson, P.J., and Martin, A. (2006). Identification of serum biomarkers for colon cancer by proteomic analysis. *Br. J. Cancer* **94**, 1898–1905.

5. Carrette, O., Demalte, I., Scherl,. A, Yalkinoglu, O., Corthals, G., Burkhard, P., Hochstrasser, D.F., and Sanchez, J.C. (2003). A panel of cerebrospinal fluid potential biomarkers for the diagnosis of Alzheimer's disease. *Proteomics* **8**, 1486–1494.

6. Florian-Kujawski, M., Hussain, W., Chyna, B., Kahn, S., Hoppensteadt, D., Leya, F., and Fareed, J. (2004). Biomarker profiling of plasma from acute coronary syndrome patients. Application of ProteinChip array analysis. *Int. Angiol.* **3**, 246–254.

7. Wetmore, B.A., and Merrick, B.A. (2004). Toxicoproteomics: proteomics applied to toxicology and pathology. *Toxicol. Pathol.* **32**, 619–642.

8. Dare, T.O., Davies, H.A., Turton, J.A., Lomas, L., Williams, T.C., and York, M.J. (2002). Application of surface-enhanced laser desorption/ionization technology to the detection and identification of urinary parvalbumin-alpha: a biomarker of compound-induced skeletal muscle toxicity in the rat. *Electrophoresis* **18**, 3241–3251.

9. White, C.N., Zhang, Z., and Chan, D.W. (2005). Quality control for SELDI analysis. *Clin. Chem. Lab. Med.* **43**, 125–126.

10. Rodland, K.D. (2004). Proteomics and cancer diagnosis: the potential of mass spectrometry. *Clin. Biochem.* **7**, 579–583.

11. Semmes, O.J., Feng, Z., Adam, B.L., Banez, L.L., Bigbee, W.L., Campos, D., Cazares, L.H., Chan, D.W., Grizzle, W.E., Izbicka, E., Kagan, J., Malik, G., McLerran, D., Moul, J.W., Partin, A., Prasanna, P., Rosenzweig, J., Sokoll, L.J., Srivastava, S., Srivastava, S., Thompson, I., Welsh, M.J., White, N., Winget, M., Yasui, Y., Zhang, Z., and Zhu, L. (2005). Evaluation of serum protein profiling by surface-enhanced laser desorption/ionization time-of-flight mass spectrometry for the detection of prostate cancer: I. Assessment of platform reproducibility. *Clin. Chem.* **51**, 102–112.

12. Coombes, K.R., Fritsche, H.A. Jr., Clarke, C., Chen, J.N., Baggerly, K.A., Morris, J.S., Xiao, L.C., Hung, M.C., and Kuerer, H.M. (2003). Quality control and peak finding for proteomics data collected from nipple aspirate fluid by surface-enhanced laser desorption and ionization. *Clin. Chem.* **49**, 1615–1623.

13. Hong, H., Dragan, Y., Epstein, J., Teitel, C., Chen, B., Xie, Q., Fang, H., Shi, L., Perkins, R., and Tong, W. (2005) Quality control and quality assessment of data from surface-enhanced laser desorption/ionization (SELDI) time-of-flight (TOF) mass spectrometry (MS). *BMC Bioinformatics* **6**, Suppl 2:S5.

14. Baggerly, K.A., Morris, J.S., and Coombes, K.R. (2004) Reproducibility of SELDI-TOF protein patterns in serum: comparing datasets from different experiments. *Bioinformatics* **20**, 777–785.

15. Liggett, W.S., Barker, P.E., Semmes, O.J., and Cazares, L.H. (2004). Measurement reproducibility in the early stages of biomarker development. *Dis. Markers* **6**, 295–307

Chapter 23

Differential Proteomics Incorporating iTRAQ Labeling and Multi-dimensional Separations

Ben C. Collins, Thomas Y.K. Lau, Stephen R. Pennington, and William M. Gallagher

Abstract

Considerable effort is currently being expended to integrate newly developed "omics"-based approaches (proteomics, transcriptomics, and metabonomics) into preclinical safety evaluation workflows in the hope that more sensitive prediction of toxicology can be achieved as reported by Waters and Fostel (Nat. Rev. Genet. 5(12):936–948, 2004) and Craig et al. (J. Proteome Res. 5(7):1586–1601, 2006). Proteomic approaches are well placed to contribute to this effort as (a) proteins are the metabolically active products of genes and, as such, may provide more sensitive and direct predictive information on drug-induced liabilities and (b) they have the potential to determine tissue leakage markers in peripheral fluids. Here, we describe a workflow for proteomic semi-quantitative expression profiling of liver from rats treated with a known hepatotoxicant using a multiplexed isobaric labeling strategy and multi-dimensional liquid chromatography.

Key words: Toxicoproteomics, iTRAQ, Proteomics, Toxicology, Liver

1. Introduction

The application of diverse proteomic approaches for differential expression profiling to pharmaceutical toxicology and safety evaluation is rapidly gaining credibility in the drug development community (1–4). Broadly speaking, the aims can be summarized as being (a) to identify biomarkers that might serve to predict toxicity early in candidate development and (b) to delineate the mechanistic details of particular toxicological events. iTRAQ (isobaric tag for relative and absolute quantitation) is a non-gel-based technique used to identify and quantify proteins derived from multiple samples in a single experiment. It utilizes isotope-coded

Jean-Charles Gautier (ed.), *Drug Safety Evaluation: Methods and Protocols*, Methods in Molecular Biology, vol. 691,
DOI 10.1007/978-1-60761-849-2_23, © Springer Science+Business Media, LLC 2011

tags to covalently modify tryptic peptides at the free amino groups of lysine residues and the N-terminus. In this protocol, proteins are extracted from the livers of rats treated daily with a known hepatotoxicant or vehicle for a maximum of 14 days. Each protein sample is then reduced, alkylated, precipitated, subjected to proteolytic digestion with trypsin, and labeled with one of the four isobaric labeling reagents (iTRAQ 114, 115, 116, or 117). The labeled samples are pooled and fractionated by offline strong cation exchange chromatography and analyzed by reversed phase liquid chromatography connected online to a quadrupole time of flight (TOF) tandem mass spectrometer. Reporter ions generated from the iTRAQ labels are used to infer relative peptide and, hence, protein concentrations from samples in a multiplex fashion (5). Although this protocol is based on measurement of protein in rat liver, it can readily be applied, with little or no modification, to other tissues or biofluids.

2. Materials

Unless otherwise stated, all reagents are purchased from Sigma–Aldrich and are of the highest grade available. All solvents are Chromasolv HPLC grade from Sigma–Aldrich. All solutions should be made up in HPLC grade water or solvents.

2.1. Protein Extraction from Tissue

1. Lysis buffer 1: 10 mM Tris, pH 7.5, 1 mM EDTA, and 0.2 M sucrose.
2. Lysis buffer 2: 7 M urea, 2 M thiourea, 4% (w/v) CHAPS, 40 mM dithiothreitol, and 20 mM spermine.
3. Nuclease: benzonase (Calbiochem).
4. Protease inhibitor: Protease Inhibitor Cocktail set III (Calbiochem).
5. Bradford reagent: Bioquant (Merck Biosciences).
6. Protein standard: 2 mg/ml bovine serum albumin (Sigma–Aldrich).

2.2. Tryptic Digestion and iTRAQ Labeling

1. Trypsin: sequencing grade trypsin (Promega).
2. Isobaric labels: iTRAQ Reagents 114, 115, 116, and 117 (Applied Biosystems) [provided in the iTRAQ reagent multiplex kit].
3. Dissolution buffer: 0.5 M triethylammonium bicarbonate (TEAB) pH 8.5 [this reagent is provided in the iTRAQ reagent multiplex kit or can be prepared in the laboratory].
4. Denaturant: 2% sodium dodecyl sulfate.

5. Reducing agent: 50 mM Tris–(2-carboxyethyl) phosphine (TCEP) [this reagent is provided in the iTRAQ reagent multiplex kit or can be prepared in the laboratory].

6. Alkylating agent: 0.5 M iodoacetamide (IAA).

2.3. Offline Strong Cation Exchange Fractionation

1. Strong cation exchange buffer A (SCX buffer A): 25% (v/v) acetonitrile, 10 mM KH_2PO_4 in HPLC grade H_2O, pH 3.0.

2. Strong cation exchange buffer B (SCX b B): 25% (v/v) acetonitrile, 10 mM KH_2PO_4, and 600 mM KCl in HPLC grade H_2O, pH 5.0.

3. Strong cation exchange column: Polysulfoethyl A, 100× 2.1 mm, 5 μm 200Å (PolyLC).

4. HPLC system: Ultimate Plus equipped with a Switchos micro-column switching module, an Ultimate UV detector, and a Probot fraction collector (LC Packings).

5. Salt clean-up columns: MacroSpin columns and Vydac silica C18 (The Nest Group).

2.4. Online Reversed Phase Liquid Chromatography– Mass Spectrometry

1. Reversed phase buffer A (RP buffer A): 0.1% formic acid, 3% (v/v) acetonitrile in HPLC grade H_2O.

2. Reversed phase buffer B (RP buffer B): 0.1% formic acid, 90% acetonitrile in HPLC grade H_2O.

3. Column: HPLC-Chip 150 mm×75 μm, Zorbax 300SB-C18 5 μm, 160 nl trap (Agilent).

4. LC–MS system: 1200 series nanoLC connected online to a 6510 Q-TOF equipped with a Chip Cube source (Agilent Technologies) (see Note 8).

5. Mass spectrometer calibrant: ES-TOF Tuning Mix (Agilent Technologies).

6. Standard protein digest: Protein mixture digest (LC Packings).

2.5. Data Processing and Interpretation

1. Software for data interpretation: Spectrum Mill MS Proteomics Workbench (Rev A.03.03.078).

3. Methods

The overall workflow for this experiment is illustrated in Fig. 1.

3.1. Protein Extraction from Tissue

This section describes the extraction of proteins from liver tissue (protocol adapted from Fella et al. (6)). In this experiment, we have used the left lateral lobe of the liver (see Note 1).

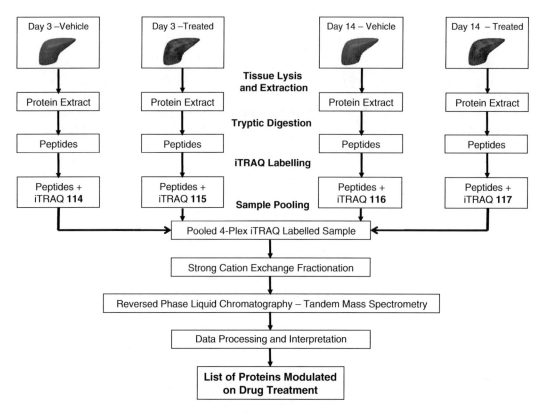

Fig. 1. Proteins are extracted from each of the four liver samples post-treatment. The protein sample is then digested by trypsin, the resulting peptides are labeled with one of the four iTRAQ labels, and the labeled samples are pooled. The multiplexed sample is then fractionated by offline strong cation exchange chromatography and each fraction is analyzed by reversed phase LC–MS/MS from which the peptide sequence and iTRAQ reporter ion ratios can be determined and relative concentrations of proteins can be inferred.

1. Add 125 µl of lysis buffer 1, 30 µl of benzonase, and 5 µl of protease inhibitor cocktail into a minifuge tube and vortex. Pour some liquid nitrogen into a mortar and add 100 mg (±50 mg) of liver tissue. Cool the end of the pestle in liquid nitrogen and pulverize the tissue into a fine powder. Take care not to let the tissue thaw. Add more liquid nitrogen to the mortar if necessary. Cool a metal spatula and transfer the powdered tissue into the minifuge tube.

2. Pipette up and down 30 times to suspend the mixture. Add 875 µl of lysis buffer 2 and pipette 30 times. Vortex the suspension and then place the tube on a rotary shaker at 500 rpm for 60 min at room temperature.

3. The extract is then ultra-centrifuged at $73,000 \times g$ for 30 min at 10°C and the supernatant is carefully transferred to a new tube, aliquoted, and stored at –80°C. This is the soluble protein extract (see Note 2).

4. The protein concentration is estimated by Bradford assay. All protein standards and samples should be prepared in duplicate. Prepare a dilution series of the BSA protein standard with HPLC grade H_2O in the following concentrations: 0, 0.05, 0.1, 0.2, 0.4, 0.6, 0.8, and 1.0 µg/µl. For each diluted protein standard, transfer 25 µl to a minifuge tube (the protein standards should also include a volume of lysis buffer equivalent to the diluted sample – this will depend on the sample dilution). The protein sample will need to be diluted such that the protein concentration is in the range of the protein standards, i.e., between 0.05 and 1.0 µg/µl (a 1 in 15 dilution is usually appropriate). Transfer 25 µl of each diluted protein sample into minifuge tubes. Add 1.25 µl of Bradford reagent to each of the sample and standard tubes, vortex, and transfer into 1.5-ml cuvettes. After 5 min, read the absorbance at 595 nm, construct a standard curve, and extrapolate the protein concentration for each sample.

3.2. Tryptic Digestion and iTRAQ Labeling

In this step, the proteins that have been extracted from tissue are digested by the proteolytic enzyme trypsin. The resulting peptides can then be labeled at the primary amine groups of the N-terminus and lysine residues with one of the four iTRAQ reagents (114, 115, 116, or 117). Before digestion, it is necessary to reduce and alkylate the cysteine residues and to clean up the sample by acetone precipitation (in particular, primary amines in the spermine and Tris contained in the lysis buffers could interfere with labeling efficiency). Particular care should be taken during these steps to minimize contamination of the samples with dust and other particulate which will lead to identification of commonly observed contaminant proteins (e.g., cytokeratin).

1. Take 100 µg from each of the four protein samples and make them up to the same volume (e.g., 20 µl) with lysis buffer 2 and vortex.

2. For efficient enzymatic digestion, it is recommended to reduce disulfides and alkylate the resulting thiol groups on cysteine residues. Add TCEP to a final concentration of 5 mM and incubate at room temperature for 20 min to reduce disulfides. Add IAA to a final concentration of 10 mM and incubate at room temperature in the dark for 30 min to alkylate thiols.

3. Dilute each sample one in two with HPLC grade water (to avoid urea precipitation on addition of cold acetone). Add six volumes of cold acetone, which has been pre-cooled to –20°C, to each sample, vortex, and incubate at –20°C for 2 h to precipitate protein. Pellet the precipitate in a centrifuge pre-cooled to 4°C at 5,000×g for 10 min. Aspirate

the acetone and allow the pellet to air dry for 5 min. Do not over-dry as resuspension will be problematic. Resuspend and dissolve the pellet in 20 μl of 0.5 M TEAB (if the pellet is difficult to dissolve, SDS can be added to a final volume of 0.1% (w/v) or the volume of TEAB can be increased – try to avoid increasing the volume above 50 μl, as this will decrease the efficiency of the labeling step).

4. Allow a vial of trypsin to come to room temperature and reconstitute it with 40 μl of TEAB and vortex. Immediately add 5 μg of trypsin (trypsin to protein ratio of 1:20) to each of the four samples and incubate overnight at 37°C.

5. Add ethanol to each sample to a final concentration of 60% (v/v).

6. Allow one vial of each iTRAQ reagent (114, 115, 116, and 117) to come to room temperature and add 70 μl of ethanol to each vial and vortex. Transfer the contents of one iTRAQ reagent vial into one of the sample tubes and repeat for each sample with a different iTRAQ reagent as indicated in Table 1.

7. Vortex the tubes and incubate for 1 h at room temperature to allow the labeling reaction to proceed (see Note 3). Combine the contents of each labeling reaction into a single tube and vortex. Speedvac the solution to dryness.

3.3. Offline Strong Cation Exchange Fractionation

This section outlines the pre-fractionation of the labeled sample by preparative strong cation exchange HPLC chromatography (see Note 4). After fractionation, the samples must be desalted by solid phase extraction with C18 spin columns before they can be introduced into the LC–MS system.

1. The HPLC should be programmed with a flow rate of 200 μl/min under the gradient conditions indicated in Table 2.

2. Install the SCX column, purge the pump, set the UV detector to 215 nm, and equilibrate the SCX column by running buffer A until the back pressure and the intensity on the UV chromatogram have stabilized. It is advisable to do two to three

Table 1
iTRAQ label sample assignment

iTRAQ reagent	Sample
114	Day 3 – vehicle
115	Day 3 – treated
116	Day 14 – vehicle
117	Day 14 – treated

Table 2
Strong cation exchange chromatography gradient table

Time (min)	% RP buffer B
0	0
10	0
50	30
60	50
65	100
70	100
85	0
90	0

blank injections of buffer A to ensure that the system is fully equilibrated (a shorter gradient can be used for this step).

3. Load a 96-well plate onto the Probot and set it to collect a fraction every 60 s. This will result in 90 fractions of 200 μl each. The Probot can be programmed to begin fraction collection on a signal from the HPLC system (this command is required in both the HPLC program and the Probot program).

4. Dilute the sample in 1,000 μl of strong cation exchange buffer A and check the pH with pH paper. If the pH is greater than 3.0, it should be carefully adjusted to pH 3.0 with 1% (v/v) formic acid.

5. Introduce the sample into the HPLC system by direct injection and start the gradient program (ensuring that the fraction collector is functioning correctly). At pH 3.0, the vast majority of the peptides will be positively charged and will bind to the negatively charged cation exchange column. The gradual increase in concentration of positively charged potassium ions in the mobile phase across the run time causes a stepwise displacement and elution of peptides dependent on their affinity for the negatively charged stationary phase. In this way, an effective fractionation of the complex peptide mixture can be achieved.

6. When the run is complete, examine the UV chromatogram to determine if the fractionation has been successful. See the example in Fig. 2 for a typical UV chromatogram from this procedure. The majority of peptides will elute between

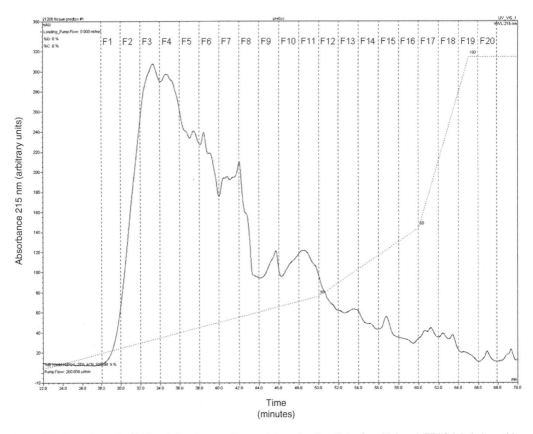

Fig. 2. UV chromatography (215 nm) for strong cation exchange fractionation of multiplexed iTRAQ labeled peptides derived from liver protein extracts. The *dashed line* shows the % of SCX buffer B. Fractions pooling should be informed by the intensity of the UV absorbance for a given time segment. The figure displays the peptide elution in 22–70 min of a 90-min total run time.

approximately 25 and 70 min. This time period corresponds to about 45 fractions in the 96-well plate. Two to three adjacent fractions are pooled to create approximately 20 samples. Fraction pooling should be informed by the intensity of the UV chromatogram. Where the UV intensity is lower (indicating a lower concentration of peptides), samples should be pooled from three fractions (see Note 5).

7. Speedvac the samples to dryness and resuspend in 100 μl of reversed phase buffer A.

8. Equilibrate a C18 MacroSpin Column (one column is required for each of the 20 samples) by loading 500 μl of RP buffer B onto the column and centrifuging at $110 \times g$ until the buffer is eluted (1–2 min). Repeat once. Load 500 μl of RP buffer A onto the column and centrifuge at $110 \times g$ until the buffer is eluted. Repeat once.

9. Load the sample onto the column and centrifuge at $110 \times g$ until the buffer is eluted. The peptides will be retained on the

column, while polar and/or ionic solutes such as salt will flow through. Wash the column 2× with 250 µl of RP buffer A.

10. Replace the collection tube with a clean one, load 250 µl of RP buffer B onto the column, and centrifuge the column at $110 \times g$ until the buffer is eluted. The high organic content of RP buffer B will elute the peptides from the column. Wash the column with a further 250 µl of RP buffer B and centrifuge, eluting the buffer into the same collection tube.

11. Speedvac the samples to dryness and resuspend the peptides in 10 µl of RP buffer A in preparation for injection onto the reversed phase HPLC system.

3.4. Online Reversed Phase Liquid Chromatography–Mass Spectrometry

After the upfront ion exchange fractionation, the sample is further separated by nano-flow reversed phase chromatography and introduced into the mass spectrometer directly by nano-electrospray. Peptides are automatically selected for MS/MS sequencing as in a normal data-dependent tandem mass spectrometry experiment. Collision induced dissociation (CID) of a peptide will also lead to the cleavage of the iTRAQ label, yielding the diagnostic iTRAQ reporter ions (114, 115, 116, and 117). As such, selection of the peptide for fragmentation should yield not only the peptide sequence but also the relative proportion of that peptide originating from each of the four samples, as illustrated in Fig. 3.

1. The HPLC capillary pump should be set with a flow rate of 3 µl/min and the nanopump should be set with a flow rate of 300 nl/min under the gradient conditions indicated in Table 3.

2. The critical settings for the mass spectrometer are as follows: the collision energy is determined depending on the precursor m/z – slope = 3 V/100 Da, offset = 2 V; precursors are prioritized by charge state in the order 2+, 3+, >3+, and unknown; the threshold for selection of precursors is set at 1,000 counts or 0.01% of the base peak; the scan rates are set at eight scans per second for MS and three scans per second for MS/MS, with six precursors selected for sequencing per cycle; ensure that the mass range for MS/MS includes the iTRAQ reporter ion region (e.g., 50–3,000); set at least one reference mass using a common background ion (for example, the protonated bis-2-ethylhexylphthalate ion at m/z 391.284286).

3. Calibrate the mass spectrometer by infusing ES-TOF Tuning Mix. Load the HPLC-Chip into the Chipcube, purge the nano and capillary pumps, and after 60 min of flow, ensure that a stable spray has been established. If the spray is not stable, adjust the cap voltage and spray tip position until a stable spray is attained. Fifty volts should be added to the voltage required to stabilies the spray on 1007. RP buffer A to guard against spray collapse during the run. Set the flush volume in the Chipcube dialog to 12 µl.

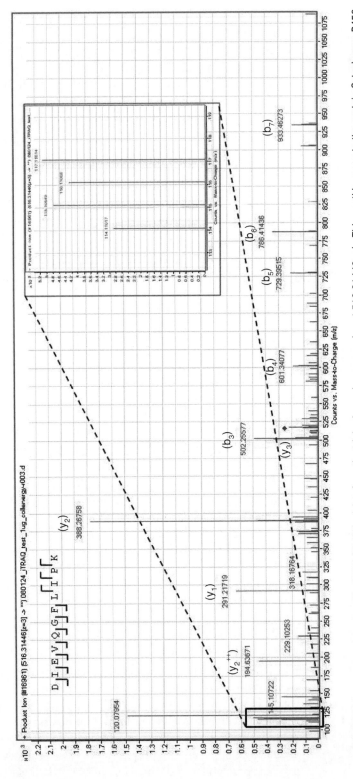

Fig. 3. MS/MS spectrum of the peptide DIEVQGFLIPK arising from the triply charged precursor ion at 516.31446 *m/z*. This peptide maps to the protein Cytochrome P450 2D3 (IPI00202580), an enzyme that is well described in terms of its role in xenobiotic-metabolism. The iTRAQ reporter ion region (114–117 *m/z*) is enlarged, the matched *b* and *y* ions are labeled, and the precursor ion is denoted with a *diamond*.

Table 3
Reversed phase chromatography gradient table

Time (min)	% RP buffer B
0	0
10	0
100	40
110	90
125	90
135	0

4. Set the injection volume to 8 µl and perform two to three blank injections using RP buffer A to ensure that the system is equilibrated (this can be done with a shorter gradient). In order to make certain that the system is performing adequately, it is recommended to inject a standard protein digest mix and verify that the chromatography and protein identifications are satisfactory (see Note 6).

5. Create a work list to inject all samples sequentially and start the sequence. When the run is complete, manually examine the chromatography and some of the mass spectra. If the quality is satisfactory, copy the .d directory for each injection and paste into a single folder in the Spectrum Mill>msdataSM directory.

3.5. Data Processing and Interpretation

The raw data must now be processed and searched against an in silico digest of a relevant protein database, and the intensity of the iTRAQ reporter ions for each identified peptide/protein must be determined. The data can then be exported for statistical analysis of the expression changes in particular peptides/proteins.

1. Open the Spectrum Mill MS Proteomics Workbench.

2. Each batch of iTRAQ reagents is supplied with a certificate of analysis that details correction factors particular to that batch which must be incorporated into the calculations. Open the *Tool Belt* page in the *Utilities* list and select *create iTraq correction factors*. Input the batch number and correction factors from the certificate of analysis and click *Create*. Select *Apply iTraq correction factors* and associate the relevant .d directories with the iTRAQ correction factors for that batch.

3. In order to reduce search time, the spectra are subjected to a data extraction procedure which serves to merge scans from the same precursor in a given time segment (improves s/n ratio), to remove spectra with low information content, and to determine precursor charge state (where possible). Open the Data *Extractor* tool and select the appropriate .d directories. Choose *Carbamidomethylation (C)* and *iTRAQ (N-term, K)* as fixed modifications. Set *merge scans with the same precursor m/z* to ±15 s, ±0.025 *m/z, similarity merging* enabled, leave the remaining parameters at the default setting, and click on *Extract*.

4. The filtered data can now be searched against an appropriate protein database, such as the International Protein Index Rat database (7), which has been digested in silico according to the known rules for trypsin. Open the *MS/MS Search* page and select the appropriate .d directories. The majority of parameters on this page can be left as default settings; however, some modifications are advised. Select the IPI Rat database and choose *Carbamidomethylation (C)* and *iTRAQ (N-term, K)* as fixed modifications. Ensure that the correct instrument is selected – *Agilent ESI-QTOF*. *Identity* mode should be selected, *dynamic peak thresholding* and *Calculate reverse database scores* should be switched on. Click *Start Search* to begin the search algorithm.

5. When the database search has been completed, the results can be viewed in the *Protein/Peptide Summary* page (see Note 7). For an overview of the data, select the *Protein Summary Details* from the *Mode* menu. Select the appropriate data directory, ensure that the *iTRAQ intensities* option is checked, select one of the reporter ions (e.g., 114) as the control in the *iTRAQ ratios control* option, and click *Summarize*. This summary provides a protein-centric view of the data where the mean and standard deviation of the iTRAQ ratios for each protein are calculated from the contributing peptides.

6. For a more statistically rigorous evaluation of the data, it must be exported for analysis using other tools (e.g., Excel, SPSS, and R). Select the *peptide* from the *Mode* menu, check the *excel export* option, and click *Summarize*. The software then offers the options to *Upload File to LIMS* or *Display Created File Below*. Right click on *Display Created File Below*, select the *save target as* option, and save the file to an appropriate directory. The file is saved in the *.ssv* (semi-colon separated value) format, which can be easily imported into Excel or other software for extended statistical analysis.

4. Notes

1. It is strongly recommended that a parallel sample be prepared from the beginning of the protocol and to "mock" iTRAQ label this sample (i.e., using ethanol; see Subheading 3.2, step 6). This will allow the investigator to check the suitability of the strong cation exchange chromatography system and the reversed phase chromatography system, as well as acquisition parameters in the mass spectrometer. Including this precaution in the protocol should help to avoid wasting iTRAQ labeling reagent and provide confidence in the final results.

2. The tissue lysis and protein extraction protocol can be modified easily (many other protocols are available), but some caution is required to avoid substances interfering with the iTRAQ labeling. For example, in the protocol above, there are two reagents containing primary amines. If the acetone precipitation clean-up step was not included, these primary amines would compete with the lysine-containing peptides for the iTRAQ label and could result in poor labeling efficiency. It is recommended to consult the iTRAQ Reagents Chemistry Reference Guide (8) before modifying the tissue lysis, tryptic digestion, or iTRAQ labeling protocols.

3. In order for the labeling reaction to proceed efficiently, a number of conditions must be satisfied. The aqueous content should not be more than 40% (v/v) and the ethanol content should be at least 60% (v/v). Avoid decreasing the protein concentration by overdilution of the sample as this will reduce labeling efficiency. Excess buffer can be removed by evaporation if required. The pH of the labeling reaction should be 8.5; this can be easily tested with pH paper and adjusted if the samples are suspected to be acidic.

4. For tissue types other than liver, or for alternate tissue lysis protocols, it may be necessary to adjust either the potassium chloride salt gradient or the concentration of salt in SCX buffer B. In order to attain an efficient fractionation by strong cation exchange chromatography, this should be optimized using an unlabeled sample, as mentioned in Note 1.

5. Strong cation exchange chromatography is the most popular and conventional method for achieving up-front fractionation in multidimensional LC–MS experiments. Recently, another approach referred to as "off-gel electrophoresis" has emerged as a possible alternative to SCX. This technique is based on preparative isoelectric focusing of peptides using standard immobilized pH gradient gel strips, with recovery of the peptides in the liquid phase. Proponents of this technique

maintain that the resolution is improved and that the peptides are more evenly distributed across fractions in comparison with that in SCX and, as a consequence, more proteins are identified (9, 10).

6. The stability of the reversed phase chromatography system and the electrospray is of paramount importance for maximizing the information content of the results. If the chromatographic resolution is not optimal, as judged by a standard digest sample, the column should be replaced. The spray stability can be improved by adjusting the position of the spray tip and by adjusting the spray voltage (Vcap) from a starting point of 1,800 V (do not go above 2,000 V as the instrument can be damaged).

7. By default, Spectrum Mill uses an *Autovalidation* function to filter for high-quality database matches based on user-defined score thresholds [*Score* – an overview score that accounts for matched fragment ions, immonium, and other marker ions, and penalizes for unaccounted peaks in a spectrum; *% Scored Peak Intensity* – the percentage of peaks in the spectrum that are explained by the database match; *Fwd – Rev Score* – this is calculated by reversing the sequence of all the peptides (excluding the end residues) in the database and scoring the spectrum versus these, and subtracting the best reverse score hit from the best forward score; *Rank 1–2 Score* – the difference between the scores of the top two hits]. The *Autovalidation* settings should be left at default values. The Spectrum Mill workflow advocates starting first with the autovalidated results and then adding further identifications to the validated group by iterative rounds of searching using variable modifications (such as oxidized methionine) and also by manual inspection of MS/MS spectra for quality. Direct measurement of the false discovery rate for identifications is not supported in Spectrum Mill at this time; however, if this is required, it can be achieved by appending a decoy database to the search database (11). DBToolkit is a useful freely available program for performing protein database manipulations such as reversal and concatenation (12).

8. Other instrumentation and software: This workflow has been described using a particular set of instrumentation and analysis tools but the iTRAQ strategy has been applied on a variety of tandem mass spectrometer types (primarily Q-TOF and TOF–TOF (13)), but more recently, ion trap-type instruments have been adapted for this purpose (14). The analysis software provided by the instrument vendors generally supports iTRAQ quantification (assuming that the instruments support the workflow) but there are also a num-

ber of freely available tools that can be used with iTRAQ data. A popular example is Libra, an element of the Trans Proteomic Pipeline created at the Institute for Systems Biology, Seattle (15).

Acknowledgments

We would like to thank all the members of the PredTox Consortium. Funding is acknowledged under the EU FP6 Integrated Project, InnoMed. The UCD Conway Institute and the Proteome Research Centre is funded by the Programme for Research in Third Level Institutions (PRTLI), as administered by the Higher Education Authority (HEA) of Ireland.

References

1. Collins, B.C., et al. (2007) Use of proteomics for the discovery of early markers of drug toxicity. *Expert Opin. Drug Metab. Toxicol.* **3(5)**, 689–704.

2. Merrick, B.A. (2006) Toxicoproteomics in liver injury and inflammation. *Ann. N. Y. Acad. Sci.* **1076**, 707–717.

3. Merrick, B.A. (2008) The plasma proteome, adductome and idiosyncratic toxicity in toxicoproteomics research. *Brief Funct. Genomic Proteomic* **7(1)**, 35–49.

4. Wetmore, B.A., and Merrick, B.A. (2004) Toxicoproteomics: proteomics applied to toxicology and pathology. *Toxicol. Pathol.* **32(6)**, 619–642.

5. Aggarwal, K., Choe, L.H., and Lee, K.H. (2006) Shotgun proteomics using the iTRAQ isobaric tags. *Brief Funct. Genomic Proteomic* **5(2)**, 112–120.

6. Fella, K., et al. (2005) Use of two-dimensional gel electrophoresis in predictive toxicology: identification of potential early protein biomarkers in chemically induced hepatocarcinogenesis. *Proteomics* **5(7)**, 1914–1927.

7. Kersey, P.J., et al. (2004) The International Protein Index: an integrated database for proteomics experiments. *Proteomics* **4(7)**, 1985–1988.

8. *iTRAQ Reagents Chemistry Reference Guide.* (2004) [http://www3.appliedbiosystems.com/cms/groups/psm_marketing/documents/generaldocuments/cms_041463.pdf]

9. Essader, A.S., et al. (2005) A comparison of immobilized pH gradient isoelectric focusing and strong-cation-exchange chromatography as a first dimension in shotgun proteomics. *Proteomics* **5(1)**, 24–34.

10. Lengqvist, J., Uhlen, K., and Lehtio, J. (2007) iTRAQ compatibility of peptide immobilized pH gradient isoelectric focusing. *Proteomics* **7(11)**, 1746–1752.

11. Elias, J.E., and Gygi, S.P. (2007) Target-decoy search strategy for increased confidence in large-scale protein identifications by mass spectrometry. *Nat. Methods* **4(3)**, 207–214.

12. Martens, L., Vandekerckhove, J., and Gevaert, K. (2005) DBToolkit: processing protein databases for peptide-centric proteomics. *Bioinformatics* **21(17)**, 3584–3585.

13. Yang, Y., et al. (2007) A comparison of nLC-ESI-MS/MS and nLC-MALDI-MS/MS for GeLC-based protein identification and iTRAQ-based shotgun quantitative proteomics. *J. Biomol. Tech.* **18(4)**, 226–237.

14. Griffin, T.J., et al. (2007) iTRAQ reagent-based quantitative proteomic analysis on a linear ion trap mass spectrometer. *J. Proteome Res.* **6(11)**, 4200–4209.

15. Keller, A., et al. (2005) A uniform proteomics MS/MS analysis platform utilizing open XML file formats. *Mol. Syst. Biol.* Article number: 1, 2005.0017. pages 1–8.

Chapter 24

NMR and MS Methods for Metabonomics

Frank Dieterle, Björn Riefke, Götz Schlotterbeck, Alfred Ross, Hans Senn, and Alexander Amberg

Abstract

Metabonomics, also often referred to as "metabolomics" or "metabolic profiling," is the systematic profiling of metabolites in bio-fluids or tissues of organisms and their temporal changes. In the last decade, metabonomics has become increasingly popular in drug development, molecular medicine, and other biotechnology fields, since it profiles directly the phenotype and changes thereof in contrast to other "-omics" technologies. The increasing popularity of metabonomics has been possible only due to the enormous development in the technology and bioinformatics fields. In particular, the analytical technologies supporting metabonomics, i.e., NMR, LC-MS, UPLC-MS, and GC-MS have evolved into sensitive and highly reproducible platforms allowing the determination of hundreds of metabolites in parallel. This chapter describes the best practices of metabonomics as seen today. All important steps of metabolic profiling in drug development and molecular medicine are described in great detail, starting from sample preparation, to determining the measurement details of all analytical platforms, and finally, to discussing the corresponding specific steps of data analysis.

Key words: Metabonomics, Metabolomics, Metabolic profiling, NMR, LC-MS, UPLC-MS, GC-MS

1. Introduction

In this chapter, the principles of metabonomics, the associated technologies, and the best practices to apply these technologies are introduced. Besides the term metabonomics, metabolomics and metabolic profiling are also often found in the literature. The reason is a historical parallel evolvement of the concept of metabolite profiling of plants mainly based on chromatographic technologies creating the term "metabolomics," and of metabolic profiling in preclinical and clinical applications primarily based on nuclear magnetic resonance (NMR) spectroscopy forming the associated term "metabonomics". Nowadays technologies have crossed the

Jean-Charles Gautier (ed.), *Drug Safety Evaluation: Methods and Protocols*, Methods in Molecular Biology, vol. 691,
DOI 10.1007/978-1-60761-849-2_24, © Springer Science+Business Media, LLC 2011

borders of these scientific fields, and both terms and the rather new term "metabolic profiling" are used interchangeably.

But what is metabonomics precisely? The most cited definition of metabonomics was published in 1999 as "the quantitative measurement of the dynamic multiparametric response of living systems to pathophysiological stimuli or genetic modification" (1). In other words, metabonomics is the systematic profiling of metabolites in biofluids or tissues of organisms and their temporal changes caused by different factors such as drug treatment, environmental influences, nutrition, lifestyle, genetic effects or diseases. Hereby, single endogenous metabolites and patterns of endogenous metabolites can be of interest. The total number of different metabolites in an organism (the so-called metabolome) is not known. Estimates based on known pathways range from several hundreds to several thousands. Yet, recently it has been shown that more endogenous metabolites exist than the number of metabolites covered by presently known pathways (2). Biochemically, metabonomics is the ultimate endpoint measurement of biological events linking genotype to phenotype and capturing the influence of nutrition, environmental influences, response to pharmaceuticals, and many more. The importance of metabonomics for assessing health and the influence of therapies is also expressed in terms of biological timing and biological probabilities: Genetics and genomics capture events that might happen, proteomics captures events that are happening, and metabonomics captures events, that have happened.

Metabonomics is often perceived as the newest of the various "-omics" technologies and is often believed to be still in its childhood. This is because a systematic profiling of as many metabolites as possible has gained broad interest only during the last decade. Yet, less systematic analyses of metabolites with gas chromatography were already proposed during the 1970s (3). In the 1980s and 1990s several applications of metabolic profiling have been reported but the broad breakthrough came along only with recent advances in analytical and computational technologies. Besides the use of metabonomics as unbiased biomarker discovery technology, measurements of small molecules in body fluids are well established and accepted in clinical biochemistry, also evident by the fact that 95% of all diagnostic clinical assays test for small molecules (4). The majority of these tests analyze single metabolites in a targeted way, and bases on typical technologies common in clinical chemistry. They are completely different from non-targeted technologies to measure and quantify numerous metabolites simultaneously. Untargeted metabonomics technologies are based on two main analytical platforms: NMR and mass spectroscopy (MS), whereby the latter is typically coupled with a chromatographic separation technology. In the field of drug development, four technologies are widely used: NMR, the combination of liquid chromatography with mass spectroscopy (LC-MS), its evolvement called ultra-performance liquid chromatography coupled to mass spectroscopy (UPLC-MS), and gas chromatography coupled to mass spectroscopy (GC-MS). Hereby, the different technologies do not compete, but complement each other in terms of types of metabolites being covered by the different technologies. Only recently, it has been shown how synergies can be created between the different analysis technologies using new data analysis methods (5). The analytical platforms generate hundreds to thousands of data points, which render multivariate data analysis methods indispensable for reducing the amount of data and to simplify complexity.

In the next section, methods for the appropriate sampling of biofluids and sample preparation steps are discussed in detail. Afterwards, the application of the different technologies is described with the focus on best practices. Particularities of data analysis, appropriate software and databases are discussed.

2. Materials

2.1. Sample Collection

1. Sample tubes: NUNC cryovials, Eppendorf Safelock tubes.
2. Metabolic cages, e.g., LabMaster Metabolic Cages from TSE Systems GmbH; Siemensstr. 21; 61352 Bad Homburg; Germany.
3. NaN_3 (sodium azide), e.g., S2002 from Sigma-Aldrich.

2.2. NMR Sample Preparation

1. TSP (sodium trimethylsilyl $[2,2,3,3\text{-}^2H_4]$ propionate).
2. NaN_3 (sodium azide).
3. D_2O, e.g., 151882 from Sigma-Aldrich.
4. NaCl 0.9% solution.
5. NMR tubes (o.d. 3 mm or 5 mm), e.g., from Wilmad, 1002 Harding Hwy Buena, NJ 08310.

2.3. LC-MS Sample Preparation

1. Methanol for extraction from serum samples.
2. Re-suspension in starting gradient: acetonitrile/0.1% formic acid 5/95.

2.4. LC-MS Analysis

1. An RP HPLC column with 2.1-mm internal diameter, normally packed with C18 material, maintained at 40°C.
2. Gradient elution: Acetonitrile/0.1% formic acid, starting from 5% to 90% organic phase.

2.5. GC-MS Sample Preparation

1. Extraction mixture: Methanol/water/chloroform (750/250/200 v/v/v).
2. Methoxymation reagent: 20 mg/ml methoxyamine hydrochloride in pyridine.

3. Silylation reagent: MSTFA (*N*-methyl-*N*-trimethylsilyltri-fluoroacetamide).

2.6. GC-MS Analysis

1. Standard GC or GC×GC instrument.

2. Standard MS with quadrupole analyzer or time of flight (TOF) analyzer.

3. DB 20 m×180 μm DB5-MS with 0.18-μm film column.

4. Helium as carrier gas.

5. Methane as reagent gas in chemical ionization (CI).

6. Lock reference using heptacosa in electron ionization (EI) or methyltriazine in CI.

2.7. Software and Databases

1. *Bio-Rad Laboratories Know-It-All*: Bio-Rad Laboratories, Informatics Division; Two Penn Center Plaza, Suite 800; 1500 John F. Kennedy Blvd.; Philadelphia, PA 19102-1737 USA; Toll-free phone (USA & Canada): +1 888 5 BIO-RAD (+1 888 524 6723); Phone (other countries): +1 267 322 6931; Fax: +1 267 322 6932; E-mail: informatics.usa@bio-rad.com.

2. *Bruker Biospin Biofluid Spectra Base*: Bruker Biospin GmbH; 76287 Rheinstetten; Phone: +49-721-5161-0; Fax: +49-721-517101; E-mail: nmr@brukerbiospin.de.

3. *Chenomx NMR Suite*: Chenomx Suite 800; 100 50112 Street; Edmonton, Alberta T5K291; Phone: +001-780-432-0033; Fax: +001-780-432-3388; http://www.chenomx.com.

---

3. Methods

3.1. Sample Collection

3.1.1. General Comments on Sample Collection

In principal, ¹H-NMR or LC-MS based metabonomics analysis can be applied on a large variety of body fluids such as blood serum or plasma, urine, cerebrospinal fluid, saliva, sinovial fluid, amniotic fluid, ascites, and all types of tissue extracts (e.g., tumors, brain, and muscle) (6). Most important for studies in animals and humans are sampling of blood serum or plasma and also urine as these samples are easy to obtain and are often drawn in parallel to clinical chemistry sampling during a human study or pre-clinical experiment with animals. Therefore, we will focus in the following on sampling of blood serum and urine.

In contrast to experiments with animals, using inbred strains with homogenous genetic background, age distribution, controlled food and water supply, and defined living conditions (caging, standardized day-night cycles) (7, 8), the situation we face working in the clinical environment is the opposite. All the above-mentioned variables have influence on the metabonomics result and influence the scatter of the effects to be measured (6, 9, 10). In human studies, some of the variables can be controlled for a certain time (11–13), but this will not be possible for a long-term or larger clinical study or trial for ethical reasons. In order to minimize variability, the sampling time and conditions should be standardized as much as possible.

3.1.2. Human Blood Sampling

1. For NMR and LC-MS methods, an aliquot of 200 µL of serum or plasma is sufficient, which means that 500 µL of whole blood have to be drawn (see Note 1).

2. Allow serum sample to clot for 30 min at room temperature or on ice.

3. Centrifuge for 15 min at $1,500 \times g$.

4. The supernatant is transferred to a sample tube for storage at −20°C or lower.

5. Prepare all the necessary aliquots for different types of measurements (NMR, LC-MS, clinical chemistry, and other biomarkers) before freezing to avoid thawing–freezing cycles of samples. Samples should always be taken from single individuals separately, pooling of individual samples should be avoided (14, 15).

3.1.3. Human Urine Sampling

1. Human urine samples should be taken in the morning hours in a clean and dry container using mid-stream urine (see Note 2).

2. Samples can be stored below −20°C for long-term storage up to 3 months (16). A minimum volume of 500 µL urine sample should be reserved for NMR- and LC-MS analysis each.

3.1.4. Animal Blood Sampling

Handling and sampling of laboratory animals should to be performed by specially trained and experienced personnel in comvpliance with the existing guidelines for good practice of laboratory animals (17–19) and in compliance with the respective regulations in the countries of the European union which may differ for special sampling techniques and the local Ethics Committees.

Blood samples can be drawn from smaller rodents (mice and rats) in conscious or, more common, anesthetized state, depending of the established techniques and experiences of the respective laboratory. For non-rodents (dogs, mini-pigs, and non-human primates), blood sampling in conscious animals is the common standard. An overview of the techniques is given in reference (20) and can also be found in the Internet (http://awic.nal.usda.gov/nal_display/index.php?info_center=3&tax_level=1&tax_subject=185. last check by the author: 2.04.08).

Blood sampling for metabonomics is ideally performed in parallel to sampling for clinical pathology, which offers the opportunity of correlation analysis of metabolite profiles to classical endpoints. In order to obtain time profiles of the response, multiple sampling of single animals could be considered. In this case, the maximal extractable blood volume per time point should be in compliance with the good practice guide (21) and should not be exceeded, not to influence and stress the experimental system by exaggerated blood sampling. This is especially important for smaller animals like rats and critical in mice. Sample volumes are discussed in the section for human sampling above.

3.1.5. Animal Urine Sampling

For non-invasive urine collection, the experimental animals, mice and rats or non-rodents, have to be transferred in metabolic cages (22) and kept for a longer time interval, in the ideal case for 24 h. Also, shorter intervals such as 8 h or 16 h have been reported in the literature, which are a compromise between circadian rhythm, animal welfare, and capturing fast metabonomic trajectories. The design of the metabolic cages should allow separate collection of feces and urine to avoid contamination (22). The metabolic response during this longer time interval reflects activity and resting phases of the animals. When the amount of urinary excretion is known to be sufficient, sampling can be fragmented in smaller intervals, e.g., 0–8, 8–16, 16–24, and 24–32 h, to study acute and late effects with higher time resolution and sensitivity (23). During the sampling interval, urine should be collected in a clean container and kept at low temperatures between 0 and 4°C by using a cooling bath or ice container, for example. To prevent metabolite degradation by bacteria, addition of NaN_3 is recommended (14).

In case of the larger non-rodent animals, it may be possible, depending on the construction of the metabolic cages, that urine is contaminated with feces or the animal has not urinated. In this case, urine collection via a catheter from the bladder can be considered to get a clean and defined urine sample.

3.2. NMR

The theory of NMR is highly developed and the dynamics of nuclear spin-systems is fully understood (24, 25). For the acquisition of a NMR spectrum, a liquid sample is placed in a static magnetic field. After irradiation with high-frequency pulses (pulse-sequences), the response of the NMR sample is detected by an induced current. The highest field strength available in 2008's NMR spectrometers is 21 Tesla corresponding to 900 MHz ^{1}H (proton) frequency. Most applications in metabolic profiling use 600 MHz (14.1 Tesla) instruments.

The amplitude response of a NMR spectrometer is perfectly linear to the concentration of the sample, which allows easy quantification of compound concentrations for metabolic profiling in the micromolar to millimolar range. All steps involved in the acquisition and processing of NMR data, including preparation and exchange of samples, can be performed fully automated for hundreds of samples without the need for manual interaction. A state-of-the-art hardware setup is shown in Fig. 1.

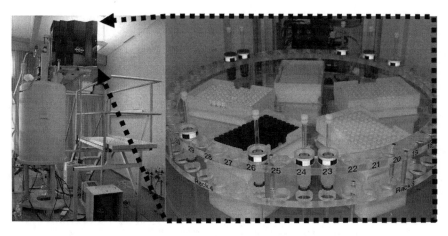

Fig. 1. A sample changing robot (Sample Jet, Bruker Fällanden Switzerland) allows fast sequential single-tube submission under temperature-controlled conditions. The system can thus efficiently handle up to 480 samples.

The sensitivity of NMR spectrometers depends primarily on the inherent sensitivity of the detection device (probehead), besides the magnetic field strength and the nucleus detected. Probeheads tailored for the highest sensitivity depending on sample concentration and amount are available with different coil sizes, ranging from 10 mm to 1 mm in diameter. Cryogenically cooled probeheads operated with 5-, 3-, or 1.7-mm NMR tubes which enhance the signal-to-noise ratio by a factor of approximately four compared to conventional room-temperature probes present an attractive compromise – flow-through inserts are available nowadays. It must be noted that a fourfold increase of sensitivity reduces experimental time 16-fold (26).

The inter-laboratory comparability of NMR data was tested for a set of samples shipped to different laboratories. Data were acquired with NMR spectrometers operated at different field strengths. Compared to any other analytical technique, NMR shows an impressive analytical reproducibility and repeatability, reflecting itself in a coefficient of variation of 2% for a study invoking a large set of spectra (25). Thus, the observed variances in NMR spectra of a biological study are highly dominated by biological effects.

NMR offers a wealth of experimental techniques tailored for extraction of structural, chemical-kinetic, structural-dynamic, and other information, especially in multidimensional applications.

Compared to more elaborate applications of NMR, pulse sequences applied in metabonomics require a relatively low level of sophistication. The application of NMR for biological samples is faced with the problem of water suppression, as the metabolites are present in micromolar or lower concentration in the presence of water at 55 M concentration. This problem is solved by several water suppression techniques (27). The method of water suppression has to be considered when combined data sets (28) from different laboratories are analyzed.

In the following solvent suppression techniques, NMR experiments and data processing procedures, which are widely employed in metabolic profiling, are briefly reviewed. For applications of HR-MAS NMR for tissue samples and rarely used heteronuclear techniques, the reader is referred to the literature (29–34). Common NMR experimental parameters are provided in Table 1.

3.2.1. NMR Sample Preparation

In contrast to other analytical techniques such as MS-based methods, metabolite profiling of biofluids by NMR requires, in general, no sophisticated sample preparation procedures (35). In most cases, adding H_2O/D_2O or buffer to account for pH variation or to reduce viscosity is sufficient as sample preparation before the NMR measurement (36). This means that one potential source of variance due to sample extraction procedures is absent.

Table 1
Parameters of NMR experiments as used in our laboratory for application to biological samples. If two rows are given in a cell, the first and second row provide values for f_2 and f_1, respectively

Description	Number of scans NS	Interscan delay day 1 [s]	Time domain TD	Spectral width SW	Processing size SI	Window function	Window function (parameters)
Noesy 1D with sign-alternating gradient prior to first pulse, preset [50 Hz] for day 1 and during 100 ms mixing time no gradient during mixing time	32	2	32 k	20 ppm	64 k	Exponential	lb 1
Gradient dqf-cosy, preset [50 Hz] during day 1	>32	1	4 k 256	20 ppm 20 ppm	4 k 1 k	Squared sine	ssb 3
TOCSY, MLEV-17 mixing time of 80 ms, preset [50 Hz] during day 1	>32	1	4 k 300	20 ppm 20 ppm	4 k 512	Squared sine	ssb 2.5
Jres, preset [50 Hz] during day 1	>8	1	16 k 64	20 ppm 40 Hz	16 k 256	Exponential sine	lb 1 ssb 0

The common sample preparation protocol for urine samples includes pH-adjustment with phosphate buffer:

1. Mix two parts of urine with one part of 0.2 M phosphate buffer (pH 7.4) containing 1 mM TSP (sodium trimethylsilyl [2,2,3,3-$^2H_4$] propionate), 3 mM sodium azide, and 15% D_2O.
2. Centrifuge at 4°C for 10 min at >10,000×g.

For plasma or serum, dilution with saline is applied:

1. Mix one part of plasma or serum with one part of 0.9% NaCl in 10% D_2O.
2. Centrifuge at 4°C for 10 min at >10,000×g.

Prepared samples are transferred to size-matched NMR tubes (o.d. 3 mm or 5 mm) or to 96-format deep-well plates from where they can be inserted in a fully automated way via a sample-changer or a flow-through probehead into the NMR spectrometer.

3.2.2. 1D ^{1}H-Spectroscopy   Most applications of NMR for metabonomics rely on one-dimensional (1D) NMR experiments based on the ^{1}H nucleus, which offers the highest detection sensitivity. Typical 1D NMR spectra of serum, urine, and CSF are shown in Fig. 2.

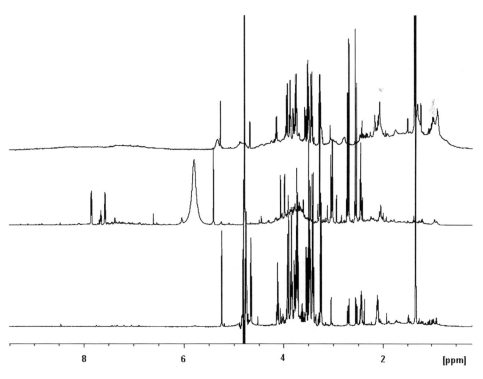

Fig. 2. 1D ^{1}H NMR spectra of serum, urine, and CSF of rat (*top to bottom*). Very different spectral signatures of the body fluids are clearly visible. The serum spectrum is dominated by broad signal background due to high molecular weight proteins and lipoproteins. The most prominent signal in urine is the urea signal around 5.9 ppm, whereas the CSF spectrum is characterized by high glucose (3–4 ppm) and lactate (1.2 ppm) content..

Spectra of these biofluids can be measured with sufficient signal-to-noise (S/N) ratio within a few minutes per sample.

The most widespread solvent suppression technique in use is presaturation (37) applied in a NMR pulse method known as noesy-presat (38). Due to the excellent chemical shift selectivity and baseline properties, the method allows a reliable quantification of signals, which resonate close to water, e.g., the anomeric proton of glucose. As a drawback, signals of hydrogen atoms interacting with water by chemical exchange (e.g., OH, NH, and NH_2) show reduced signal intensities. This is, for example, seen for urea in urine, which cannot be quantified if water presaturation is applied.

Alternatively, the WET (39) sequence is used for water suppression. Here, effects due to analyte–water interaction are less serious. The drawback of the method is a reduced performance with respect to chemical shift selectivity. WET allows for accurate absolute value quantification.

3.2.3. Editing Techniques

NMR signals of rigid, high molecular weight molecules experience fast decay due to relaxation. This property is exploited in metabonomics for selective removal of signals of proteins and lipoproteins. These large biomolecules are found at high concentration in blood serum, plasma (40, 41, 59), or tissue samples. Complementary information focusing on high molecular weight compounds can be obtained by removal of signals from small molecules by employing diffusion editing methods (42–44). Applications in metabonomics research with biofluids and tissues can be found in the literature (45, 46).

3.2.4. 2D NMR

The use of 2D NMR in metabonomics is limited to small sample arrays as the measuring time is up to several hours per sample. Nevertheless, examples can be found in the literature (47). The 2D techniques unfold their full power if an unknown structure of a newly found biomarker has to be elucidated in a biological sample (48). All 2D experiments applied so far depend on the detection of highly sensitive hydrogen nuclei.

In *J-resolved spectroscopy*, the J-coupling information is separated into a second dimension orthogonal to the chemical shift axes in the spectrum. This technique was applied to body fluids including urine (49), CSF (50), seminal fluid (51), and blood plasma (52). From the J-resolved spectrum, a so-called chemical shift spectrum of reduced complexity can be extracted, which can be used for simplified quantification by use of a spectral reference database (53).

In *correlation* (COSY) and *total correlation* (TOCSY) spectroscopy (54), a correlation signal is obtained if two spins belong to a homonuclear J-coupling network (55–57). Metabonomics applications for liquids are described in (58). A combination of total correlation spectroscopy with diffusion editing has also been reported (59).

3.2.5. NMR Raw Data Processing

Fourier transformation (FT) of the NMR signal (FID) leads to the NMR spectrum. Prior to FT, data are multiplied by a window function (60) to achieve an ideal compromise between high spectral resolution and S/N in the spectrum. Often used window functions in metabonomics involve exponentially decaying functions adding one Hz of additional line width to the data, and squared cosine-shaped windows for multidimensional data. After FT, the spectra have to be phased and baseline corrected by subtraction of a tailored polynom (see Note 3). The whole process is summarized in Fig. 3 and more information can be found in ref. (61).

3.2.6. Data Pre-processing

Data pre-processing technologies in metabonomics based on NMR aim at reducing variances and influences interfering with data analysis. This variance can be attributed to NMR-specific effects (incorrect phases, and baselines), biological effects (different dilutions of samples, different osmolality), or combined effects that induce shifting peaks in the spectra. Pre-processing of NMR spectra for metabonomics involves three steps described in the following.

3.2.6.1. Excluding Spectral Regions

The first step of NMR data pre-processing is the exclusion of spectral regions, which contain non-reproducible information, or which are dominated by drug metabolites, which are not of interest in metabonomics. In particular, the following exclusion steps are performed:

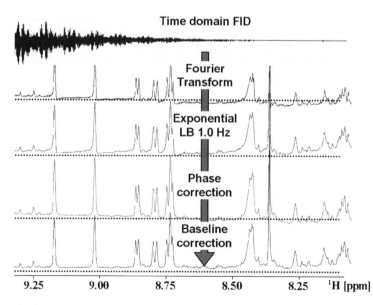

Fig. 3. Processing of a time-domain NMR signal (*at the top*). The frequency domain result after Fourier Transformation (FT) of this signal is shown with low signal-to-noise ratio, baseline-offset, and dispersive contribution. Application of an exponential window function of 1 Hz LB prior to FT results in the trace with substantially improved signal-to-noise ratio. Other artifacts remain. A spectrum suited for metabonomics interpretation is obtained after phase and baseline correction. The last two steps have to be inspected visually.

1. Usually, the spectrum outside the window of 0.2–10 ppm is excluded, since this region in most cases contains only noise and artifacts.

2. The water region between 4.6 and 5.0 ppm is removed, as this region does not contain quantitative information due to solvent suppression used.

3. In case of urine, the amplitude of the strong urea signal is falsified due to proton exchange with water and is excluded (see Note 4).

4. The exclusion of regions covered by drug metabolites and vehicles is a study- and drug-specific process. In single-dose studies, related signals can be best identified in spectra collected directly after administration of drugs (e.g., 0–8 h post-dosing). To ensure compatibility of spectra between studies, these regions are often not excluded, but replaced by representative spectra of normal subjects.

3.2.6.2. Peak Shifts, Binning of Spectra, and Peak Alignments

Small changes of individual chemical shift of signals of the same metabolite in different samples (variation of the matrix) is the major obstacle for data analysis and peak assignment of NMR signals in biofluids. The matrix of biofluids, and in particular, of urine varies highly. This influences the local environment of protons and consequently related chemical shifts. Variation of the matrix is caused by change of the pH (0.1 unit difference is seen easily in NMR), variation of salt concentrations and composition, overall dilution, relative concentration of interacting metabolites, and many more (39). All these effects are reduced but never controlled completely by sample preparation (buffering and addition of EDTA).

Consequently, an appropriate algorithm to reduce these effects is highly beneficial for data analysis and interpretation. Three different mathematical methods are discussed in the following:

1. Equidistant binning: In this most widely used method, spectra are integrated within a defined number of small equidistant spectral regions, which are called "bins" or "buckets." As long as peaks shift only within the borders of these bins, subsequent data analysis procedures are not affected. In the de facto standard of ^{1}H-NMR metabonomics, the spectrum is split into evenly spaced integral regions with a spectral width of 0.04 ppm (see Note 5).

2. Non-equidistant binning: To prevent signal shift between and intersection of signals by boundaries of bins, non-equidistant binning can be used. In one approach, the boundaries of an equidistant 0.04 ppm binning are shifted to nearby minima in a sum or a skyline projection of a set of spectra (62).

3. Automated peak alignment is an alternative to account for peak shifts. Hereby, each spectrum is segmented into regions, which are shifted, stretched, and shrunken to maximize the correlation between the segments in a test and a target spectrum. Overlaps are deleted and gaps are interpolated (63). In another approach, peaks are identified by shape analysis. These peaks are shifted to an a-priori defined average frequency (64). Although for both methods promising first results have been demonstrated, they have not reached a broad application in the scientific community until now.

Although binning and peak alignment methods are beneficial for an automated data analysis, the resulting reduced spectra – especially in the case of binning – suffer from a high loss of information. A stimulus-induced correlated change of a low-concentrated metabolite will be hidden by an uncorrelated change of a high-concentrated metabolite if signals of both compounds contribute to the same bin. As a consequence, recent developments have focused on analyzing spectra at full resolution using spectroscopic correlation methods (STOCSY) or orthogonal projection to latent structures (O-PLS) (65, 66). In any case, a manual inspection of the high-resolution spectra is indispensable to validate if observed differences are artifacts and to find subtle differences in spectra, which analyses of low-resolution spectra or automated analyses might have missed.

3.2.6.3. Normalization of Spectra

Normalization is performed to account for variations in the overall concentration of samples. This is of high importance for homoeostatically not controlled liquids such as urine. Urine of humans and animals typically vary in concentration by a factor of 4–5, but in case of disease, food deprivation, or drug treatment (e.g., diuretics such as furosemide), concentration differences up to a factor of 10 between normal subjects and affected subjects are observed. Further factors, that will influence numeric signal amplitudes can be attributed to dilution induced by sample preparation or differences in NMR hardware in use.

In contrast to changes in the overall concentration of samples, metabolic responses typically influence only a limited number of metabolites. These metabolic changes have to be identified on the background of a varying overall concentration of the sample influencing all metabolites coherently. To achieve this normalization, in the methods, dilution is compensated by multiplication with a calculated scaling factor (which is the dilution). This factor must not be influenced by the metabolic changes investigated.

The following normalization methods are used in the field of metabonomics: Creatinine, integral, and quotient normalization. All normalization steps are usually applied after the pre-processing steps described above.

3.2.6.3.1. Creatinine Normalization

This normalization was the first normalization method to be applied in metabonomics (67). It originates from clinical chemistry, where it is common practice to normalize urinary parameters to the concentration of urinary creatinine (68, 69). The assumption behind this is the constant production of creatinine in the body and its constant excretion into urine. In case of NMR-based metabonomics, this normalization can be performed as follows:

1. Integrate the creatinine peaks at 3.05 and 4.05 ppm.
2. Divide each point of the spectrum or alternatively each bin by the creatinine integral value.

Practical application of creatinine normalization is faced by several problems. Metabolites, that have peaks overlapping with those of creatinine will interfere with step (1).

The 4.05-ppm peak of creatinine is prone to pH-induced shift, rendering a peak-picking procedure necessary for step 1.

The most problematic challenge is, however, the biological factor: It has been shown in several studies that the excretion of creatinine into urine can be modulated as a metabolic response or due to nephrotoxicity (70). In that case, the creatinine normalization is worthless. As a consequence, the creatinine normalization was very soon replaced by integral normalization in the field of metabonomics.

3.2.6.3.2. Integral Normalization

Integral normalization has been the standard method in NMR metabonomics for the last two decades (71–73). The primary assumption behind the integral normalization is that the integral of a spectrum is primarily a function of the total concentration of the corresponding sample, as the integral of a spectrum is a function of the concentrations of all NMR-visible metabolites of a sample. The influence of specific changes of a few metabolites on the total integral of the spectrum is assumed to be negligible compared to a change of overall concentration. The different steps of the integral normalization are as follows:

1. Calculate the total integral of the complete spectral region analyzed.
2. Divide each data point of a full-resolution spectrum or each bin of a binned spectrum by the total integral.
3. Multiply the result by 100. This step is not needed, but it is a convention to use a total integral of 100.

Though being the de facto standard, the integral normalization produces artifacts if the above-mentioned assumptions are not valid, for example, when changes of single metabolites dominate the overall picture of the spectrum.

Quotient normalization has been recently introduced to overcome limitations of integral normalization (74). If the integral of the spectrum is substantially influenced by the concentration of interesting metabolites, the variation of these metabolites falsifies the calculated normalization factor. It has been observed in metabonomics studies that single metabolites can be excreted at very high concentrations. An example is glucosuria, where the peaks of glucose account for a very high proportion (50–90%) of the total integral of the spectrum. Obviously, this will result in a wrong integral normalization.

Similar to the integral normalization, the quotient normalization also assumes that dilution of a sample affects all metabolites, whereas specific metabolic responses only affect a limited number of metabolites, but here a most probable concentration quotient between a spectrum and a reference spectrum is calculated as normalization factor. This most probable quotient is derived from the distribution of the quotients of each bin/data point of a spectrum divided by the corresponding bins/data points of a reference spectrum. The median of this distribution has been proven as a very robust method for estimation of the most probable quotient (see Note 6).

The single steps of the quotient normalization can be summarized as follows:

1. Perform an integral normalization of all spectra.
2. Calculate a reference spectrum as median spectrum of all control subjects (each data point/bin is the median value of the data points of the spectra of all control subjects).
3. Calculate the quotients of all data points/bins of the test spectrum with corresponding data points/bins of the reference spectrum.
4. Calculate the median of the quotients.
5. Divide all data points/bins of the test spectrum by this median.

The quotient normalization can be applied to binned or to full-resolution spectra. When applying the method to full-resolution spectra, data points in spectral regions that do not contain peaks should be excluded, as the noise in these spectral regions is not subjected to sample dilution.

Besides this caveat, it has been shown that the quotient normalization is superior to other methods, as it is not influenced by strong metabonomics responses.

3.3. LC-MS

LC coupled with electrospray ionization mass spectrometry (ESI-MS) is the most common MS-based method for metabonomics investigations. Other ionization strategies for LC coupled to MS, such as nanospray ESI, atmospheric pressure chemical ionization (APCI), and atmospheric pressure photoionization

(APPI) (75) are less frequently used for non-targeted analyses of biofluids. Robust high-resolution separation methods such as high performance liquid chromatography (HPLC), RR-LC, and UPLC are able to reduce the complexity of biofluid samples significantly. Therefore, they are ideal methods to be coupled to MS, especially with ESI interfaces, to investigate biological samples. Separation of hundreds to thousands of endogenous metabolites present in biofluids by high-resolution LC reduces the degree of co-elution to a great extent. Thus the major drawback of ESI, ion suppression, is significantly decreased whereas sensitivity and reproducibility are improved (76). Other approaches such as hydrophilic liquid interaction chromatography (HILIC) were recently applied in metabonomics studies as a complementary tool to study polar metabolites (77). However, until now HILIC has not reached the level of reliability, stability, and reproducibility of HPLC or UPLC methods.

3.3.1. LC-MS Sample Preparation

Blood plasma or serum is a complex mixture containing a wide variety of chemically diverse high and low molecular weight components. For LC-MS investigations of the low molecular plasma or serum metabolome, it is of key importance to remove proteins selectively before analysis without affecting the low molecular weight metabolome. This is mandatory to reduce signal suppression of low abundance compounds and to avoid protein precipitation under reversed phase (RP) liquid chromatography conditions. Several procedures for deproteinization exist, such as extraction of low molecular weight compound by organic solvents, acids, or denaturation of proteins by heat (78–80). With regard to reproducibility, number of metabolic features detected and robustness, extraction by methanol proved to be the best method. A common extraction method is as follows:

1. Mix one part of plasma or serum with two parts of methanol and incubate for at least 20 min at –20°C.
2. Centrifuge at 4°C for 10 min at $>10,000 \times g$.
3. Evaporate supernatant to dryness.
4. Re-suspend in one part of chromatographic starting conditions, e.g., acetonitrile/0.1% formic acid 5/95 (v/v).

For LC-MS metabolic profiling, urine is a challenging matrix. Especially the high salt content, the complex composition, and the varying dilution of urine oppose its advantage of easy and non-invasive collection to special analytical requirements. To overcome this problems, urine samples are normally desalted before LC-MS analysis by solid phase extraction (81) or column switching procedures (82) (see Note 7). High-resolution chromatographic separation techniques such as rapid resolution (RR)-LC or UPLC are applied. In some cases, small injection volumes of neat urine were used with UPLC-MS analysis (83).

3.3.2. LC-MS Analysis

A generic LC method (84) for metabonomic investigations of biofluids comprises

1. 2.1-mm internal diameter RP HPLC column, normally packed with C_{18} material, maintained at 40°C.

2. Gradient elution with acetonitrile/0.1% formic acid starting from 5 to 90% organic phase within 10–60 min and with flow rates between 250 and 400 μL/min.

3. Injections of 5–10 μL of extract/desalted sample.

The most common mass analyzers for metabolomics studies are quadrupole and TOF-based analyzers and hybrids thereof (85, 86). In addition, also ion traps, Fourier transform (FT), and Orbitrap instruments were used. Quadrupole mass spectrometers are robust, flexible, and have a high linear dynamic range, but are limited in full scan data acquisition due to long duty cycles. Benefits of ion trap instruments are their capability to perform progressive fragmentation steps (MS^n), compact size, and fast full scanning but at low resolution. Linear ion traps quadrupole hybrid instruments (Q TRAP or QqLIT) combine the MS^n capabilities of ion trap instruments with the neutral loss and precursor ion scan capabilities of triple quadrupole instruments. Therefore, the shortcomings of both approaches are overcome. TOF instruments excel in fast scanning capabilities, wide mass range, and high resolution. Quadrupole TOF (Q-TOF) hybrid instruments combine the stability and robustness of the quadrupole analyzer with TOF features and allow for MS-MS experiments.

Non-targeted metabolite profiling approaches require a sensitive full scan mode and exact masses. Therefore, Q-TOF instruments or linear ion trap FT-MS instruments are advantageous. In contrast, for targeted analysis of selected metabolites, triple quadrupole instruments and Q TRAP instruments with their capability for multiple reaction monitoring are frequently used (see Note 8).

3.4. GC-MS

A prerequisite for GC-MS analysis is to obtain volatile compounds. But the physical–chemical properties of endogenous metabolites in metabonomics analysis are highly variable in complex biological matrices, e.g., (plant) tissue extracts, urine, and blood, etc. Therefore, an extraction procedure that maximizes the number and amounts of metabolites combined with a derivatization that converts polar compounds (e.g., sugars, amino acids, organic acids, etc.) into volatile compounds is necessary before GC/MS analysis (see Note 9). There are many methods of extraction and derivatization available. Most methods are based on the extraction of Bligh and Dyer's (87–89) with little variations and optimization combined with two-stage derivatization methods (28, 90, 91). In the first step, a methoxymation converts aldehyde and keto groups into oximes using hydroxylamines or alkoxyamines to reduce the number of tautomeric forms (due to the limited rotation along the

C=N bond). The second step of silylation then derivatizes polar functional groups (e.g., –OH, –SH, and –NH) into trimethylsilyl groups (TMS ethers, TMS sulfides, and TMS amines) resulting in more volatile compounds.

After these extraction and derivatization steps, GC is normally performed with a non-polar column, whereas for the MS, an EI or (CI) can be used depending on the results that are favored. With EI, the molecules break down in different fragments that give some structural information of the molecules. On the contrary, CI is a less energetic process and often results in less fragmentations and the formation of the molecular ion species to access the mass of the molecules. Besides normal GC-MS, 2D GC×GC-MS techniques can be used to increase the resolution of peaks in complex mixtures (92, 93). Also in GC, the mass analyzers can be a quadrupole analyzer or a TOF analyzer for the determination of the exact mass of a molecule (see Note 10).

3.4.1. Sample Extraction and Derivatization

1. The sample (plants, organs, tissue, blood, urine, or cell culture) of 100–200 mg is homogenized with a mixture of hydrophilic and lipophilic solvents, e.g., with 800 μl of an extraction mixture of methanol/water/chloroform (750/250/200 v/v/v).

2. After extraction, the samples are centrifuged at 13,000 rpm for 10 min.

3. The supernatant containing the aqueous phase (methanol and water) is then separated from the lipophilic phase (chloroform).

4. A volume of 180 μl of the aqueous extract is evaporated to dryness.

5. The residue is methoxymated with 30 μl of 20 mg/ml methoxyamine hydrochloride in pyridine for 17 h and silylated with 30 μl of MSTFA (*N*-methyl-*N*-trimethylsilyltrifluoroacetamide) for 1 h.

3.4.2. GC-MS Analysis

Some typical GC-MS conditions include the following parameters.

1. Inject 1 μl (with a 5:1 split) of the extracted and derivatized samples into the GC-MS. The column of the GC can be a 20 m×180 μm DB5-MS with 0.18-μm film column. Use a typical temperature gradient from 70°C to 320°C, increasing by 15°C/min with a flow of 1 ml/min of helium.

2. For the MS, an EI or a CI can be used with methane as the reagent gas in CI.

3. If a TOF analyzer is used, the lock reference can be heptacosa in EI or methyltriazine in CI.

4. The mass range that is recorded should be 50–1,000 Da.

3.5. Data Pre-processing

The extraction of relevant information and de-noising from full-scan metabolic profiles is an important step when analyzing LC-MS data from complex samples such as serum, plasma, or urine. It is a prerequisite for statistical analysis to apply data alignment procedures and to reduce variance between samples that is not attributed to true differences. For GC-MS and especially LC-MS non-linear shifts in retention time, peak overlap, and m/z shifts are the major source of such variances. In general, three preprocessing strategies are followed for LC-MS data sets:

1. Alignment of spectra along the chromatographic and spectral axis.

2. Reduction of dimensionality by binning or bucketing procedures.

3. Automatic detection and quantification of significant peaks.

Several commercial and open source routines for automatic alignment, de-noising, deconvolution, and extraction of peak have been published and are reviewed by Katajamaa et al. (94).

3.6. Databases and CROs

1. NMR: The assignment of metabolites in high-resolution ^{1}H-NMR spectra is the fundamental basis for the correct biological interpretation of metabonomics data. As pointed out in the previous chapter, metabolite assignment can be performed on the relevant peaks or bins in the spectra or binned data sets responsible for differences between groups of interest derived from multivariate analysis. This step requires to go back to the high-resolution spectra and compare the signals in the respective chemical shift areas with spectra of the corresponding biofluid from reference examples in the literature for example (95). Naturally, this work should be performed by an experienced NMR spectroscopist. This manual assignment of metabolites in each spectrum of a study is a tedious and time-consuming process, especially when up to hundreds of spectra in a study have to be analyzed. Thus, easier and less time-consuming assignment technologies are indispensable. This "must have" need of the community was taken up by software providers in NMR spectroscopy by developing metabolite data basis during the last years with reference spectra of relevant metabolites at different pH values and connection to biological information databases. Currently, there are three software modules available, which differ in size, number, and type of metabolites, as well as mode of assignment and, of course, the price:

   (a) Bio-Rad Laboratories Know-It-All

   (b) Bruker Biospin Biofluid Spectra Base

   (c) Chenomx NMR Suite

2. LC/MS and GC/MS: For the biological interpretation, the assignment of unknown metabolites is an important step in metabonomics analysis. There are different non-commercial and commercial databases, software, and web sites available of metabolites with information such as MS, MS/MS spectra, chromatographical information, and other meta data, and the number of databases and compounds is still growing. Weckwerth et al. published a list of some of these databases (96), which is also summarized in Table 2.

Table 2
Non-commercial and commercial databases, software and websites for assignment of unknown metabolites

Name	Publisher	Homepage	Application
AnalyzerPro	MatrixAnalyzer Spectralworks	http://www.spectralworks.com	High-throughput LC-MS and GC-MS data processing engine
ArMet	University of Wales, Aberystwyth	http://www.armet.org/	Framework for the description of plant metabolomics experiments
Automated Mass US National Institute of Standards (AMDIS)	US National Institute of Standards and Technology	http://chemdata.nist.gov/mass-spc/amdis/	GC mass spectral library
CHEBI (Chemical Entities of Biological Interest)	European Bioinformatic Institute (EBI)	http://www.ebi.ac.uk/chebi/	Database dictionary of small chemical compounds
Component Detection Algorithm (CODA)	ACD Labs	www.acdlabs.com	Prediction of mass spectral, fragmentation for LC, Simulation of LC and GC chromatograms
CSBDB	Max Planck Institute of Plant Physiology	http://csbdb.mpimp-golm.mpg.de/	Access to public mass spectra libraries and metabolite profiling experiments
Human Metabolome Database	Genome Alberta and Genome Canada (not-for-profit organization)	http://www.hmdb.ca/	Database with chemical, clinical, and molecular/biochemistry data

(continued)

**Table 2
(continued)**

Name	Publisher	Homepage	Application
KEGG: Kyoto Encyclopedia of Genes and Genomes	Kanehisa Laboratories in the Bioinformatics Center of Kyoto University and the Human Genome Center of the University of Tokyo	http://www.genome.jp/kegg/	Database of biological systems (genes, proteins, metabolites, and pathways)
Madison Metabolomics Consortium Database	National Magnetic Resonance Facility at Madison	http://mmcd.nmrfam.wisc.edu/	Database with NMR and MS data
MassFrontier	Thermo Electron	http://www.highchem.com/	Management, interpretation, and evaluation of mass spectra
MetAlign	Plant Research International PRI	http://www.metalign.nl/UK/	Analysis, alignment, and comparison of GC-MS or LC-MS datasets
METLIN: Scripps Center for Mass Spectrometry	Siuzdak and Abagyan groups and Center for Mass Spectrometry at The Scripps Research Institute	http://metlin.scripps.edu/	Repository for mass spectral metabolite data
MeT-RO	UK Centre for Plant and Microbial Metabolomic Analysis	http://www.metabolomics.bbsrc.ac.uk/MeT-RO.htm	Primary and secondary metabolite profiling approach
NIST Standard Reference Database	National Institute of Standards and Technology	http://www.nist.gov/srd/nist1.htm	Mass spectral reference library
Wiley Mass Spectral Library	Wiley	http://www.wiley.com	Library and comprehensive collections in mass spectrometry

3. Commercial CROs: Currently, several contract research organizations (CROs) offer commercial services in the field of metabolic profiling. Most of the CROs summarized in Table 3 have a strong focus on MS-based metabolic profiling. Complementary information on NMR-based metabolic profiling is offered only rarely (see Note 11).

Table 3
CROs offering expertise and services for metabolic profiling (metabolomics/metabonomics) and/or data evaluation. The list was compiled from publicly available information and from the authors' scientific networks

Company name	Company name	Company name
Amphioxus Cell Technologies, 11222 Richmond Ave., Suite 180, Houston, TX, USA. 77082-2646, Phone: 281-679-7900, http://www.amphioxus.com	Keio University[a], Institute for Advanced Biosciences, Tsuruoka City, Yamagata, Japan. Phone: +81 235 29 0534, Officetck.keio.ac.jp, http://www.iab.keio.ac.jp	Metabolon, Inc.[a], 800 Capitola Drive, Suite 1, Durham, NC, USA, 27713. Phone: 919-572-1711, http://www.metabolon.com
Avestha Gengraine Technologies Pvt. Ltd., International Technology Park Ltd., Whitefield Road, Bangalore, India, 560066. Phone: 91-80-2841-1665, http://www.avesthagen.com	Kiadis, Zerninkepark 6-8, Groningen, Netherlands, 9747 AN. Phone: 31-0-50-547-42-70, http://www.kiadis.com	Phenomenome Discoveries Inc.[a], 204-407 Downey Road Saskatoon, Saskatchewan, Canada, S7N 4L8. Phone: 306-244-8233, http://www.phenomenome.com
BIOCRATES Life Sciences GmbH[a], Innrain 66/2, Innsbruck, Austria, 6020. Phone: +43-512-57-98-23, http://www.biocrates.at	Lipomics[a], 3410 Industrial Boulevard, Suite 103, West Sacramento, CA 95691, USA. Phone: +1 916 669 0475, http://www.lipomics.com	Quest Pharmaceutical Services, 3 Innovation Way, Suite 240, Newark, DE, USA, 19711. Phone: 302-369-5601, http://www.questpharm.com
BG Medicine (partnering with TNO Pharma)[a], 40 Bear Hill Road, Waltham, MA 02451, USA. Phone: +1 781 890 1199, http://www.bg-medicine.com	Linden Bioscience, 35A Cabot Road, Woburn, MA, USA. 01801. Phone: 781-933-2769, http://www.lindenbioscience.com	Sidmap, 2990 S. Sepulveda Blvd. #300B, Los Angeles, CA, USA, 90064. Phone: 310-478-1424, http://www.sidmap.com
Cantata Pharmaceuticals, Inc. (Private), 300 Technology Square, 5th Floor, Cambridge, MA, USA, 02139. Phone: 617-225-9009. http://www.cantatapharm.com	METabolic Explorer, Biopole Clermont-Limagne, Saint-Beauzire, France, 63360. Phone: 33-473-334300, http://www.metabolic-explorer.com	SurroMed,Inc., 1430 O Brien Drive, Menlo Park, CA, USA, 94025-1435. Phone: 650-470-2300, http://www.surromed.com
CHENOMX Inc.[a], 10050 112 Street, Edmonton, Alberta, Canada, T5K 2J1. Phone: 780-432-0033, http://www.chenomx.com	Metabometrix Ltd[a], RSM, Prince Consort Road, London, UK, SW7 2BP. Phone: 44-0-20-7594-6595, http://www.metabometrix.com	Shimadzu Biotech, 7102 Riverwood Drive, Columbia, MA, USA, 21046. Phone: 925-417-2097, http://www.shimadzu-biotech.net

(continued)

**Table 3
(continued)**

Company name	Company name	Company name
CombiSep Inc, 2711 South Loop Drive, Suite 4200, Ames, IA, USA, 50010. Phone: 1-888-822-7949, http://www.combisep.com	Minkon Biotechnology, 15875 Gaither Drive, Gaithersburg, MD, USA, 20877. Phone: 240-683-5851, http://www.minkon.com	Target Discovery, Inc., 4030 Fabian Way, Palo Alto, CA, USA, 94303. Phone: 1-650-812-8100, http://www.targetdiscovery.com
ESA, Inc, 22 Alpha Road, Chelmsford, MA, USA, 01824. Phone: 978-250-7000, http://www.esainc.com	Metanomics Health[a], Tegeler Weg 33, Berlin, 10589, Germany. Phone: +49 030 34807-111, http://www.metanomic.de	TNO Pharma (partner of BG-Medicine)[a], PO Box 6064, Delft, Netherlands, 2600 JA. Phone: 31-15-269-69-00, http://www.tno.nl/kwaliteit_van_leven/index.xml

[a]Companies that have previously been collaborating with the authors

3.7. Challenges and Opportunities of Data Analysis of Metabonomics Data Sets

For the data analysis of spectra recorded with NMR and LC-MS spectrometers, several methods have been proposed. Most of the methods come from the informatics discipline of pattern recognition and the chemometrics discipline of multivariate data analysis. Among the various methods, principal component analysis (PCA) and projection to latent structures (PLS) play the predominant role, especially as these methods are implemented in a variety of commercial and free data analysis software. Other less-often used analysis methods comprise k-nearest neighbors (KNN), hierarchical cluster analysis (HCA), Batch-PLS, orthogonal signal correction (OSC) combined with PCA, and different implementations of neural networks. In most cases, these methods are sensitive to peak shifts between the different spectra of a study to be analyzed. Therefore, these data analysis methods have been applied to reduced spectra (binned spectra) in most cases. The consequences are that small metabolic changes are often missed due to two factors. The first factor is the reduction of information contained in spectra. As a consequence, strong changes of low-concentrated metabolites can be masked by small changes of highly concentrated metabolites if these metabolites have adjacent or overlapping peaks (see Subheading 3.1.5, step 2 for more details). The second factor can be attributed to the multivariate projection methods/data composition methods themselves (e.g., PCA and PLS). These methods focus on the strongest variations in the data and rotate the new coordinate system in a way that the first new coordinates (components) are dominated by these variations. Consequently, more subtle but important changes represented by higher components are often neglected by the data miner, or are distributed over several components not visible to the data miner any more. Experienced data miners circumvent this situation by the following rather tedious approach of analyzing the data:

1. A multivariate analysis of the complete data set is performed.

2. The most important changes in the multivariate model are identified and the metabolites behind the corresponding peaks are assigned to the peaks. This assignment often raises the need to go back to the original high-resolution spectra to confirm the tentative assignment of peaks to metabolites.

3. The data points/bins of these identified metabolites are removed from the data set and the multivariate analysis is repeated.

4. Steps 1–3 are repeated until only noise is identified as the most significant variance in the multivariate model.

Recently introduced new methods for analyzing metabonomics data render these tedious data analyses unnecessary, as these methods can be applied to full-resolution spectra, such as O-PLS (72), or statistical correlation methods such as the statistical total correlation spectroscopy (STOCSY) (73). These new methods (especially the correlation methods) also identify small but significant changes and significant changes of low-concentrated metabolites in the presence of changes of high-concentrated metabolites. STOCSY is based on the computation of correlation statistics between all data points in a set of complex mixture spectra. In this way, the connectivity of signals from molecules, which vary in concentration between samples, is visible in 2D plots similar to spectra of 2D NMR methods. STOCSY has not only been applied to correlate NMR spectra, but also for LC-NMR (97) data. Moreover, the method was used to calculate "virtual coupling spectra" between NMR and UPLC-MS data recorded for the same samples (5). In this case, SHY (statistical heterospectroscopy) is used as an acronym. Here, attention has to be paid to the fact that only metabolites will be identified, which are detected by both methods or which are correlated with metabolites detected by the other method. Therefore, when using these recent offsprings of metabonomics data analysis, a careful manual inspection of the high-resolution spectra is highly advised.

Another source of discussion is the scaling of spectra. Scaling of spectra means that each data point/bin is divided by its total variance (univariate scaling) or by the square root of its variance (pareto scaling) calculated along the complete data set. Scaling of spectra has been primarily used with data decomposition/projection methods such as PCA and PLS. In this context, scaling renders the influence of each bin/data point on the multivariate model equally important. Therefore, the above-described dominance of highly concentrated metabolites on projection methods is diminished. Yet, scaling spectra also have a number of disadvantages:

1. Scaled spectra are highly distorted and do not reflect the concentration–intensity relationship. Therefore, it is not visible in these spectra if changes of peaks correspond to strong or weak changes of the corresponding metabolite. These spectra are not usable for a quantification of metabolites.

2. Scaling also modulates noise. Areas of spectra, that are dominated by noise can be rendered artificially "important."

Therefore, scaling of spectra might only be advisable for subsequent analyses by projection/data decomposition methods such as PCA and PLS. The same holds true for centering spectra. Hereby, the average of the bin/data point calculated for the complete study is subtracted from the corresponding bin/data point of each spectrum, ending up in an average intensity of zero of each bin over the complete data set. This helps in the context of data decomposition/projection methods to reduce the number of components needed by a factor of one. Yet, these centered spectra are distorted and cannot be used for a direct quantification of the metabolites behind the peaks. A further disadvantage is the fact that the physical constraint of non-negativity of the signal is removed, which is often used by certain data analysis procedures, including 3D data decomposition methods and peak-fitting algorithms. In summary, it can be said that centering and scaling should only be used if absolutely necessary for data analysis. The results of these analyses should be inspected manually with care.

4. Notes

1. Ideally, blood serum samples should be taken in the early morning hours in an empty stomach state (fasted). The syringe equipment should not contain gel enhancer to avoid contamination of the sample or other additives such as EDTA or citrate, which would result in additional signals in the ^{1}H-NMR spectrum.

2. Human urine can be kept at room temperature for 24 h without significant changes in metabolite composition. Fast cooling and freezing of the sample under standardized conditions is advantageous.

3. Correct phase and baseline correction is a critical step in NMR data processing. Parameters of phase and baseline correction have to be carefully determined for each individual spectrum manually, as reliable automation is missing for these procedures.

4. To account for water and urea, it is common practice for urine to exclude the complete region between 4.50 and 5.98 ppm.

By this procedure, some peaks of metabolites of interest are also excluded (e.g., α-anomeric proton of glucose at 5.24 ppm).

5. For equidistant binning, it is common practice to sum up bins covering the citrate doublets (two bins each) into two super-bins. One typically transfers a highly resolved NMR spectrum to a data vector of 210 components. This vector is, however, a lot more suited for multivariate data analysis methods to identify significantly changed spectral regions. Low resolution does not allow for an interpretation of single peaks anymore. A recourse to non-binned spectra is needed after multivariate analysis for assignment of individual signals and related metabolites.

6. For the calculation of quotients for quotient normalization, a reference spectrum is needed. This can be a single "golden" spectrum of the study, or a calculated spectrum derived from a subset. Simulations have demonstrated that taking a median spectrum of control animals or control subjects is the most robust approach. It is also recommended to perform an integral normalization prior of applying quotient normalization to scale spectra of different studies (NMR hardware) to the same absolute magnitude.

7. To overcome problems with urine in LC-MS analysis such as high salt content, the complex composition, and the varying dilution, urine samples are normally desalted before LC-MS analysis by solid phase extraction or column switching procedures.

8. Non-targeted metabolite profiling with LC-MS requires a sensitive full-scan mode and exact masses; therefore, often Q-TOF or linear ion trap FT-MS instruments are used. For targeted analysis of selected metabolites, triple quadrupole instruments and Q TRAP instruments with their capability for multiple reaction monitoring are frequently used.

9. Physical–chemical properties of endogenous metabolites in complex biological matrices (e.g., (plant) tissue extracts, urine, and blood) are highly variable. Therefore, an extraction procedure that maximizes the number and amounts of metabolites combined with a derivatization that converts polar compounds (sugars, amino acids, organic acids, etc.) into volatile compounds is necessary before GC/MS analysis.

10. For GC-MS analysis, EI or CI can be used depending on the result that is favored. EI breaks down the molecules in different fragments to give some structural information. The less energetic process of CI often results in less fragmentations and the formation of the molecular ion species to access the mass of the molecules. Also, the use of a TOF analyzer helps to determine the exact masses of the molecules.

11. The assignment of metabolites from NMR-, LC-MS, and GC-MS spectra is the fundamental basis for the correct biological interpretation of metabonomics data. For this, several non-commercial and commercial databases, software tools, or CROs are available.

References

1. Nicholson, J.K., Lindon, J.C., and Holmes, E. (1999) "Metabonomics": understanding the metabolic responses of living systems to pathophysiological stimuli via multivariate statistical analysis of biological NMR spectroscopic data. *Xenobiotica* **29**, 1181–1189.

2. Dieterle, F., Schlotterbeck, G., Binder, M., Ross, A., Suter, L., and Senn, H. (2007) Application of metabonomics in a comparative profiling study reveals N-Acetylfelinine excretion as a biomarker for inhibition of the Farnesyl pathway by bisphosphonates. *Chem. Res. Toxicol.* **20**, 1291–1299.

3. Pauling, L., Robinson, A.B., Teranishi, R., and Cary, P. (1971) Quantitative analysis of urine vapor and breath by gas-liquid partition chromatography. *Proc. Natl. Acad. Sci. U. S. A.* **68**, 2374–2376.

4. Wishart, D.S. (2007) Proteomics and the human metabolome project. Expert Rev. Proteomics **4**, 333–335.

5. Crockford, D.J., Holmes, E., Lindon, J.C., Plumb, R.S., Zirah, S., Bruce, S.J., Rainville, P., Stumpf, C.L., and Nicholson, J.K. (2006) Statistical heterospectroscopy, an approach to the integrated analysis of NMR and UPLC–MS data sets: application in metabonomic toxicology studies. *Anal. Chem.* **78**, 363–371.

6. Bollard, M.E, Holmes, E., Lindon, J.C., Mitchell, S.C., Branstetter, D., Zhang, W., and Nicholson, J.K. (2001) Investigations into biochemical changes due to diurnal variation and estrus cycle in female rats using high resolution 1H NMR spectroscopy of urine and pattern recognition. *Anal. Biochem.* **295**, 194–202.

7. Bell, J.D., Sadler, P.J., Morris, V.C., and Levander, O.A. (1991) Effect of aging and diet on proton NMR spectra of rat urine. *Magn. Reson. Med.* **17**, 414–422.

8. Phipps, A.N., Steward, J., Wright, B., and Wilson, I.D. (1998) Effect on diet on urinary excretion of hippuric acid and other dietary-derived aromatics in the rat. A complex interaction between diet, gut microflora and substrate specificity. *Xenobiotica* **28**, 527–537.

9. Bollard, M.E., Stanley, E.G., Lindon, J.C., Nicholson, J.K., and Holmes, E. (2005) NMR-based metabonomic approaches for evaluating physiological influences on biofluid composition. *NMR Biomed.* **18**, 143–162.

10. Griffin, J.L., Walker, L.A., Garrod, S., Holmes, E., Shore, R.F., and Nicholson, J.K. (2000) NMR spectroscopy based metabonomic studies on the comparative biochemistry of the kidney and urine of the blank vole (*Clethrionomys glareolus*), wood mouse (*Apodemus sylvaticus*), white toothed shrew (*Crocidura suaveolens*), and the laboratory rat. *Comp. Biochem. Physiol.* **127**, 357–367.

11. Van Dorsten, F.A., Daykin, C.A., Mulder, T.P.J., and Duynhoven, J.P.M. (2006) Metabonomic approach to determine metabolic differences between green tea and black tea consumption. *J. Agric. Food Chem.* **54**, 6929–6938.

12. Stella, C., Beckwith-hall, B., Cloarec, O., Lindon, J.C., Powell, J., van der Ouderaa, F., Bingham, S., Cross, A.J., and Nicholson, J.K. (2006) Susceptibility of human metabolic phenotype to dietary modulation. *J. Proteome Res.* **5**, 2780–2788.

13. Solanky, K.S., Bailey, N.J.C., Beckwith-Hall, B., Davies, A., Bingham, S., Holmes, E., Nicholson, J.K., and Cassidy, A. (2003) Application of biofluid ^{1}H nuclear resonance-based metabonomic technique for the analysis of biochemical effects of dietary isoflavones on human plasma profiles. *Anal. Biochem.* **323**, 197–204.

14. Beckonert, O., Keun, H.C., Ebbels, T.M.D., Bundy, J., Holmes, E., Lindon, J.C., and Nicholson, J.K. (2006) Metabolic profiling and metabonomics procedures for NMR spectroscopy or urine, plasma and serum and tissue extracts. *Nat. Protoc.* **2** (**11**), 2692–2703

15. Teahan, O., Gamble, S., Holmes, E., Waxman, J., Nicholson, J.K., Bevan, C., and Keun, H.C. (2006) Impact of analytical bias in metabonomic studies of human blood serum and plasma. *Anal. Chem.* **78** (**13**), 4307–4318.

16. Maher, A.D., Zirah, S.F., Holmes, E., and Nicholson, J.K. (2007) Experimental and analytical variation in human urine in 1H NMR spectroscopy-based metabolic phenotyping studies. *Anal. Chem.* **79** (**14**), 5204–5211.

17. European Convention for the Protection of Vertebrate Animals used for Experimental and

Other Scientific Purposes Strasbourg, 18.III. 1986 Text amended according to the provisions of the Protocol (ETS No. 170) as of its entry into force on 2 December 2005.

18. EEC Directive. Council Directive of November 24, 1986 on the approximation of laws, regulations and administrative provisions of the Member States regarding the protection of animals used for experimental and other scientific purposes 86/609/EEC. Official Journal of the European Community No. L 358 of 18 December 1986.

19. Good Laboratory Practice Regulations for Nonclinical Laboratory Studies of the United States Food and Drug Administration (21 CFR Part 58).

20. Morton, D.B., Abbot, D., Barclay, R., Close, B.S., Ewbank, R., Gask, D., Heath, M., Mattic, S., Poole, T., Seamer, J., Southee, J., Thompson, A., Trussell, B., West, C., and Jennings, M. (1993) Removal of blood from laboratory mammals and birds. *Lab. Anim.* **27**, 1–22.

21. Diehl, K.H., Hull, R., Morton, D., Pfister, R., Rabemampianina, Y., Smith, D., Vidal, J.M., and Van den Vorstenbosch, C. (2001) A good practice guide to the administration of substances and removal of blood, including routes and volumes. *J. Appl. Toxicol.* **21**, 15–23.

22. Robertson, D.G., Reily, M.D., Lindon, J.C., Holmes, E., and Nicholson, J.K. (2002) Metabonomic Technology as a Tool for Rapid Throughput *In Vivo* Toxicity Screening. In *Comprehensive Toxicology.* **14**, 583–610.

23. Nicholls, A., Nicholson, J.K., Haselden, J.N., and Waterfield, C.J. (2000) A metabonomics approach to the investigation of drug-induced phospholipidosis: an NMR spectroscopy and pattern recognition study. *Biomarkers* **5 (6)**, 410–423.

24. Ernst, R.R., Bodenhausen, G., and Wokaun, A. (1990) Principles of Nuclear Magnetic Resonance in One and Two Dimensions, Oxford University Press, Oxford.

25. Goldman, M. (1991) Quantum Description of High-Resolution NMR in Liquids, Oxford University Press, Oxford.

26. Kovacs, H., Moskau, D., and Spraul, M. (2005) Cryogenically cooled probes – a leap in NMR technology. *Prog. Nucl. Magn. Reson. Spectrosc.* **46**, 131–155.

27. Prince, W.S. (1999) Water signal suppression in NMR spectroscopy. *Ann. Rep. NMR Spectrosc.* **38**, 289–354.

28. Potts, B.C., Deese, A.J., Stevens, G.J., Reily, M.D., Robertson, D.G., and Theiss, J. (2001) NMR of biofluids and pattern recognition: assessing the impact of NMR parameters on the principal component analysis of urine from rat and mouse. *J. Pharm. Biomed. Anal.* **26**, 463–476.

29. Schlotterbeck, G., Ross, A., Dieterle, F., and Senn, H. (2006) Metabolic profiling technologies for biomarker discovery in biomedicine and drug development. *Pharmcogenomics* **7**, 1055–1075.

30. Ross, A., Schlotterbeck, G., Dieterle, F., and Senn, H. (2007) NMR Spectroscopy Techniques for Application in Metabonomics. In *The Handbook of Metabonomics and Metabolomics* (Lindon, J.C., Nicholson, J.K., and Holmes, E., eds.), Elsevier, Amsterdam, pp. 55–112.

31. Chen, J.H., and Singer, S. (2007) High-Resolution Magic Angle Spinning NMR Spectroscopy. In *The Handbook of Metabonomics and Metabolomics* (Lindon, J.C., Nicholson, J.K., and Holmes, E., eds.), Elsevier, Amsterdam, pp. 113–148.

32. Keun, H.C., Beckonert, O., Griffin, J.L., Richter, C., Moskau, D., Lindon, J.C., and Nicholson, J.K. (2002) Cryogenic probe ^{13}C NMR spectroscopy of urine for metabonomic studies. *Anal. Chem.* **74**, 4588–4593.

33. Boros, L.G., Brackett, D.J., and Harrigan, G.G. (2003) Metabolic biomarker and kinase drug target discovery in cancer using stable isotope-based dynamic metabolic profiling (SIDMAP). *Curr. Cancer Drug Targets* **3**, 445–453.

34. Ben-Yoseph, O., Badar-Goffer, R.S., Morris, P.G., and Bachelard, H.S. (1993) Glycerol 3-phosphate and lactate as indicators of the cerebral cytoplasmic redox state in severe and mild hypoxia respectively: a ^{13}C- and ^{31}P-NMR study. *Biochem. J.* **291**, 915–919.

35. Lindon, J.C., Nicholson, J.K., Holmes, E., and Everett, J.E.R. (2000) Metabonomics: metabolic processes studied by NMR spectroscopy of biofluids. *Concepts Magn. Reson.* **12**, 289–320.

36. Keun, H.C., Ebbels, T.M.D., Antti, H., Bollard, M.E., Beckonert, O., Schlotterbeck, G., Senn, H., Niederhauser, U., Holmes, E., Lindon, J.C., and Nicholson, J.K. (2002) Analytical reproducibility in 1H NMR-based metabonomic urinalysis. *Chem. Res. Toxicol.* **15**, 1380–1386.

37. Hoult, D.I. (1976) Solvent peak saturation with single phase and quadrature fourier transformation. *J. Magn. Reson.* **21**, 337–347.

38. Kumar, A., Ernst, R.R., and Wüthrich, K. (1980) A two-dimensional nuclear overhauser enhancement (2D NOE) experiment for the elucidation of complete proton-proton

cross-relaxation networks in biological macro-molecules. *Biochem. Biophys. Res. Commun.* **95**, 1–6.

39. Ogg, R.J., Kingsley, P.B., and Taylor, J.S. (1994) WET, a T_1- and B_1-insensitive water-suppression method for *in vivo* localized 1H NMR spectroscopy. *J. Magn. Reson.* **104B**, 1–10.

40. Lenz, E.M., Bright, J., Wilson, I.D., Morgan, S.R., and Nash, A.F.P. (2003) A ^{1}H NMR-based metabonomic study of urine and plasma samples obtained from healthy human subjects. *J. Pharm. Biomed. Anal.* **33**, 1103–1115.

41. Meiboom, S., and Gill, D. (1958) Effects of diffusion on free precession in nuclear magnetic resonance experiments. *Rev. Sci. Instrum.* **29**, 688–691.

42. Gibbs, S.J., and Johnson, Jr. C.S. (1991) A PFG NMR experiment for accurate diffusion and flow studies in the presence of Eddy currents. *J. Magn. Reson.* **93**, 395–402.

43. Wider, G., Dötsch, V., and Wüthrich, K. (1994) Self-compensating pulsed magnetic-field gradients for short recovery times. *J. Magn. Reson.* **108A**, 255–258.

44. Morris, K.F., and Johnson, Jr. C.S. (1992) Diffusion-ordered two-dimensional nuclear magnetic resonance spectroscopy. *J. Am. Chem. Soc.* **114**, 3139–3141.

45. Griffin, J.L., Williams, H.J., Sang, E., and Nicholson, J.K. (2001) Abnormal lipid profile of dystrophic cardiac tissue as demonstrated by one- and two-dimensional magic-angle spinning 1H NMR spectroscopy. *Magn. Reson. Med.* **46**, 249–255.

46. Garrod, S., Humpfer, E., Spraul, M. et al. (1999) High-resolution magic angle spinning ^{1}H NMR spectroscopic studies on intact rat renal cortex and medulla. *Magn. Reson. Med.* **41**, 1108–1118.

47. Dumas, M.E., Canlet, C., André, F., Vercauteren, J., and Paris, A. (2002) Metabonomic assessment of physiological disruptions using ^{1}H-^{13}C HMBC-NMR spectroscopy combined with pattern recognition procedures performed on filtered variables. *Anal. Chem.* **74**, 2261–2273.

48. Günther, H. (1992) NMR Spectroscopy, Wiley & Sons Inc. New York.

49. Holmes, E., Foxall, P.J.D., Spraul, M., Farrant, R.D., Nicholson, J.K., and Lindon, J.C. (1997) 750 MHz ^{1}H NMR spectroscopy characterization of the complex metabolic pattern of urine from patients with inborn errors of metabolism: 2-Hydroxyglutaric aciduria and maple syrup urine disease. *J. Pharm. Biomed. Anal.* **15**, 1647–1659.

50. Sweatman, B.C., Farrant, R.D., Holmes, E., Ghauri, F.Y., Nicholson, J.K., and Lindon, J.C. (1993) 600 MHz ^{1}H-NMR spectroscopy of human cerebrospinal fluid: effects of sample manipulation and assignment of resonances. *J. Pharm. Biomed. Anal.* **11**, 651–664.

51. Lynch, M.J., Masters, J., Pryor, J.P., Lindon, J.C., Spraul, M., Foxall, P.J.D., and Nicholson, J.K. (1994) Ultra high field NMR spectroscopic studies on human seminal fluid, seminal vesicle and prostatic secretions. *J. Pharm. Biomed. Anal.* **12**, 19–25.

52. Nicholson, J.K., and Foxall, P.J.D. (1996) 750 MHz ^{1}H and ^{1}H-^{13}C NMR spectroscopy of human blood plasma. *Anal. Chem.* **67**, 793–811.

53. Viant, M.R. (2003) Improved methods for the acquisition and interpretation of NMR metabolomic data. *Biochem. Biophys. Res. Commun.* **310**, 943–948.

54. Bax, A., and Davis, D.G. (1985) MLEV-17-based two-dimensional homonuclear magnetization transfer spectroscopy. *J. Magn. Reson.* **65**, 355–360.

55. Bax, A., and Freeman, R. (1981) Investigation of complex networks of spin-spin coupling by two-dimensional NMR. *J. Magn. Reson.* **44**, 542–561.

56. Derome, A., and Williamson, M. (1990) Rapid-pulsing artifacts in double-quantum-filtered COSY. *J. Magn. Reson.* **88**, 177–185.

57. Ancian, B., Bourgeois, I., Dauphin, J.F., and Shaw, A.A. (1997) Artifact-free pure absorption PFG-enhanced DQF-COSY spectra including a gradient pulse in the evolution period. *J. Magn. Reson.* **125A**, 348–354.

58. Nicholls, A.W., Holmes, E., Lindon, J.C., et al. (2001) Metabonomic investigations into hydrazine toxicity in the Rat. *Chem. Res. Toxicol.* **14**, 975–987.

59. Liu, M., Nicholson, J.K., and Lindon, J.C. (1996) High-resolution diffusion and relaxation edited one- and two-dimensional ^{1}H NMR spectroscopy of biological fluids. *Anal. Chem.* **68**, 3370–3376.

60. Traficante, D.D., and Rajabzadeh, M. (2000) Optimum window function for sensitivity enhancement of NMR signals. *Concepts Magn. Reson.* **12**, 83–101.

61. Hoch, J.C., and Stern, A.S. (1997) NMR Data Processing. John Wiley & Sons Inc. New York.

62. Lefebvre, B., Golotvin, S., Schoenbachler, L., Beger, R., Price, P., Megyesi, J., and Safirstein, R. (2004) Intelligent bucketing for

metabonomics – Part 1, Poster http://www.acdlabs.com/download/publ/2004/enc04/intelbucket.pdf.

63. Forshed, J., Schuppe-Koistinen, I., and Jacobssen, S.P. (2003) *Anal. Chim. Acta* **487**, 189.

64. Stoyanova, R., Nicholls, A.W., Nicholson, J.K., Lindon, J.C., and Brown, T.R. (2004) *J. Magn. Reson.* **170**, 329.

65. Cloarec, O., Dumas, M.E., Trygg, J., Craig, A., Barton, R.H., Lindon, J.C., Nicholson, J.K., and Holmes, E. (2005) Evaluation of the orthogonal projection on latent structure model limitations caused by chemical shift variability and improved visualization of biomarker changes in 1H NMR spectroscopic metabonomic studies. *Anal. Chem.* **77**, 517–526.

66. Cloarec, O., Dumas, M.E., Craig, A., Barton, R.H., Trygg, J., Hudson, J., Blancher, C., Gauguier, D., Lindon, J.C., Holmes, E., and Nicholson, J. (2005) Statistical total correlation spectroscopy: an exploratory approach for latent biomarker identification from metabolic 1H NMR data sets. *Anal. Chem.* **77**, 1282–1289.

67. Holmes, E., Foxall, P.J.D., Nicholson, J.K., Neild, G.H., Brown, S.M., Beddell, C.R., Sweatman, B.C., Rahr, E., Lindon, J.C., Spraul, M., and Neidig, P. (1994) Automatic data reduction and pattern recognition methods for analysis of 1H nuclear magnetic resonance spectra of human urine from normal and pathological states. *Anal. Biochem.* **220**, 284–296.

68. Fauler, G., Leis, H.J., Huber, E., Schellauf, C., Kerbl, R., Urban, C., and Gleispach, H. (1994) Determination of homovanillic acid and vanillylmandelic acid in neuroblastoma screening by stable isotope dilution GC-MS. *J. Mass Spectrom.* **32**, 507–514.

69. Encyclopedia.com, Creatinine, http://www.encyclopedia.com/doc/1O39-creatinine.html.

70. Shockcor, J.P., and Holmes, E. (2002) Metabonomic applications in toxicity screening and disease diagnosis. *Curr. Top. Med. Chem.* **2**, 35–51.

71. Antti, H., Bollard, M.E., Ebbels, T., Keun, H., Lindon, J.C., Nicholson, J.K., and Holmes, E. (2002) Batch statistical processing of H-1 NMR-derived urinary spectral data. *J. Chemometr.* **16**, 461–468.

72. Keun, H.C., Ebbels, T.M.D., Antti, H., Bollard, M.E., Beckonert, O., Holmes, E., Lindon, J.C., and Nicholson, J.K. (2003) Improved analysis of multivariate data by variable stability scaling: application to NMR-based metabolic profiling. *Anal. Chim. Acta* **490**, 265–276.

73. Brindle, J.T., Nicholson, J.K., Schofield, P.M., Grainger, D.J., and Holmes, E. (2003) Application of chemometrics to 1H NMR spectroscopic data to investigate a relationship between human serum metabolic profiles and hypertension. *Analyst* **128**, 32–36.

74. Dieterle, F., Ross, A., Schlotterbeck, G., and Senn, H. (2006) Probabilistic quotient normalization as robust method to account for dilution of complex biological mixtures. Application in 1H NMR metabonomics. *Anal. Chem.* **78**, 4281–4290.

75. Wang, G., Hsieh, Y., and Korfmacher, W.A. (2005) Comparison of atmospheric pressure chemical ionization, electrospray ionization, and atmospheric pressure photoionization for the determination of cyclosporin A in rat plasma. *Anal. Chem.* **77**, 541–548.

76. Want, E.J., Nordström, A., Morita, H., and Siuzdak, G. (2007) From exogenous to endogenous: the inevitable imprint of mass spectrometry in metabolomics. *J. Proteome Res.* **6**, 459–468.

77. Idborg, H., Zamani, L., Edlund, P.O., Schuppe-Koistinen, I., and Jacobsson, S.P. (2005) Metabolic fingerprinting of rat urine by LC/MS Part 1. Analysis by hydrophilic interaction liquid chromatography–electrospray ionization mass spectrometry. *J. Chromatogr. B* **828**, 9–13.

78. Want, E.J., O'Maille, G., Smith, C.A., Brandon, T.R., Uritboonthai, W., Qin, C., Trauger, S.A., and Siuzdak, G. (2006) Solvent-dependent metabolite distribution, clustering, and protein extraction for serum profiling with mass spectrometry. *Anal. Chem.* **78**, 743–752.

79. Boernsen, K.O., Gatzek, S., and Imbert, G. (2005) Controlled protein precipitation in combination with chip-based nanospray infusion mass spectrometry. An approach for metabolomics profiling of plasma. *Anal. Chem.* **77**, 7255–7264.

80. Trygg, J., Gullberg, J., Johansson, A.I., Jonsson, P., Antti, H., Marklund, S.L., and Moritz, T. (2005) Extraction and GC/MS analysis of the human blood plasma metabolome. *Anal. Chem.* **77**, 8086–8094.

81. Wagner, S., Scholz, K., Sieber, M., Kellert, M., and Voelkel, W. (2007) Tools in metabolomics: an integrated validation approach for LC-MS metabolic profiling of mercapturic acid in human urine. *Anal. Chem.* **79**, 2918–2926.

82. Waybright, T.J., Van, Q.N., Muschik, G.M., Conrads, T.P., Veenstra, T.D., and Issaq, H.J. (2006) LC-MS in metabonomics: optimization of experimental conditions for the analysis of metabolites in human urine. *J. Liq. Chromatogr. Related Technol.* **29**, 2475–2497.

83. Wilson, I.D., Plumb, R., Granger, J., Major, H., Williams, R., and Lenz, E.M. (2005) HPLC-MS-based methods for the study of metabolomics. *J. Chromatogr. B* **817**, 67–76.

84. Pham-Tuan, H., Kaskavelis, L., Daykin, C.A., and Janssen, H.G. (2003) Method development in high-performance liquid chromatography for high-throughput profiling and metabonomic studies of biofluid samples. *J. Chromatogr. B* **789**, 283–301.

85. Dunn, W., and Ellis, D.I. (2005) Metabolomics: current analytical platforms and methodologies. Trends *Analyt. Chem.* **4**, 285–294.

86. Ackermann, B.L., Hale, J.E., and Duffin, K.L. (2006) The role of mass spectrometry in biomarker discovery and measurement. *Curr. Drug Metab.* **7**, 525–539.

87. Bligh, E.G., and Dyer, W.J. (1959) A rapid method of total lipid extraction and purification. *Can. J. Biochem. Physiol.* **37**, 911–917.

88. Peña-Alvarez, A., Díaz, L., Medina, A., Labastida, C., Capella, S., and Vera, L.E. (2004) Characterization of three *Agave* species by gas chromatography and solid-phase microextraction-gas chromatography-mass spectrometry. *J. Chromatogr. A* **1027**, 131–136.

89. Le Belle, J.E., Harris, N.G., Williams, S.R., and Bhakoo, K.K. (2002) A comparison of cell and tissue extraction techniques using high-resolution 1H-NMR spectroscopy. *NMR Biomed.* **15**, 37–44.

90. Gullberg, J., Jonsson, P., Nordström, A., Sjöström, M., and Moritz, T. (2004) Design of experiments: an efficient strategy to identify factors influencing extraction and derivatization of *Arabidopsis thaliana* samples in metabolomics studies with gas chromatography/mass spectrometry. *Anal. Biochem.* **331**, 283–295.

91. Schröder, N.W., Schombel, U., Heine, H., Göbel, U.B., Zähringer, U., and Schumann, R.R. (2003) Acylated cholesteryl galactoside as a novel immunogenic motif in *Borrelia burgdorferi sensu stricto. J. Biol. Chem.* **278**, 33645–33653.

92. Shellie, R.A., Welthagen, W., Zrostlikovà, J., Spranger, J., Ristow, M., Fiehn, O., and Zimmermann, R. (2005) Statistical methods for comparing comprehensive two-dimensional gas chromatography-time-of-flight mass spectrometry results: metabolomic analysis of mouse tissue extracts. *J. Chromatogr. A* **1086**, 83–90.

93. Van Mispelaar, V.G., Tas, A.C., Smilde, A.K., Schoenmakers, P.J., and van Asten, A.C. (2003) Quantitative analysis of target components by comprehensive two-dimensional gas chromatography. *J. Chromatogr. A* **1019**, 15–29.

94. Katajamaa, M., and Oresic, M. (2007) Data processing for mass spectrometry-based metabolomics. *J. Chromatogr. A* **1158**, 318–328.

95. Lindon, J.C., and Nicholson, J.K. (1999) NMR Spectroscopy of Biofluids. In *Annual Reports in NMR Spectroscopy* (Webb, G.A., ed.) **38**, 2–78.

96. Weckwerth, W., and Morgenthal, K. (2005) Metabolomics: from pattern recognition to biological interpretation. *Drug Discov. Today* **10**, 1551–1558.

97. Cloarec, O., Campbell, A., Tseng, L.H., Braumann, U., Spraul, M., Scarfe, G., Weaver, R., and Nicholson, J.K. (2007) Virtual chromatographic resolution enhancement in cryoflow LC-NMR experiments via statistical total correlation spectroscopy. *Anal. Chem.* **79**, 3304–3311.

Chapter 25

Absolute Quantification of Toxicological Biomarkers by Multiple Reaction Monitoring

Thomas Y.K. Lau, Ben C. Collins, Peter Stone, Ning Tang, William M. Gallagher, and Stephen R. Pennington

Abstract

With the advent of "–omics" technologies, there has been an explosion of data generation in the field of toxicology, as well as in many others. As new candidate biomarkers of toxicity are being regularly discovered, the next challenge is to validate these observations in a targeted manner. Traditionally, these validation experiments have been conducted using antibody-based technologies such as Western blotting, ELISA, and immunohistochemistry. However, this often produces a significant bottleneck as the time, cost, and development of successful antibodies are often far outpaced by the generation of targets of interest. In response to this, recently there have been several developments in the use of triple quadrupole (QQQ) mass spectrometry (MS) as a platform to provide quantification of proteins by multiple reaction monitoring (MRM). This technology does not require antibodies; it is typically less expensive and quicker to develop, and has the opportunity for more accessible multiplexing. The speed of these experiments combined with their flexibility and ability to multiplex assays makes the technique a valuable strategy to validate biomarker discovery.

Key words: Catalase, Mass spectrometry, Multiple reaction monitoring, Quantification, Proteomics, Biomarkers

1. Introduction

There are currently several different ways to perform mass spectrometry (MS)-based absolute quantification (1, 2), each having a unifying principle that a labeled standard peptide is designed against a proteotypic peptide of the protein(s) of interest. A proteotypic peptide is a (typically tryptic) peptide with a sequence unique to that protein (3). Labeled standards consist of biologically or chemically produced peptides that have mass

Jean-Charles Gautier (ed.), *Drug Safety Evaluation: Methods and Protocols*, Methods in Molecular Biology, vol. 691, DOI 10.1007/978-1-60761-849-2_25, © Springer Science+Business Media, LLC 2011

shifts produced by the incorporation of isotopically labeled amino acids. These mass shifts allow the standard to be differentiated from the native peptide while maintaining its chromatographic properties. Here, we describe a workflow for the absolute quantification of catalase by peptide multiple reaction monitoring (MRM). In MRM mode, the mass spectrometer filters for a specific precursor mass in the first quadrupole and then another specific fragment ion in the second. This allows for high selectivity even in complex samples matrices. Catalase is an enzyme with a well-established background in removal of reactive oxygen species (ROS) and thus is important to the study of ROS-induced toxicology. Catalase was selected for this proof-of-principle experiment due to its toxicological relevance. The ability to quantify increases in the expression of catalase may indicate oxidative stress and associated toxicological responses. Specifically, we describe in this chapter the selection and design of appropriate stable isotope-labeled synthetic peptide standards, protein extraction from rat liver tissue followed by tryptic digestion, sample spiking with synthetic peptide standards, acquisition of data using reverse phase liquid chromatography (LC) coupled online to a triple quadrupole mass spectrometer, and processing and interpretation of data. The different steps of the workflow are illustrated in Fig. 1.

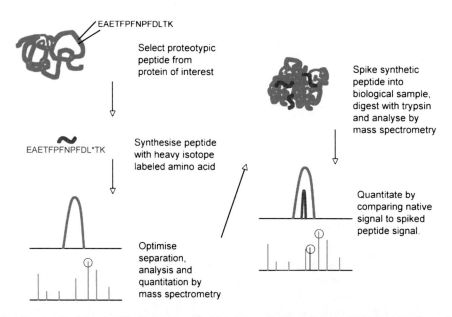

Fig. 1. Workflow for absolute quantification using spiked labeled synthetic peptides by MRM. Proteotypic peptides are chosen and then synthesized with an isotope label to differentiate them from endogenous peptides. Quantification is made possible by comparing the ratio of the peak areas between a spiked standard of known concentration to the endogenous peptide.

2. Materials

Unless otherwise stated, all reagents are purchased from Sigma–Aldrich and are of the highest grade available. All solvents were Chromasolv HPLC grade solvents from Sigma–Aldrich. All solutions should be made up in HPLC grade water or solvents.

2.1. Sample Preparation

1. Mortar and pestle.
2. Liquid nitrogen.
3. Tissue lysis buffer: 9.8 M urea, 4% CHAPS, 5 µl/ml Protease Inhibitor Cocktail Set III, final concentration 500 µM AEBSF HCl, 0.4 µM aprotinin, 25 µM bestatin, 7.5 µM E-64, 10 µM leupeptin hemisulfate, and 5 µM pepstatin A (Merck).
4. Reagents for Bradford method.
5. Tris-2-carboxyethyl-phosphine (TCEP) is used for denaturing.
6. Iodacetamide (IAA) for alkylation.
7. Acetone.
8. Ammonium bicarbonate, 100 mM.
9. Rapigest 0.1% (w/v) (Waters), an acid-labile surfactant, aids the solubilization of proteins and increases digestion efficiency.
10. Trypsin (sequencing-grade modified porcine) (Promega) for tryptic digestion.
11. Formic acid 2% (v/v).

2.2. Liquid Chromatography and Mass Spectrometry

1. Gradient buffer A: H_2O with 0.1% formic acid.
2. Gradient buffer B: 90% acetonitrile with 0.1% formic acid.
3. Column HPLC-Chip 150 mm × 75 µm, Zorbax 300SB-C18 5 µm, and 160 nl trap (Agilent).
4. LC–MS systems: 1200 series nano-LC connected online to a 6510 Q-TOF equipped with a Chip Cube source (Agilent).
5. 1200 series nano-LC connected online to a 6410 Triple Quadropole equipped with a Chip Cube source (Agilent).
6. Mass spectrometer calibrant: ESI-Tuning Mix (Agilent).
7. Synthetic peptides synthesized with C13 and N15 leucine, thus creating a 7-Da mass shift with respect to the endogenous peptide. Synthetic peptides were synthesized at Peptide Protein Research, UK.

2.3. Softwares

1. Spectrum Mill peptide selector (Agilent).

2. MassHunter qualitative and quantitative analysis software (Agilent).

3. Methods

3.1. Choice and Design of Proteotypic Peptides

As described earlier, a proteotypic peptide is a (typically tryptic) peptide that is unique to a particular protein. Typically, a protein will have several proteotypic peptides. However, not all of these peptides will be equally amenable for MS-based quantification, as their abundance and chemical properties may make them unsuitable for detection using traditional LC and MS. In our experiments, we first used a bioinformatic approach to select peptides that were both unique to catalase and likely to be detected by a mass spectrometer by using the software Peptide Selector, as illustrated in Fig. 2.

1. The SwissProt accession number for catalase (*Rattus norvegicus*) is found at http://www.expasy.org.

2. This SwissProt number (P04762) is entered in Spectrum Mill peptide selector (Agilent Technologies).

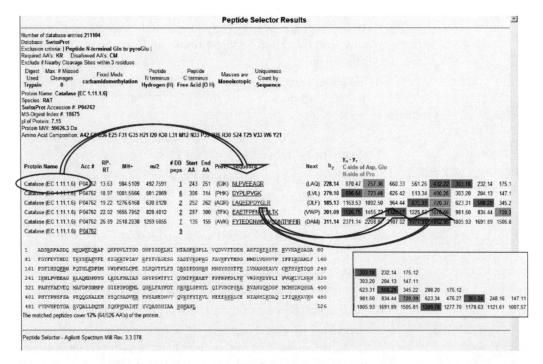

Fig. 2. Search result with peptide selector. Peptide selector performs an in silico tryptic digest and suggests proteotypic peptides and the corresponding fragment ions. It predicts the mass of the ions and which ions will give the best signal and, therefore, be good choices to perform MRM quantification on.

3. The results suggest proteotypic peptides and their likely fragmentation ions in MS/MS.

4. Choose proteotypic peptides that have good predicted ionization and strong predicted fragment ions. In general, it is best to choose peptides that do not contain residues such as cysteine and methionine that are prone to modification during the sample preparation and digestion procedures. Even a sub-stoichiometric modification would cause a portion of the endogenous peptide to be unobservable by this type of targeted approach and could lead to a significant bias in results (see Notes 1 to 5 and 8 for more information on peptide selection).

3.2. Sample Preparation

In this study, we analyzed liver tissue from rats having drug-induced toxicity. Parallel studies have indicated that catalase is up-regulated in high doses of the drug.

1. Pulverize 50–100 mg of frozen tissue using a pestle and mortar and liquid nitrogen.

2. Dissolve powdered tissue in 1,000 µl of tissue lysis buffer.

3. Vortex for 30 s and pipette up and down 30 times.

4. Put the samples on an orbital shaker (~1,000 rpm) for 60 min at RT.

5. Centrifuge at $13,000 \times g$ for 5 min.

6. Determine protein concentration (using Bradford method).

7. Dilute 100 µg of proteins from each sample to 20 µl with tissue lysis buffer and vortex briefly.

8. Reduce disulfide bonds with 5 mM (final concentration) TCEP , i.e., add 2 µl of 50 mM TCEP and incubate for 60 min.

9. Alkylate reduced thiols with 10 mM (final concentration) IAA, i.e., add 1 µl of 200 mM IAA and incubate at RT in the dark for 30 min.

10. Precipitate proteins using 6 volumes of acetone (stored at –20°C) for 3 h.

11. Pellet the precipitate by centrifugation for 10 min at $5,000 \times g$ at 4°C (pre-cool the centrifuge) and aspirate acetone.

12. Resuspend the pellet in 20 µl of 100 mM ammonium bicarbonate and 0.1% (w/v) of Rapigest. It may be necessary to increase the volume of this solution or the concentration of Rapigest to achieve complete solubilization of proteins.

13. Add 5 µg of trypsin and incubate for 18–24 h at 37°C.

14. Add formic acid to a concentration of 2% (v/v) and incubate for 4 h at 37°C to degrade the Rapigest surfactant.

The surfactant hydrolysis products are insoluble and are pelleted by centrifugation at $13,000 \times g$ for 30 min. The supernatant is then removed and stored at −80°C until further analysis (see Notes 7–9 for more information on tryptic digestion).

3.3. Test Run of Tissue Lysate Sample

To ensure the presence of the catalase proteotypic peptide and correct digestion of the sample, the digested tissue lysate sample was run on full-scan mode on an Agilent QQQ.

1. Calibrate the mass spectrometer using an ESI-Tuning Mix and purge the LC lines. Set the nano-pump to run at 0.3 μl/min and the capillary pump to run at 3 μl/min. Check that the source is receiving a good stable electrospray.

2. Set the gradient timetable for the LC as indicated in Table 1.

3. Set the mass spectrometer to run in full-scan mode.

4. Run a blank sample of HPLC·H$_2$O to clear and check the system.

5. Assuming that the blank sample ran without issues (see Note 6), inject 5 μl of the sample.

6. Open the data results in Spectrum Mill. Using an "Easy MS/MS" search, one should be able to detect the catalase proteotypic peptide and also see which fragment ions are the strongest, as illustrated in Fig. 3.

3.4. External Calibration of Synthetic Peptides

Before performing the relative quantification typically used in these experiments, we must first optimize the experiment by creating a calibration curve and selecting the best collision energy and fragmentor values for each MRM transition.

1. Purge the LC system and calibrate the instrument using the ESI-Tuning mix.

**Table 1
LC gradient timetable
for lysate test run**

Minutes	Percentage B
0	2
40	42
45	90
48	90
48.1	3

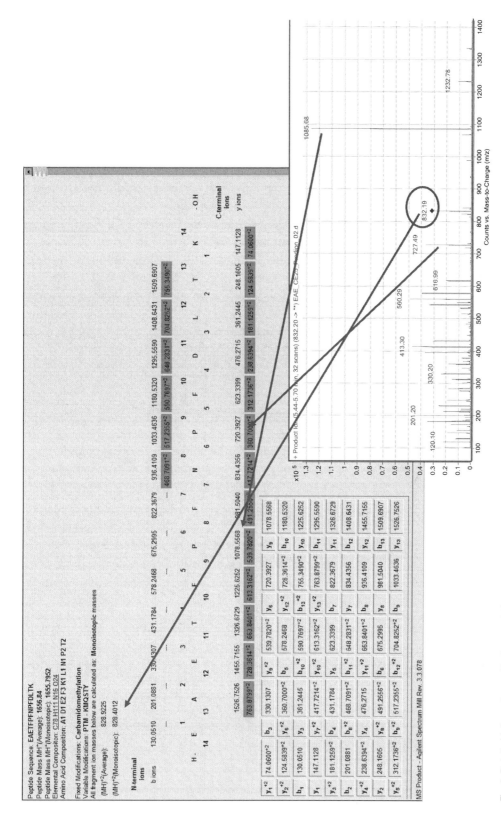

Fig. 3. Detailed information on the fragmentation pattern of the peptide helps select the optimal MRM transitions. Spectrum Mill peptide selector can provide in-depth detail of the fragmentation pattern of a peptide. A side-by-side comparison highlights that the in silico predictions can be reasonably accurate when compared to data acquired from Fig. 3. (Continued) the mass spectrometer. The ions detected on the mass spectrometer are matched with predicted masses with *arrows*, including the precursor, which is marked with an *asterisk*.

2. Resuspend the lyophilized synthetic peptides in 3% acetonitrile with 0.1% formic acid and make dilutions to correspond to 100 fg, 1 pg, 10 pg, 100 pg, 1 ng, and 10 ng in a pool of the tissue lysate digests.

3. Set the mass spectrometer to detect the MRM transitions under different collision energies and fragmentor values.

4. Run a test sample of tissue with a spike of 1 ng of synthetic peptide using the LC gradient indicated in Table 2.

5. Using MassHunter qualitative analysis software, assess which collision energy and fragmentor values gives the strongest MRM signal for the spiked peptide.

6. Once the collision energy has been optimized, run the tissue lysate with spiked peptides (using the same method as previously described) with at least triplicate injections and in order of increasing concentrations of spiked synthetic peptides.

7. Using MassHunter quantitative analysis software, import the data generated and assign the appropriate concentration values and MRM transitions for peak integration and generation of a calibration curve as illustrated in Figs. 4 and 5.

8. The calibration curve should have an R-squared value close to 1.

3.5. Relative Quantification

1. Prepare the mass spectrometer and LC systems as described for the external calibration curve (see Subheading 3.4). Set the mass spectrometer to monitor the MRM transitions of both the synthetic peptide and the native proteotypic peptide.

2. Run the tissue lysate sample as before but with the addition of a single 1-ng spike of the synthetic peptide.

3. Import the data into the MassHunter quantitative analysis software. Assign the synthetic peptide as an internal standard. Integrate the MRM peaks and the software will provide calculated concentrations, as illustrated in Table 3.

Table 2
LC gradient timetable for MRM run

Minutes	Percentage B
0	0
35	35
40	90
50	90
54	3

External quantitation curve of catalase peptide EAETFPFNPFDL*TK from 60 amol to 6000 fmol

Sample				EA E* Method		EA E* Results					Qualifier (727.5)	
Name	Type	Level	Data File	Exp.Conc.	Units	RT	Resp.	S/N	Calc.Conc.	Accuracy	Ratio	S/N
Blank	Sample		SeqA_01-r001.d		fMol	33.561	12372.84	189.341	17.4715506		23.43	68.499
Catalase_Spike_100fg	Cal	1	SeqA_02-r001.d	0.06	fMol	33.44	592.8869	9.32415	0.03967831	66.13052	19.4	2E+308
Catalase_Spike_100fg	Cal	1	SeqA_02-r002.d	0.06	fMol	33.437	632.7031	8.47097	0.09865951	164.4325	18.1	4.8002
Catalase_Spike_1pg	Cal	2	SeqA_03-r001.d	0.6	fMol	33.095	679604.1	1415.03	951.487127	158581.2	23.31	151
Catalase_Spike_1pg	Cal	2	SeqA_03-r002.d	0.6	fMol	33.115	527471.6	800.281	746.997854	124499.6	22.85	446.86
Catalase_Spike_10pg	Cal	3	SeqA_04-r001.d	6	fMol	33.442	4341.728	56.666	5.59114253	93.18571	23.03	35.992
Catalase_Spike_10pg	Cal	3	SeqA_04-r002.d	6	fMol	33.47	4322.859	88.2939	5.56320925	92.72015	20.61	41.86
Catalase_Spike_100pg	Cal	4	SeqA_05-r001.d									
Catalase_Spike_100pg	Cal	4	SeqA_05-r002.d									
Catalase_Spike_1ng	Cal	5	SeqA_06-r001.d									
Catalase_Spike_1ng	Cal	5	SeqA_06-r002.d									
Catalase_Spike_10ng	Cal	6	SeqA_07-r001.d									
Catalase_Spike_10ng	Cal	6	SeqA_07-r002.d									
Catalase High Dose	Sample		SeqA_08-r001.d									

RSD < 5%

Fig. 4. Quantification of MRM peaks. This figure shows the output following peak integration using the MassHunter quantification software, which automatically calculates the response of the peptide in the mass spectrometer. The table gives information such as signal-to-noise (*S/N*) ratio, response, and accuracy for the different concentrations of the standard. The arrow indicates that a well-defined peak at low concentrations such as 60 amol can be detected and integrated. The adjoining image has overlaid the peaks from different concentrations. The quantification is reliable with a relative standard deviation (RSD) of less than 5%.

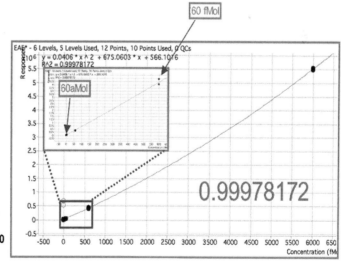

External quantitation curve of catalase peptide EAETFPFNPFDL*TK from 60 amol to 6000 fmol

Fig. 5. External calibration curve. The calibration curve shows good linear response over six orders of magnitude and sensitivity reaching the amol range. This is important where one might be quantifying biomarkers with very low abundance and/or large dynamic changes in quantity. The coefficient of correlation is indicated at the bottom right and is approximately 1.

Table 3
The results table gives information on the retention time (RT), response (Resp), and signal-to-noise (*S/N*) ratio

Sample	Results				Qualifier 1		Qualifier 2		ISTD	
	RT	Resp	*S/N*	Calc conc	Ratio	*S/N*	Ratio	*S/N*	RT	Resp
Lysate replicate 1	33.394	11,551	296.85	3,063.939	20.65	113.38	25.73	20.79	33.436	3,770
Lysate replicate 2	33.446	12,059	249.95	4,599.204	19.16	216.6	23.03	17.85	33.42	2,622

A ratio is calculated from the known spiked synthetic peptides (internal standard, ISTD). This is compared to two MRM responses for the native peptide (qualifiers 1 and 2) to produce a calculated concentration

4. Notes

1. When selecting proteotypic peptides, as well as choosing peptides that do not have methionine and cysteines, it may also be necessary to exclude peptides next to multiple cleavage sites and peptides with chemically reactive residues (such as D–G, N–G, and end terminal N and E).

2. To further validate the quantification, it is suggested that at least three or four peptides be used so that the calculated concentrations can be compared between different peptides.

3. For each peptide, several (at least two) MRM transitions should be used for the same reason of comparing consistency of quantification. In addition, the ratio of these qualifier transitions to the primary MRM can be used as a quality control measure to detect a potential interfering MRM. This ratio, within an acceptable error, as determined with the standard peptides should be consistent for the endogenous peptide, and this will be flagged in the quantitative analysis software if this is not the case.

4. Peptide MS repositories such as the Global Proteome Machine Database (5) and the Peptide Atlas (6) can be very useful when selecting peptides that will be observable by MS. In addition, a computational tool for predicting observable peptides from physicochemical properties based on empirical data is available (7).

5. Absolute quantification experiments via MRM are very amenable to multiplexing (naturally, this will require the synthesis of additional synthetic peptides). The limit of the multiplex capability is related to the duty cycle of the mass spectrometer. As additional MRMs are added, the duty cycle

will increase and the number of points for each MRM across the chromatographic peak will be reduced (at least 10–12 data points are required for each MRM). As the dwell time for each MRM is decreased, a loss of sensitivity and signal-to-noise ratio will be observed.

6. Standard LC–MS practices to minimize carryover should be utilized, i.e., running blanks, run samples in increasing concentrations, etc.

7. All samples should be kept at 4°C while being used. Otherwise, the samples should be stored at –20°C.

8. The premise of using a tryptic peptide as a surrogate measure of the concentration of a protein is completely dependent on effective digestion of the parent protein by trypsin. Particular attention should be paid to following the digestion protocol. If modification of the protocol is required, a recent article details a number of tryptic digestion protocols and associated issues (4).

9. The efficiency of the tryptic digestion tends to decrease with increasing volume. It is recommended to keep the volume below 50 µl, where possible.

Acknowledgments

The authors would like to thank Agilent Technologies, Santa Clara, for generating much of the data and figures used in this example. We would also like to thank all members of the PredTox Consortium. Funding is acknowledged under the FP6 Integrated Project, InnoMed. The UCD Conway Institute and the Proteome Research Centre is funded by the Programme for Research in Third Level Institutions (PRTLI), as administered by the Higher Education Authority (HEA) of Ireland.

References

1. Gerber, S.A., et al. (2003) Absolute quantification of proteins and phosphoproteins from cell lysates by tandem MS. *Proc. Natl Acad. Sci. U. S. A.* **100(12)**, 6940–6945.

2. Anderson, L. and Hunter, C.L. (2005) Quantitative mass spectrometric multiple reaction monitoring assays for major plasma proteins. *Mol. Cell. Proteomics* **5(4)**, 573–588.

3. Kuster, B., et al. (2005) Scoring proteomes with proteotypic peptide probes. *Nat. Rev. Mol. Cell. Biol.* **6(7)**, 577–583.

4. Chen, E.I., et al. (2007) Optimization of mass spectrometry-compatible surfactants for shotgun proteomics. *J. Proteome Res.* **6(7)**, 2529–2538.

5. Craig, R., Cortens, J.P., and Beavis, R.C. (2004) Open source system for analyzing, validating, and storing protein identification data. *J. Proteome Res.* **3(6)**, 1234–1242.

6. Desiere, F., et al. (2006) The PeptideAtlas project. *Nucleic Acids Res.* **34** (Database issue), D655–D658.

7. Mallick, P., et al. (2007) Computational prediction of proteotypic peptides for quantitative proteomics. *Nat. Biotechnol.* **25(1)**, 125–131.

INDEX

Jean-Charles Gautier (ed.), *Drug Safety Evaluation: Methods and Protocols*, Methods in Molecular Biology, vol. 691
DOI 10.1007/978-1-60761-849-2, © Springer Science+Business Media, LLC 2011